Home Health Care Practice

Second Edition

Edited By:
Patrick N. Catania, Ph.D.
Professor and Chairman
Department of Pharmacy Practice
School of Pharmacy
University of the Pacific
Stockton, CA

Martin M. Rosner, Ph.D.
President
Health Markets Research
Palo Alto, CA

Home Health Care Practice, Second Edition

851 Moana Court
Palo Alto, CA 94306
(415) 948-1960

Library of Congress Catalog Card Number 93-079105
ISBN: 0-9627640-4-3

Layout: The Pocket Press, Sacramento, CA
Printing: Bookcrafters, Chelsea MI

Indications, adverse reactions, and dosing schedules for drugs are included in this book. However, the reader must confirm all product information with the manufacturer.

Contributing Authors
Home Health Care Practice
Second Edition

Richard R. Abood, J.D.
Professor of Pharmacy Administration
School of Pharmacy
University of the Pacific
Stockton CA

Michael P. Akahoshi, Pharm.D.
Consultant Pharmacist
Home Health Care
Lake Forest CA

Steven F. Bauwens, Pharm.D., FASCP
Director, Education and Scientific Affairs
The Center for Long Term Care
Research and Education
Chesapeake VA

Barbara C. Bolinger, Pharm.D.
Clinical Pharmacist, Ambulatory Care
Assistant Professor of Clinical Pharmacy
USC Norris Cancer Hospital
Los Angeles CA

Todd A. Brown, B.S. Pharmacy
Clinical Assistant Professor of Pharmacy Practice
College of Pharmacy
Northeastern University
Boston MA

Richard Bulich, Pharm.D.
Director of Pharmacy
Critical Care America
Monterey CA

Thomas J. Cali, Pharm.D., FASCP
Director, Clinical Affairs
The Center for Long Term Care
Research and Eduction
Chesapeake VA

Patrick N. Catania, Ph.D., RPh
Professor and Chairman
Department of Pharmacy Practice
School of Pharmacy
University of the Pacific
Stockton CA

Thomas M. Chamberlain, Pharm.D., FASCP
Executive Director, Center for Long Term Care
Research and Education
Chesapeake VA

Ronald R. Conte, Pharm.D.
Senior Clinical Associate
Total Pharmaceutical Care
Santa Rosa CA

Jan Cuzzell, R.N., M.A.
Director, The Wound Care Center
Sherman Oaks Hospital and
Medical Center
Sherman Oaks CA

Norm Enriquez, Pharm.D.
Vice President, Clinical Pharmacy Services
Total Pharmaceutical Care
Santa Barbara CA

William E. Fassett, Ph.D., RPh
Associate Professor of Pharmacy
School of Pharmacy
University of Washington
Seattle WA

Madeline Feinberg, Pharm.D.
Assistant Professor
School of Pharmacy
University of Maryland
Baltimore MD

Barbara Fotheringill, B.A.
Manager
Allcare Medical, Inc.
Bellevue WA

Julie Wilson Ganz, Pharm.D.
Assistant Clinical Professor
Director, Home Therapy Services
School of Pharmacy
University of California, San Francisco
San Francisco CA

Jeff A. Keimach, Pharm.D.
President
Jeff A. Keimach & Associates
Irvine CA

Michael L. Kleinberg, M.S., FASHP
Director, Professional Services
Immunex Corporation
Seattle WA

Jane W. Kwan, B.S. Pharmacy, M.P.H.
Coordinator, Pharmacy Alternate Delivery Programs
M.D. Anderson Cancer Center Pharmacy
Houston TX

Peter P. Lamy, Ph.D., Sc.D.
Professor and Director
The Center for the Study of Pharmacy and Therapeutics for the Elderly
School of Pharmacy
University of Maryland at Baltimore
Baltimore MD

Julio R. Lopez, Pharm.D.
Director, Drug Information Center
Veterans Administration Northern California Clinics
Martinez CA

Robert A. Louie, Pharm.D.
Director, Ambulatory Pharmaceutical Services
USC Norris Cancer Hospital
Assistant Professor of Clinical Pharmacy
University of Southern California
Los Angeles CA

Mary Lynn McPherson, Pharm.D., BCPS
Assistant Professor
School of Pharmacy
University of Maryland
Baltimore MD

David M. Melikian, Pharm.D.
National Pharmacy Services Manager
HOMEDCO, INC.
Fountain Valley, CA

Randell K. Miyahara, Pharm.D.
Associate Professor
Mercer University
Southern School of Pharmacy
Atlanta GA

Patricia B. New, Pharm.D.
Clinical Coordinator
Watsonville Hospital
Formerly Senior Clinical Pharmacist
Critical Care America
Monterey CA

Diane Nykamp, Pharm.D.
Associate Professor of Pharmacy Practice
Mercer University
School of Pharmacy
Atlanta GA

Martin M. Rosner, Ph.D.
President
Health Markets Research
Palo Alto CA

Charles C. Schraa, Pharm.D.
Clinical Instructor
School of Pharmacy
Medical College of Virginia
Virginia Commonwealth University
Richmond VA

Ralph E. Small, Pharm.D.
Professor of Pharmacy and Medicine
School of Pharmacy
Medical College of Virginia
Virginia Commonwealth University
Richmond VA

Rene Steffen, B.S., RRT, RCP
Clinical Supervisor
Abbey Medical
Stockton CA

Virginia Tobiason, R.N., M.B.A.
Abbott Home Infusion Services
Abbott Park IL

Beverly Yachmetz, Pharm.D., CDE
Clinical Director
Health Connections, Inc.
Baltimore MD

Ilene H. Zuckerman, Pharm.D.
Associate Professor
School of Pharmacy
University of Maryland
Baltimore MD

Editorial Advisory Board

Table of Contents

Preface

Our goals in preparing the second edition of Home Health Care Practice were the same as those for the first edition. Its audience is pharmacists and pharmacy students who wish to enter home health care or to expand their practice into this important health care alternative. Our book is designed to provide the requisite clinical and technical knowledge to help pharmacists and pharmacy students become reliable sources of information on home health care products and services. In addition, we believe that pharmacists need to practice in an environment that will allow them to provide home health care products and services in a profitable manner. Because of this belief, we supplemented technical and clinical information with sections on promotion, market analysis, and operational management.

From the outset we wanted Home Health Care Practice to reflect accurately the unique nature of pharmacy practice in home health care settings. The term home health care practice, home care, home health care are synonymous—referring to the deliver of health and medical care to patients in their homes. We recruited as contributing authors home health care pharmacy practitioners, and supplemented their input with that of other recognized experts in specialized areas of health care. Our book could not have been written without the dedicated efforts of the authors and reviewers. We hope that the deep appreciation that we have for our contributing authors and members of our editorial advisory board is transmitted by this note. They took time from their very busy schedules to write, review, and rewrite the chapters. We extend a special note of appreciation for their response to our sincere effort to publish Home Health Care Practice in a timely manner.

In preparing the second edition, we requested the help and advice of representatives of the American Pharmaceutical Association (APhA), American Society of Hospital Pharmacists (ASHP), and the American Society of Consultant Pharmacists (ASCP). Special thanks are extended to Susan Cantrell, M.S., ASHP Director of Managed Care and Home Care Departments; Laura Lawson, APhA Director of Special Projects; and Marie A. Smith, Pharm.D., ASHP Director, Special Projects Division. The suggestions of APhA's 1992 Academy Publications Committee and the cooperation of ASCP's Catherine M. Burdette are gratefully acknowledged. These individuals' collective wisdom, along with the insightful comments of the leading home health care wholesaler, Herb Gray, President of Suburban Ostomy, contributed to the success of our project.

Home Health Care Practice could not have been completed without the assistance of Sydne Heidrich, who spent many hours at her desk deciphering the manuscripts from the various authors. Eddy Shimizu was in charge of final copy editing and layout and did an excellent job in preparing camera-ready copy. Last but not least, our book could not have been completed without the support of our wives, Harriet Catania and Judy Rosner, whose patience helped us with this challenging and, at times, trying project.

We hope our book facilitates the provision of pharmaceutical care in home health care settings. Whatever shortcomings the manuscript has should be attributed to the editors.

Patrick N. Catania
Stockton California

Martin M. Rosner
Palo Alto California

October 1993

1 Introduction to Home Health Care

Patrick N. Catania, Ph.D., RPh

Home health care (HHC) is a health care alternative that has been the subject of various definitions and descriptions. However, there is no consensus among practitioners, regulatory entities, and third party payers on the choice of "home health care", "home care", or "homecare" as the proper phrase to describe the services and products provided to patients in their homes. In its broadest definition, HHC is synonymous with home care and consists of medical, nursing, pharmaceutical, and other care provided to patients in their places of residence.[1] HHC services are generally classified as skilled or personal care services. Skilled services are provided by health care professionals, while personal care services are provided by technical or supportive personnel. In many cases, the specific products and services that are provided are determined by the third party payer. As a result, the insurance company may define home health services for health care providers seeking reimbursement for services rendered.

From a pharmaceutical care perspective, HHC includes a wide variety of pharmaceutical and biomedical products and services provided by pharmacists to patients in their homes. Products such as home medical equipment (HME), convalescent aids and accessories, therapeutic agents administered parenterally, along with the requisite clinical services associated with the provision of these products, are part of HHC pharmacy practice. For the purpose of this book, a variety of self-care products and services for specialized patient prototypes are also included within the framework of HHC. The needs of the elderly patient, diabetic patient, the AIDS patient, ostomy patient, hospice patient, and other patients at home with short term and long term needs of pharmaceutical caregivers are included.

The successful HHC pharmacist has expertise as a clinician, educator, product and equipment manager, and drug therapy consultant. A commitment to patient care and a concern for positive patient outcomes are needed to insure quality care at home. In addition, a strong working knowledge of legal and regulatory issues, accreditation requirements, and financial and reimbursement strategies are needed to facilitate succeeding in the current economic climate. (See also Chapters 2 - 4.) Lastly, the successful HHC pharmacist works with other HHC practitioners to coordinate care and insure the continuity of care of the patients referred to them. (See also Chapter 7.)

HOME HEALTH CARE DEFINITIONS

A variety of health-related terms are in common usage among HHC providers. These terms may be defined by individual state regulations or laws, the funding agency for services and products, or the practitioners involved with the provision of the service or product. Pegels[2] provided a succinct set of definitions related to HHC. HOME HEALTH SERVICES are services provided to acutely or chronically ill or injured patients at their residence according to a plan of treatment prescribed by a physician. Home health services may include nursing care, medical social services, home health aide care, nutritional and dietary services, medical supplies and equipment, drug therapy, physical therapy, speech therapy, occupational therapy, and other specialized services. SUPPORT SERVICES are social and maintenance services that enable an incapacitated or otherwise disabled person to live at home. Support services may include housekeeping chores, personal care, transportation, shopping, laundry services, and pastoral services. CERTIFIED HOME HEALTH AGENCIES meet federal and state requirements for certification/licensure. Certified agencies provide nursing service and at least one of the following: physical therapy, occupational therapy, speech therapy, nutrition services, and medical social services. To receive reimbursement for services provided to Medicare or Medicaid patients, a home health agency must be certified. MEDICAL SOCIAL SERVICES include services provided by a qualified social worker. HOME HEALTH AIDE SERVICES include assistance with simple health care tasks, personal hygiene, light housekeeping, and other related supportive tasks. A home health aide is usually required to complete a formalized training program. HOMEMAKER SERVICES include assistance and instruction in managing and maintaining a household and in dressing, feeding, and incidental household tasks.[1,2]

HHC, Self Care, and Long Term Care

Present day HHC includes products, services, and responsibilities that may overlap with self care and long term care.[3] HHC products are generally provided and/or prescribed and/or administered by a health care professional. In many cases HHC is provided after a period of hospitalization. Typical HHC products include catheters, wound dressing material, oxygen equipment, wheelchairs, and parenteral drug therapy. Home care services include nursing care, physical or occupational therapy, drug therapy monitoring, and respiratory care.

Self care products are those items used by health-conscious individuals who are usually well, and have an interest in promoting or monitoring their own health. Decisions about the purchase and use of self care products tend to be made by the individuals themselves, although sometimes on the advice of a health care provider. In some situations self care products relate to a chronic illness rather than a state of well-being, such as blood glucose monitoring devices for diabetic patients. Typical self care products include blood pressure monitors, home pregnancy kits, blood glucose and fecal monitoring products, and stethoscopes.[3] (See also Chapters 11 - 17.)

Long term care is usually associated with chronic care services provided in intermediate care and skilled nursing facilities. Long term care has a twenty year tradition of providing consultant pharmacy services in these settings. In most instances, these services are provided to geriatric patients in institutional settings. (See also Chapter 6.)

TRENDS IN HHC

For much of the past two decades, HHC has been the subject of increased interest as a novel health care alternative. However, HHC is not a new concept. As originally designed hundreds of years ago, care of the ill at home consisted of nursing care. In the late nineteenth century, nursing services for patients at home were available in cities such as Boston, Philadelphia, and New York City. Clearly, the earliest providers of HHC services were members of the nursing profession.[1]

According to Spiegel,[4] home nursing care became a part of the benefits offered by life insurance companies in the early part of the twentieth century. The preferences of patients to remain at home during periods of illness were slowly being accommodated. However, the major impetus to the development of present day HHC was given by the 1965 changes to the Social Security Act, which established HHC definitions within Medicare.[5] In 1966 there were approximately one thousand home health agencies (HHA) in the United States certified to provide services to Medicare patients. As initially defined, HHA were required to provide nursing care and at least one additional service such as physical therapy, occupational therapy, speech therapy, medical social services, or home health aide services. This "nursing plus one" requirement served as an important guideline that served as a template for the home nursing industry. The provision of pharmaceuticals was not included in the services provided by HHA in the 1960's.[4,5]

Major changes began to appear in the delivery of HHC services in the 1970's. These changes included the significant increase in the scope and sophistication of services, and inclusion of parenteral therapies at home as an increasingly common treatment alternative. As suggested by Strandell,[5] these changes have occurred as a result of societal, economic, technologic and political forces. Factors proposed by Strandell that have affected the changing trends in HHC include:

1. the increased number of frail elderly who are ambulatory patients with multiple chronic diseases;

2. the advances in medical science that have resulted in increased survival rates among trauma patients;

3. the availability of medical equipment designed for use in the home;

4. the increased mobility of society, which has reduced the traditional caregiver support historically provided by family members;

5. the employment patterns of women, who are often no longer available to care for ill family members;

6. the increased demand for health care services paid for by Medicare, Medicaid, and private third party payment programs;

7. cost containment programs such as prospective payment plans which result in patients who are discharged from hospitals "quicker and sicker"; and

8. the preference of patients to receive HHC as the treatment of choice because it is less threatening, more convenient, and easier for family members.[5]

In response to the above changing trends, the number of HHA has increased from approximately 1,000 in 1966, to over 10,000 in 1992.[6] HHA may be organized as a for-profit or tax exempt entity, as a single site or multiple site agency. Most multiple site HHA provide a variety of HHC services, ranging from the "nursing plus one" approach to the full array of services that are normally reimbursable through third party payers. Some HHA are also licensed as pharmacies and provide intravenous infusion therapy as their primary HHC service. The ten largest HHA that also serve as pharmacies are listed in Table 1-1.[6]

The HHC industry is increasingly dominated by for-profit agencies. The average number of patient visits per agency in 1992 was 380.[6] To accommodate this patient load, the HHC industry employed approximately 650,000 in 1992, an increase of 10% from 1991. Gross revenues for the industry were more than $31 billion in 1992, of which Medicare provided 53%. Private insurance provided 14.5% and Medicaid, approximately 11%.[6]

THE HHC PATIENT

Various descriptions may be used to classify HHC patients. Demographic data, medical diagnostic category, and type of care needed, are useful in defining the prototypical HHC patient. Typically,

Table 1-1 The Largest HHC Pharmacies[6]

NAME (a)	Headquarters	No. of Offices	No. of States	No. of Employees	Average No. of Employee/ Office
HOMEDCO	Fountain Valley, CA	200	42	4,200	21.0
OPTION CARE	Chico, CA	180	40	3,214	17.9
CAREMARK	Lincolnshire, Il	85	42	3,500	41.2
HOOPER HOLMES, INC.	Basking Ridge, N.J	70	24	9,000	128.6
NMC HOMECARE	Waltham, MA	63	23	1,400	22.2
TOKOS MEDICAL CORP.	Santa Ana, CA	61	34	1,046	17.2
CRITICAL CARE AMERICA	West Borough, MA	51	24	2,278	44.7
TOTAL PHARMACEUTICAL CARE, INC.	Torrence, CA	40	17	800	20.0
HOME INTENSIVE CARE	N. Miami Beach, FL	36	20	1,400	38.9
HMSS, INC.	Houston, TX	29	16	700	24.1

(a) Ranking is based upon the total number of offices or pharmacies in the United States.

HHC patients are classified as acute care or chronic care patients. Acute care patients may receive parenteral medication at home. The chronic care patient usually has multiple diseases that do not require high technology HHC. Rather, chronic care patients will be maintained on multiple oral medications. Many HHC patients are in need of chronic care, and are termed long term care patients. (See also Chapter 6 and 7.)

The typical HHC patient is usually a geriatric female who requires HHC service for more than 30 days. In addition, one-half of HHC patients in 1992 needed two or three weekly visits by HHA personnel. In general HHC patients have medical or social needs that require care or supervision, but lack the physical capabilities to seek traditional ambulatory care.[6,7]

Classifying patients by diagnostic category, e.g., diabetes, infection, is the standard, medical approach. From the diagnosis, the physician prescribes therapy, and clinical measures would be used to assess outcomes. In addition, patients may be classified on the basis of the type of care needed, e.g., acute, chronic, terminal. In practice, a combination of these approaches are used to categorize patients and their needs, as well as to assess patients in terms of their suitability for home care. Table 1-2 lists typical categories of patients who receive HHC services from HHA.[6,7]

HOME INFUSION THERAPY PATIENT

Infusion therapy consists of the administration of a drug, nutrient solution, or other fluid into the patient through a needle or catheter. Infusion therapy is usually provided via the intravenous route of administration; however, subcutaneous and other routes of administration may be used.[8] (See also Chapter 19.)

Table 1-2 Percentage of Patients with Specific Conditions [7]

Patient Condition	Government	Type of HHA (a)		VNA (b)
		Hospital	For Profit	
Ambulatory	86	78	73	71
Bedridden	14	22	27	29
Living alone	48	34	39	39
Living with spouse	48	59	54	54
Living with friend	4	7	7	7
Alzheimer's	6	6	12	8
Other dementia	16	9	17	15
AIDS	2	3	10	4
Chronic illness	66	51	48	52
Decubitus	10	8	13	13
Incontinent	18	21	27	24
Terminal	8	11	13	15
Post surgical	15	23	17	21
Paraplegic	6	3	6	8

(a) Home health agency

(b) Visiting nurse association

Because of the technological advancements associated with infusion therapy, home infusion therapy has become one of the most important HHC alternatives provided by pharmacists.[9] The heavy reliance on technologically sophisticated parenteral equipment led to the use of the phrase, "high tech HHC" to describe home infusion therapy. The use of "high tech" as a descriptor of home infusion therapy is a misnomer, in that technological advances have affected all sectors of HHC, not just infusion therapy.

Home infusion therapy patients are typically more acutely ill than the average HHC patient. Because of the inherent risk of providing drug therapy by the parenteral route of administration in the patient's home, sophisticated HHC pharmacist services are warranted. The home infusion therapy pharmacist provides three major patient care functions, namely, initial patient evaluation; compounding and dispensing of drugs, solutions, and nutrients; and ongoing clinical monitoring. (See also Chapters 18 - 25.)

THE PHARMACIST'S ROLE IN HHC[a]

HHC services are provided by pharmacists in association with hospitals, community pharmacies, HHA, and specialized home infusion companies. To assist pharmacists in defining their role, the American Society of Hospital Pharmacists (ASHP) has developed ASHP Guidelines on the Pharmacist's Role in Home Care.[10] These Guidelines refer to the provision of pharmaceutical products and clinical monitoring for patients in the home including, but not limited to, "home infusion therapy and other injectable drug therapy and enteral nutrition therapy."[10]

Although the Guidelines use home infusion therapy as the primary focus, much of the content is applicable to all types of pharmaceutical care provided by HHC pharmacists. Because of the similarity in the scope of responsibility of HHC pharmacists to all HHC patients, the ASHP Guidelines are included as follows.

Initial Patient Assessment

The pharmacist should ensure that each patient referred for HHC is assessed for appropriateness on the basis of formal, predetermined admission criteria, including the following:

- Patient, family, and caregiver agreement with services being provided in the home;
- Ability and willingness of the patient or caregiver to be trained to properly administer medications;
- Home environment conducive to the provision of home care services (e.g., electricity, running water, cleanliness);
- Reasonable geographical access to the patient by the home care provider;
- Psychosocial and family support (e.g., caregiver counseling, financial assistance and counseling, suitable family environment);
- Ongoing prescriber involvement in the assessment and treatment of the patient;
- Medical condition and prescribed medication therapy suitable for home care services and prognosis with clearly defined outcome goals;
- Appropriate indication, dose, route, and method of administration of medications; and
- Appropriate laboratory tests for monitoring patient response to medications ordered.

Before the start of HHC services, patients should be informed of their rights and responsibilities. These should be explained in detail and given to the patient, family member, or other caregiver in writing.

When the first dose of medication is to be given in the home, the pharmacist should use clinical judgment in determining, in conjunction with the prescriber, home care nurse, and patient or caregiver, whether home administration of the first dose is appropriate. Policies and procedures should define parameters to be used in making this decision and precautions necessary when first doses are administered in the home (e.g., emergency medications, monitoring and observation, presence of health care professional).[11]

Once a patient is accepted for HHC service but before the initiation of therapy, the pharmacist should assess the patient's current status and develop a thorough patient database in order to provide a basis for ongoing drug therapy monitoring and an evaluation tool for measuring patient outcomes.

The complete patient database should be documented in the patient's HHC record. This database should include, at a minimum:

- Patient's name, address, telephone number, and date of birth;

[a] From: Anon. ASHP Guidelines on the Pharmacist's Role in Home Care. Modified with Permission. Am J Hosp Pharm. 1993; 50:1940; Copyright 1993. Reprinted with permission (R93173).

- Person to contact in the event of an emergency and contact information;
- Patient's height, weight, and sex;
- Location and type of intravenous access, when necessary;
- Pertinent medical history and physical findings; drug related problem list;
- An accurate history of allergies;
- Initial and ongoing pharmaceutical assessment;
- A detailed medication profile including all medications (prescription and nonprescription), home remedies, investigational and nontraditional therapies the patient is receiving;
- Prescriber's name, address, telephone number, and any other pertinent information (e.g., Drug Enforcement Administration (DEA) number);
- Other agencies and individuals involved in the patient's care and directions for contacting them;
- Medication history;
- Goals and expected duration of therapy;
- Desired outcome indicators;
- Patient education provided;
- Any functional limitations the patient has; and
- Any pertinent social history or findings (e.g., alcohol consumption, tobacco use).

In obtaining this information, the pharmacist may use the past medical record, laboratory test results, direct communication with the patient, nurse, and prescriber, and direct observation. When the pharmacist cannot directly observe the patient, the patient's HHC nurse may provide the results of direct observation and physical assessment. If a shared service agreement exists between multiple providers, the pharmacist should ensure that this agreement specifies the responsibilities of each provider for obtaining and sharing pertinent patient information.

Patient Education, Training, And Counseling

The pharmacist is responsible for ensuring that the patient or caregiver receives appropriate education, training, and counseling regarding the patient's drug therapy. Other health care professionals may be involved. A HHC pharmacist should be readily accessible in the event that questions or problems arise.

Professional judgment should be employed in determining what information should be included in patient education and training. The following should be considered, where applicable, based upon the type of drug therapy:

- Description of drug therapy including drug, dose, dosing interval, and duration of therapy; goals of drug therapy;
- Importance of compliance in following the therapy plan;
- Proper aseptic technique; proper care of the catheter and catheter site;
- Proper administration of medications;
- Inspection of medications, containers, and supplies before use;
- Equipment use, maintenance, and troubleshooting;
- Home inventory maintenance and procedures for securing additional supplies and medications when needed;
- Potential adverse effects, drug-drug interactions, and drug-nutrient interactions, and their management;
- Special precautions for the preparation, storage, handling, and disposal of the drug, supplies, and biomedical waste;
- Information on contacting health care providers involved in the patient's care; and
- Emergency procedures.

Guidelines on patient counseling and education are available elsewhere.[12,13] Patient counseling and education should be performed in accordance with applicable state regulations and documented in the patient's HHC record.

Product, Device, And Ancillary Supply Selection

The pharmacist, in collaboration with other health care professionals and the patient, is responsible for the selection of infusion devices, ancillary drugs (e.g., heparin flush, 0.9% sodium chloride), and ancillary supplies (e.g., dressing kits, syringes, administration sets). Pharmacists should be thoroughly trained and knowledgeable in the selection and use of these devices, drugs, and supplies. Factors involved in the selection of devices and ancillary supplies may include the following:

- Stability and compatibility of prescribed medication(s) in infusion device reservoirs;
- Ability of an infusion device to accommodate the appropriate volume of medication and diluent and to deliver the prescribed dose at the appropriate rate;
- Ability of patient or caregiver to learn to operate an infusion device;
- Potential for patient complications and noncompliance;

- Patient convenience;
- Nursing or caregiver experience with therapy and selected devices;
- Prescriber preference;
- Cost considerations; and
- Safety features of infusion devices.

The HHC pharmacist in consultation with the prescriber should determine when emergency medications and supplies (e.g., anaphylaxis kits) should be dispensed to HHC patients. When standing orders for ancillary drugs or supplies or standardized treatment protocols are used, the pharmacist should review each protocol to determine its appropriateness for the patient. Information on the selection of infusion devices and catheters is available elsewhere.[14-16] (See also Chapter 19.)

Development Of Pharmaceutical Care Plans

The pharmacist, in collaboration with the patient or caregiver and other health care professionals, is responsible for developing an appropriate pharmaceutical care plan for each patient. The pharmaceutical care plan should be developed as part of the patient's overall care plan. The pharmaceutical care plan should be based on information obtained from the nurse, prescriber, patient, and caregiver. At a minimum, the pharmaceutical care plan should include the following:[17]

- Actual or potential drug therapy problems and their proposed solutions;
- Desired outcomes of drug therapy provided;
- A monitoring plan specifying objective and subjective parameters (e.g., vital signs, laboratory tests, physical findings, patient response) for monitoring outcomes and drug therapy-related problems (e.g., toxicity, adverse reactions, noncompliance); and
- Frequency for proactive monitoring of the above parameters.

The pharmaceutical care plan should be developed at the initiation of therapy and reviewed and updated on a regular basis. The degree of detail of the pharmaceutical care plan should be based on the complexity of drug therapy and the patient. The Joint Commission on Accreditation of Healthcare Organizations Accreditation Manual for Home Care includes examples of pharmaceutical care plans for various therapies.[18]

The pharmacist is responsible for communicating the pharmaceutical care plan to other health care professionals involved in the care of the patient and regularly communicating any updates as they occur. The pharmaceutical care plan and updates should be a part of the patient's HHC record.

Patient Clinical Monitoring

The pharmacist is responsible for ongoing clinical monitoring of the patient's drug therapy according to the pharmaceutical care plan developed, and for appropriately documenting and communicating the results of all monitoring activities to other health care professionals involved in the patient's care. The pharmacist is also responsible for ensuring that relevant information is obtained from the patient, caregiver, and other health care professionals and documenting this information in the patient's home care record.

Pharmacists may wish to develop clinical monitoring protocols, in collaboration with prescribers and others, for various therapies. In most HHC practice sites, the pharmacist is responsible for obtaining the medication order from the prescriber. Pharmacists may receive laboratory results before other health care providers. In such cases, the pharmacist is responsible for communicating the laboratory test results to the prescriber and other health care providers. The pharmacist should provide an interpretive analysis of the information and recommendations for dose adjustments, continuation, or discontinuation of drug therapy. The pharmacist should ensure that sufficient laboratory test results are readily available for monitoring the patient's therapy. In shared services arrangements, clinical monitoring responsibilities should be delineated.

Effective Communication With Prescribers, Nurses, And Other Health Care Personnel

Effective communication among pharmacists, prescribers, nurses, and other health care personnel is critical to the care of the patient. The pharmacist should ensure that effective channels of communication regarding the care of the patient are in place, including shared services arrangements (e.g., pain assessments, laboratory test data). Both oral and written communication methods may be used for communicating patient information. Confidentiality of patient information and pertinent federal and state regulations should be considered by the pharmacist. All relevant clinical communication should be documented in the patient's home care record. It is recommended that personnel involved in the care of the patient (e.g., nurses, pharmacists, dietitians, delivery representatives, reimbursement coordinators) meet regularly (e.g., weekly patient rounds) to discuss the clinical status of the patient and any operational issues related to the care of the patient.

The patient, family, caregiver, and all health care personnel involved in the care of the patient should have access to a pharmacist 24 hours a day. Before transferring patient care responsibilities, the pharmacist is responsible for providing a summary of all relevant clinical information to another pharmacist providing coverage for that patient (e.g., on-call pharmacist).

Direct Communication With The Patient And Caregiver

The HHC pharmacist should establish free and open channels of communication with the patient or caregiver. The pharmacist should contact the patient or caregiver as soon as the patient is accepted for service to

- Obtain information needed for the initial, pharmacy assessment;
- Provide supplemental patient education and counseling as needed;
- Assess drug therapy compliance;
- Inform the patient how to contact the pharmacist when needed; and
- Assess drug therapy problems (e.g., side effects, adverse drug reactions, noncompliance).

All patient contacts should be documented in the patient's HHC record.

Coordination Of Drug Preparation, Delivery, Storage and Administration

The pharmacist is responsible for ensuring the proper acquisition, compounding, dispensing, storage, delivery, and administration of all medications and related equipment and supplies. Compounding of sterile products should comply with applicable practice standards, accreditation standards, and pertinent state and federal regulations. If these services are being provided by another pharmacy, the pharmacist should have reasonable assurance that these standards are being met by the pharmacy providing the service. Pharmacists may administer medications to patients in the home setting unless prohibited by applicable statutes and regulations.

The pharmacist should ensure that the delivery of medications and supplies to the patient occurs in a timely manner to avoid inappropriate interruption in drug therapy. Further, the pharmacist should ensure that storage conditions during the delivery process and in the patient's home be consistent with the recommendations for storage of the product and expiration dating. The temperature of home refrigerators or freezers in which medications are stored should be within acceptable limits and should be monitored by the patient or caregiver regularly. The pharmacist should ensure that an adequate inventory of medications and ancillary supplies are available in the patient's home. It may be appropriate to provide additional inventory for unforeseen circumstances where extra doses or supplies may be required (e.g., wastage, breakage, emergencies).

Employee And Patient Safety And Universal Precautions

A HHC organization is responsible for assisting in the education and training of employees, patients, family members, and caregivers in appropriate safety and universal precautions[18] as mandated by the Occupational Safety and Health Administration (OSHA). The pharmacist should ensure that the HHC organization provides appropriate instruction and training for its employees and patients, including appropriate disposal and handling of medical waste, procedures for prevention and management of needle sticks, handling of cytotoxic and hazardous medications,[19,20] and Material Safety Data Sheets (MSDSs). The pharmacist should be a key resource in the development of such training programs. The pharmacist should assume an active role in the HHC organizations' infection control activities.[21] For high-risk patients, it may be advisable to consider using a system or device (e.g., needleless system) to minimize the potential for needle sticks.

Documentation In The HHC Record

A HHC record should be developed and used for documenting the HHC services provided to each patient. Written organizational policies and procedures should address the security of HHC records and specify personnel who have the authority to review and make entries in HHC records. The confidentiality of patient information should be stressed to all personnel.

The pharmacist is responsible for documenting all pharmacy clinical activities in the patient's HHC record in a timely manner. To minimize duplication of information, general clinician-oriented forms are preferred over specific nursing, pharmacy, or other health care professional forms.

It may be advisable for organizations that provide multiple HHC services (e.g., pharmacy, nursing, respiratory services) to use a single HHC record for documenting all clinical information regarding each patient. The HHC record should be accessible at all times to authorized personnel involved in the care of the patient.

Adverse Drug Reaction Reporting

The HHC pharmacist should assist in the development of a program for reporting and monitoring all adverse drug and device related events. Such activities should be consistent with the ASHP Guidelines on Adverse Drug Reaction Monitoring and Report.[22] The pharmacist should ensure that the prescriber is notified promptly of any suspected adverse drug reaction.

Adverse drug reactions should serve as outcome indicators of quality, and the monitoring of adverse drug reactions should be a part of the organizations' ongoing quality improvement program. To improve patient outcomes, relevant adverse drug reaction trends should be integrated into staff development and inservice education programs for pharmacists and nurses. Serious adverse drug reactions should be reported promptly to the manufacturer or Food and Drug Administration.[23]

Participation In Clinical Trails In The Home

The pharmacist should play a key role in the development of policies and procedures for handling investigational drugs in the HHC setting. The ASHP Guidelines for the Use of Investigational Drugs in Organized Health Care Settings[24] may be used as a guideline for the development of such policies and procedures. When patient participation in an investigational drug study is initiated in the institutional setting or other setting before the patient's transfer to the HHC setting, it is important that the HHC pharmacist obtain and keep on file sufficient information about the investigational protocol and drugs. If an investigational drug is dispensed or administered by the HHC organization, a copy of the informed consent form signed by the patient should be placed in the patient's HHC record. The HHC pharmacist should review the protocol before the patient is admitted to the HHC service to determine whether treatment of the patient in the home is appropriate. When investigational drug inventories are maintained in the HHC pharmacy, the pharmacist is responsible for accurate record keeping. The pharmacist should be an active participant in coordinating and monitoring investigational drug studies in HHC.

Participation In Quality Improvement Activities

Pharmacists and other members of the pharmacy staff (e.g., technicians) should be active participants in quality improvement activities in their organizations. A quality improvement program for HHC should monitor patient satisfaction and outcomes. Aspects of care that may be monitored include unscheduled inpatient admissions, unexpected discontinuation of infusion therapy, interruption of infusion therapy, development of infection(s), reported adverse drug and device related reactions, medication errors, and medication related problems. The quality improvement program should also include appropriate quality control measures for the compounding of sterile products and other activities.

Policies And Procedures

The HHC pharmacist should be an active participant in the development of organizational policies and procedures. The organization should maintain current policies and procedures on all aspects of patient care and quality assurance. Activities that should be addressed in policies and procedures include, but are not limited to, criteria for patient acceptance to HHC services, patient training and education, drug preparation and dispensing, equipment maintenance, quality control and quality assurance in sterile product compounding, infection control, and documentation in patients' home care records.

Licensure And Accreditation

Pharmacies providing HHC services should be licensed by the state board of pharmacy and other appropriate regulatory agencies. Some states require special licensure for pharmacies preparing sterile products to be dispensed to outpatients. Pharmacists dispensing medications to patients who reside in other states may also be subject to applicable regulations in those states; additional licensure may be necessary. Accreditation of the organization by the Joint Commission on Accreditation of Healthcare Organizations or the Community Health Accreditation Program (CHAP) is recommended. The pharmacist should be knowledgeable of all applicable laws, regulations, and standards.

Continuing Education And Training

Pharmacists should receive training in the provision of HHC services. Pharmacists should participate in ongoing continuing education activities as defined in the ASHP Statement on Continuing Education[25] to improve knowledge and skills related to home care. When appropriate, pharmacists should assist in training and education programs for other HHC personnel. Whenever possible, pharmacists should participate in the provision of student clerkship, externship, and internship training, as well as postgraduate residency training.

COMPETITORS IN HHC PHARMACY

In a very real sense, pharmacists have been in the business of HHC longer than any other group selling prescription and over-the-counter drugs for use at home.[10] With the establishment of the Medicare definition of HHC, pharmacy products and services were provided by a relatively small group of independent pharmacy practitioners. As HHC expanded as a viable health care alternative, independent practitioners were faced with a variety of competitors. These competitors include pharmacies, both independent and chain; independent HHC centers; national and regional HHC pharmacies such as OPTION Care and Caremark; oxygen or respiratory therapy supply dealers; rehabilitation therapy dealers; traditional medical and surgical supply retailers; mass merchandisers such as Sears; mail order retailers such as the American Association of Retired Persons; and health care providers such as home health agencies, visiting nurse association, hospitals, and physicians.[3]

However, it is misleading to state that all of these entities compete against each other. Rather, the list of competitors shows that HHC is not a single market, but a number of different markets serving the multidimensional HHC patient. It is clear, for example, that HOMEDCO's total parenteral nutrition services do not compete directly with the local Sears store. However, the pharmacy that provides blood pressure monitoring equipment is certainly in competition with the mass retailer that also markets this equipment.

Hospitals And Physicians As Competitors

In addition to being one of the most promising areas in health care today, HHC is one of the most competitive. One of the most significant aspects of competition in HHC in recent years has been the expanded involvement of hospitals and physicians. In the late 1970's hospitals and physicians had taken a casual approach to HHC, leaving HHC responsibility to a discharge planner and independent HHC practitioners. In recent years, however, because hospitals had come under increasing pressure to discharge patients earlier, as well as to find new diversification opportunities, HHC has been given a high priority by many institutions. Carefully planned and marketed HHC programs are now a routine part of many hospital ventures.[3]

Hospital-based HHC programs serve several functions. Referral patterns may become streamlined and consolidated when a full array of inpatient and outpatient services are offered. A HHC program serves the hospital as a patient management tool, helping it to move patients out of an expensive inpatient setting to a less expensive HHC environment.

Hospitals have a significant advantage in HHC because they have immediate access to the captive referral, the inpatient waiting to go home. It is convenient to many patients who are about to be discharged from the hospital, to turn to that very same hospital for HHC products and services.[3]

The role of physicians in HHC has followed the same pattern as that of hospitals. Initially, most physicians ignored HHC opportunities and concentrated on traditional hospital and office-based care. Today, however, increasing numbers of physicians view HHC as an opportunity to extend their scope of service and to diversify in response to changing reimbursement pressures.

Physicians share with hospitals concerns over the loss of patient control and revenue that are now a part of ongoing cost containment activity. Physicians may view their patients as potential captive referrals, for office-based therapies such a parenteral antibiotics, chemotherapy, and pain management. These products can become a lucrative supplement to an existing office practice.

A LESS COSTLY ALTERNATIVE

In comparing the cost of HHC with that of traditional hospital-based care, HHC has been viewed as a less costly alternative. The emphasis on cost containment in health care has served as an important stimulus to the expansion of HHC. Demonstrating the cost-benefit of HHC has been accomplished by emphasizing the daily room charge for acute hospitalization and related hospital-based charges, that are not included in the typical set of charges for HHC products and services.

A major thrust in marketing HHC to third party payers and referral sources has been that HHC is inexpensive. However, McAllister cautioned nearly ten years ago that the biggest threat to HHC is gluttony, in the form of overcharging, kickbacks, and inappropriate patient selection.[11] Recently, Abramowitz[12] reported on two main controversies in HHC: concern that HHC bills are excessive, and potential conflicts of interest by physicians who refer patients to HHC companies. (See also Chapter 2.)

In spite of the risk of fiscal abuse associated with the provision of HHC, these products and services will continue to be a less costly alternative for the homebound patient who needs acute or chronic care. To minimize further the risk of fiscal abuse, increased controls on reimbursement by third party payers will occur. Conversion to managed cared and managed competition will also have an impact on HHC as a less costly alternative. (See also Chapter 3.)

REFERENCES

1. Lamy PP. Introduction to Home Health Care. In: Catania PN and Rosner MM, eds. Home Health Care Practice. Palo Alto, Health Markets Research, 1986.
2. Pegels CC. Health Care and the Older Citizen. Rockville, Aspen Publishers, Inc. 1988.
3. Cassak DJ. Competitors in Home Health Care. In: Catania PN and Rosner MM, eds. Home Health Care Practice. Palo Alto, Health Markets Research, 1986.
4. Spiegel AD. Home Health Care, 2nd ed. Owings Mills, Rynd Communications, 1987.
5. Strandell C. Home Health Care Nursing. Rockville, Aspen Publishers, Inc., 1989.
6. Anon. Manager Care Digest: Long Term Care Edition. Kansas City, Marion Merrell Dow, 1993.
7. Winter RW, et al. Home Infusion Therapy. Washington DC, National Alliance For Infusion Therapy, 1992.
8. Anon. Report Provides Profile of home infusion services. Am J Hosp Pharm 1993; 50:846.
9. Catania PN. Parenteral Therapy as a Home Health Care Service. Parenterals 1987; 5:1.
10. Anon. ASHP Guidelines on the Pharmacist's Role in Home Care. Am J HospPharm. 1993; 50:1940-1944.
11. McNulty TJ. Initiation of antimicrobial therapy in the home. Am J Hosp Pharm. 1993; 50:773-4.
12. American Society of Hospital Pharmacists. ASHP statement on the pharmacist's role in patient education programs. Am J Hosp Pharm. 1991; 48:1780.
13. American Society of Hospital Pharmacists. ASHP guidelines on pharmacist-conducted patient counseling. Am J Hosp Pharm. 1993; 50:505-6.
14. American Society of Hospital Pharmacists. ASHP statement on the pharmacist's role with respect to drug delivery systems and administration devices. Am J Hosp Pharm. 1989; 46:2342-3.
15. Kwan J. High-technology i.v. infusion devices. Am J Hosp Pharm. 1991; 48(Suppl 1):S36-S51.
16. Bowles C, McKinnon BT. Selecting infusion devices. Am J Hosp Pharm. 1993; 50:1228-30.
17. Hepler CD, Strand LM. Opportunities and responsibilities in pharmaceutical care. Am J Hosp Pharm. 1990; 47:533-43.
18. Joint Commission on the Accreditation of Healthcare Organizations. Accreditation Manual for Home Care. Oakbrook Terrace, IL. Joint Commission on the Accreditation of Healthcare Organizations. 1993.
19. American Society of Hospital Pharmacists. ASHP technical assistance bulletin on handling cytotoxic and hazardous drugs. Am J Hosp Pharm. 1990; 47:1033-49.
20. Schaffner A. Safety precautions in home chemotherapy. Am J Nurs. 1984; 84:356-7.
21. American Society of Hospital Pharmacists. ASHP statement on the pharmacist's role in infection control. Am J Hosp Pharm. 1986; 43:2006-8.
22. American Society of Hospital Pharmacists. ASHP guidelines on adverse drug reaction monitoring and reporting. Am J Hosp Pharm. 1989; 46:336-7.
23. Draft form for reporting suspect adverse events and product problems with medications and devices; notice. Fed Regist. 1993; 58:11768-73.
24. American Society of Hospital Pharmacists. ASHP guidelines for the use of investigational drugs in organized health care settings. Am J Hosp Pharm. 1991; 48:315-9.
25. American Society of Hospital Pharmacists. ASHP statement on continuing education. Am J Hosp Pharm. 1990; 47:1855.
26. Catania PN and Rosner MM. Pharmacy Services for Home Health Care Patients. Continuing Care. 1987; 6:22.
27. McAllister III JC. Hospital Pharmacist's Guide to Home Health Care. Bethesda, American Society of Hospital Pharmacists. 1986.

2 Legal Aspects of Home Health Care Pharmacy Practice

Richard R. Abood, J.D.

Engaging in a home health care (HHC) practice exposes pharmacists to many of the same legal issues of a traditional pharmacy practice, as well as to other significant legal issues. This chapter will focus on those issues which have been of most concern to pharmacists in HHC practice over the past years. These issues include professional liability, products liability, liability for employees, Medicare/Medicaid law, antitrust law and legal issues involving the compounding of pharmaceuticals.

Although there are a substantial number of legal problems associated with the offering of any professional services or products, pharmacists should not view potential legal problems with fear, but rather respect. In no way should fear of legal issues become a reason not to engage in a legitimate professional activity. Awareness of legal requirements and potential legal problems should be used by pharmacists to tailor their practices accordingly, not avoid them.

PROFESSIONAL LIABILITY OF PROVIDERS

There are several reasons why HHC practice may present a greater risk of professional liability compared to traditional pharmacy practice, but two reasons in particular stand out. First, patients requiring HHC are often sicker than the average ambulatory patient. Sick patients obviously require extra care and attention and run a greater risk of not improving or getting worse. Moreover, HHC patients will likely be sent home even sicker in the future as hospitals, pressured by both governmental and private insurers to contain costs, discharge patients even earlier. Second, the technology of many HHC products has become very complex, requiring pharmacists to be skilled not only in using the products, but in educating patients in their use as well.

NEGLIGENCE

A pharmacist who provides professional services in a substandard manner which subsequently cause injury to a patient may be liable under the tort liability theory of negligence. The following case study can serve as an example.

Case Study

A physician telephoned an IV antibiotic prescription order to the pharmacist for a HHC patient. The patient had never used IV medications in the home before, so the pharmacist delivered the medication personally with the HHC nurse. The pharmacist briefly counseled the patient as to the nature of the drug, some of the adverse effects the patient might experience and what things the patient should avoid. The patient took the drug for two weeks and developed irreversible kidney damage. She sued the pharmacist, among other providers, contending the pharmacist was negligent not to warn her that this drug could cause nephrotoxicity. She further alleged that she had a physical condition which predisposed her to the drug's danger of nephrotoxicity and that the pharmacist was aware of this physical condition. Is the pharmacist negligent?

One cannot determine whether the pharmacist is legally negligent without knowing what constitutes negligence. To prevail in a negligence lawsuit, a plaintiff must establish four elements: (1) that the pharmacist owed the plaintiff a duty; (2) that the pharmacist breached his or her standard of care; (3) that this breach caused the injury; and (4) the amount of injury and monetary damages sought. Failure to prove any one of these elements will defeat the plaintiff's case. Most negligence cases focus on the standard of care and causation.

Standard of Care

Traditionally in duty to warn cases, courts

have generally held that pharmacists owe no duty to warn patients; that this is the physician's responsibility.[1] However, after the enactment of the federal Omnibus Budget Reconciliation Act of 1990 (OBRA-90), every state has now passed some form of law or regulation mandating that pharmacists counsel or offer to counsel patients; maintain patient profiles; and screen prescriptions for potential drug therapy problems.[2] The counseling must include advising the patient of the drug's common, severe adverse effects, if in the pharmacist's professional discretion these warnings are warranted. It is likely that courts will shift their focus from whether a duty to warn exists, to whether the pharmacist violated the appropriate standard of care. This will require the court to examine the scope of the standard of care owed including whether the pharmacist advised the patient of the particular adverse effect, and if not, why.

In determining the appropriate standard of care of a pharmacist, the court will compare the pharmacist's behavior to that of a hypothetical average, prudent pharmacist in the same or similar circumstances. More than likely the court will hear the testimony of pharmacists serving as expert witnesses for both the plaintiff and the defendant, giving their opinions as to whether the pharmacist should have warned the patient of the adverse effect. Several factors may enter into the standard of care determination by the court and probably most importantly will be the manner in which the pharmacist exercised his or her professional judgment. Questions a court might ask include: Did the pharmacist recognize the potential problem? Did the pharmacist refer to references to determine the probability of the adverse effect occurring and the potential magnitude of harm? Did the pharmacist contact the prescriber and what was the result of the discussion? Did the pharmacist violate a state statute or regulation? Did the pharmacist violate an accreditation standard?

Some courts find that if a statute or regulation establishes a standard of care, violation of that statute or regulation is per se negligence. This could be a significant liability factor for pharmacists who intentionally ignore state counseling and screening laws and regulations. In cases where the pharmacist screens in good faith, detects the problem and contacts the prescriber, the pharmacist will generally have met the standard of care if the prescriber then tells the pharmacist he or she is aware of the potential problem, but to dispense the drug anyway. However, in situations where the probability and/or magnitude of harm is very great to the patient, the pharmacist would be wise to ask the physician to cite support for the decision; and if the pharmacist is unsatisfied, refuse to dispense the medication and counsel the patient accordingly.

It might not be enough for a pharmacist to establish that the standard of care he or she met is indeed the local standard. Most courts have evolved from applying local standards to national standards. This does not necessarily mean that a rural pharmacist, for example, will be held to the same standard as that of a pharmacist working with the latest technology in a medical center. It does mean that the rural pharmacist must meet the same standards as other rural pharmacists across the country. Thus, pharmacists in HHC must ensure that their skills and knowledge are comparable to pharmacists in other areas. If a court determines that the standard of care established by the profession is too low, it could impose its own standard.[3] Pharmacists should have knowledge of how other HHC pharmacists undertake their professional tasks.

It is important to note that medication errors such as dispensing the wrong drug, the wrong dosage, improperly preparing a drug, or other errors of a mechanical nature will likely be considered negligence per se by a court. In these cases the standard of care allows for no mistakes. Only when professional judgment or discretion is involved will courts seek to determine the standard of care.

Causation

A negligent act by the defendant is not enough to warrant a verdict for the plaintiff. The plaintiff must also show that the pharmacist's negligent act or omission caused the injury to occur. Another way of stating this is that the plaintiff must show that "but for" the pharmacist's act or omission, the injury would never have occurred. In the hypothetical case above, the plaintiff must reasonably establish that the drug caused the nephrotoxicity. The defendant will attempt to prove that the nephrotoxicity would have occurred regardless of the drug. Assuming that the plaintiff does establish that the drug caused the injury, the plaintiff must also show that if the pharmacist had warned of the adverse effect it would have changed the outcome. Thus the plaintiff must show that she would have altered her behavior in some manner which would have prevented the adverse outcome, e.g., by asking for a different drug, or more closely monitoring her symptoms.

Is The Pharmacist Liable?

In this post-OBRA 90 era of mandatory screening, counseling and patient profiling, pharmacists may no longer be able to hide behind previous judicial decisions which have declared that pharmacists have no duty to detect potential drug problems and take appropriate action. This is especially true in this case and in similar situations. Many of the decisions which have found that pharmacists have no duty to detect or warn of adverse drug effects were based on the fact that the pharmacists did not have access to the patent's medical history, as does the physician. Pharmacists today, especially HHC pharmacists who dispense IV products, may be expected to know relevant information from a patient's medical history. HHC pharmacists may be expected to monitor the patient's progress, either personally or through HHC nurses. In this case, the pharmacist had, or should have had, prior knowledge of the patient's condition which put her at greater risk. The court may find that the pharmacist had a duty first to be aware of the potential danger and second to discuss with the physician the appropriateness of the drug and explore safer alternatives. Assuming the physician insisted on the drug, the court could well find that the pharmacist had a duty to counsel the patient as to the possible adverse effect and what symptoms to look for which could signal that the drug should be discontinued. Absent these actions, a court might very well conclude that the pharmacist was negligent.

PRODUCTS LIABILITY

In addition to negligence for professional activities, pharmacists who lease or sell HHC products must be concerned with product liability claims. When a patient is injured because of the use of a product, three theories of liability become potentially applicable: negligence, breach of warranty under contract law, and strict tort liability. Although plaintiffs have asserted breach of warranty and strict liability claims against pharmacists on numerous occasions for injuries caused by prescription drugs, fortunately courts have consistently rejected these claims.[4] However, breach of warranty and strict liability are allowed in lawsuits involving most other products.

Case Study

Assume the following hypothetical situation: A HHC pharmacy supplies home infusion pumps to patients when needed to administer their parenteral drugs. The pharmacy is very careful to completely check the pumps when they are returned from the patient and before they are sent to a new patient. Every six months the pharmacy also sends the pumps to a company to be serviced and cleaned. Every patient is instructed carefully and completely in the use of the pump and what to do in the event the pump should fail. The patient is told a warning will sound and is given a number to call anytime day or night. Despite all of these precautions, a pump malfunctions allowing an overdose of the drug to be administered. No warning is sounded and the patient is severely injured from the overdose. As a result of the injury the patient brought a lawsuit against the manufacturer of the pump, the distributor and the pharmacy based on the allegation that the pump was a defective product. Is the pharmacy liable for the patient's injury?

As indicated, in the suit against the pharmacy the patient might assert all three theories of products liability in the same complaint.

Negligence

Applying the negligence theory, the patient would allege that the pharmacy breached the standard of care which it owed to its patients by not properly inspecting the pump; or, not properly preparing the pump for use; or, not properly instructing the patient on how to use the pump and what to do if it malfunctions. A court would consider many of the same factors previously discussed under professional liability. Of particular importance to a court might be whether there were any applicable accreditation standards for the care and inspection of the product. Pharmacists must insure these standards are met so it is evidence used in their favor, rather than against them. In the case study, let us assume that the pharmacist met all accreditation standards. The facts in the case would then seem to indicate that the pharmacist exercised the standard of care of a reasonable, prudent pharmacist. Absent some other fact which would indicate that the pharmacist should have known that the pump could fail, it would not appear that the pharmacist was negligent.

The danger of product liability for a seller, however, is that the patient need not rely on only a negligence action for success, as the other two theories of product liability, breach of warranty and strict liability, are not fault based.

Breach Of Warranty

Breach of warranty is contract based liability. Whenever a product is sold or leased a contract is created, either expressly or impliedly, between the buyer and seller. An injured plaintiff bringing a breach of warranty action is obligated to prove the existence of a warranty, that the product was defective and that the defective product breached the warranty causing the injury. It is important to observe that under warranty theory and strict tort liability, fault or negligence are of no concern. Two types of warranties may arise from a sale, express and implied.

Breach of Express Warranty

Let us assume that the patient in the case study asked the pharmacist whether the pump was safe and error free. If the pharmacist asserted to the patient that the pump was perfectly safe and would not malfunction or would not be a danger to the patient, the pharmacist may have created an express warranty.[5] If the patient then relied on the pharmacist's statement in his use of the pump, as he did in this case, a breach of express warranty might exist. Pharmacists selling any products, including prescription drugs, must be careful not to make any promises or guarantees. In the case study, the pharmacist would have been better served to truthfully remark that the pumps hardly ever malfunction; and he has never known of a case where if a pump has malfunctioned, the alarm has failed to sound.

Breach of Implied Warranties

Not making an express warranty does not necessarily protect a pharmacist from liability under warranty theory, however. Implied warranties are created by law and unless disclaimed by the seller flow with the sale. Two types of implied warranties are possible, implied warranty of merchantability and implied warranty of fitness for a particular purpose.[6] The first type of implied warranty is more applicable to the pump example. Under an implied warranty of merchantability the seller warrants that the product is fit for the ordinary purpose for which it is sold. An infusion pump which malfunctions would not likely be fit for the ordinary purpose for which it was sold, since a reasonable consumer might not expect this occurrence. Merchantability could become an issue whenever any device or product malfunctions and causes injury to a patient.

The second type of implied warranty is not applicable to the case study, but would be applicable to the sale of some HHC products especially durable medical equipment. A breach of implied warranty of fitness for a particular purpose could occur whenever a pharmacist exercises his or her professional judgment in the selection of a particular type, size or model of a product, the patient relies on the pharmacist's judgment and is injured because of that reliance. For example, assume that a pharmacist determines that a patient would best be fitted with a particular type of leg brace. The leg brace is free of any defects and functions perfectly. However after a few weeks of use the patient's leg becomes very painful. It is ultimately determined that the patient has suffered permanent nerve damage because he was fitted with the wrong type of brace for the patient's condition and the patient's size.

In this example, there would be no breach of implied warranty of merchantability, since the brace had no physical defects. However, there may be a breach of implied warranty of fitness for a particular purpose since the patient has relied upon the skill and judgment of the pharmacist, who has selected the wrong product. Negligence on the part of the pharmacist would also be an issue in this situation.

Implied warranties may be specifically disclaimed by the seller prior to sale. A statement by the seller to the effect that the product is sold "as is", or that the seller asserts "no warranties or guaranties" would suffice. Absent any disclaimers, implied warranties will exist by law. Needless to say it would not inspire much confidence in a patient if a pharmacy sold or leased complicated, life dependent devices and issued a statement that the products are sold "as is with no warranties or guarantees." It is also unlikely that such disclaimers would be effective as a defense in court when these types of products are involved. A disclaimer on these types of products might violate social policy because of the nature of reliance between the provider and the patient.

Strict Liability

Strict liability in tort developed primarily because it was often difficult or impossible for a plaintiff to establish negligence against the seller. In many product liability cases brought today, the courts will often merge breach of warranty allegations into a strict tort liability analysis. To be successful the plaintiff must show that the product is defective, unreasonably dangerous and that the defect caused the injury.[7] Courts take different liberties in defining defective and unreasonably dangerous, but generally impose liability if the product is dangerous beyond that contemplated by an ordinary consumer.

Policy reasons for imposing strict liability against sellers include the following: the seller can better distribute the loss to the public through price increases and insurance than can an injured plaintiff; the public is relatively helpless against those who manufacture and sell defective products and thus deserve additional legal protection; and the greater risk of liability to the seller will assure that the seller sells the safest product possible.

Retailers in particular have been held accountable under strict liability because: (1) they are often the only visible party to whom an injured party can seek redress; (2) retailers play a major role in insuring that a product is safe and may be able to influence manufacturers to that end; and (3) retailers can seek indemnity against the manufacturer. Some jurisdictions, however, have fashioned what is known as the sealed container doctrine. Under this doctrine a retailer is not liable for selling a defective product which causes injury when the product is sold in the manufacturer's sealed container. As a general rule, however, retailers are liable under strict liability for selling a defective product even though they had no way of knowing that the product was defective. The retailer's recourse is to seek indemnity or contribution from the manufacturers or to be insured.

In the infusion pump example, if the court determines that the pump is unreasonably dangerous, which would seem fairly apparent, liability may be imposed against the pharmacy. Needless to say, strict liability constantly looms as a danger to product sellers and it cannot be disclaimed.

DEFENSES TO PROFESSIONAL AND PRODUCTS LIABILITY

Various defenses do exist to professional negligence and products liability actions. These include contributory negligence, comparative negligence, assumption of the risk and abnormal use of the product. Under the theories of contributory and comparative negligence, the patient is expected to act as a reasonably prudent patient to avoid the harm. For example, assume that a pharmacist refilled a patient's prescription with large, red tablets, when previously the patient's medication had been small, green capsules. The patient took the large, red tablets and suffered injury. The pharmacist was negligent in dispensing the wrong medication, but the patient would probably be contributorily negligent in not noticing that the medications looked different.

Contributory negligence is a complete bar to the plaintiff's case. To mitigate this effect on the plaintiff, many states have passed laws establishing the doctrine of comparative negligence. Under comparative negligence, the relative fault of each party is compared. If the plaintiff's fault is less than the defendant's, the plaintiff will be awarded an amount as determined by his or her degree of fault.

Assumption of the risk arises as a defense to negligence and product liability claims when the plaintiff knew of the risk yet voluntarily continued to use the product, or encounter the risk in some manner. For example, the defendant might raise this defense as an issue in the nephrotoxicity case study, if the patient was aware that her physical condition predisposed her to nephrotoxicity from the drug's use, but took the drug anyway. A defense to products liability may also exist when patients fail to heed directions or warnings supplied with the product, or improperly use the product, or use it for a purpose for which it was not intended.

Strict liability and breach of warranty apply to the sale of products, not professional services.[8] This could be a defense in several HHC situations since courts have generally held that strict liability does not apply when the sale of a product is incidental to the provision of a service. For example, in one case a dentist was sued under strict liability when the hypodermic needle he used broke in the patient's jaw.[9] The court held that even though the needle may have been defective, the dentist could only be tried under negligence since the needle was simply part of a professional service.

EXERCISING RISK MANAGEMENT

The risk of professional and products liability can be mitigated. With respect to products, the more complex the product, the more preparation required by the pharmacist, the more that the product is involved in a life sustaining function, and the more that a defect in the product might cause serious injury to the patient, the greater the risk of a products liability action. To minimize the risk of products liability actions, pharmacists should inventory HHC products from reputable manufacturers only. Products with a history of breakdowns, or products of questionable workmanship and quality should be avoided, despite their "bargain" appeal. Pharmacists and non-pharmacist employees should not sell or render advice about HHC products unless they are familiar with them. With respect to products such as parenteral preparations, pharmacists must make certain that they have the proper equipment and knowledge to prepare these products accurately and in an unadulterated manner. Also, administration and monitoring procedures for parenterals must be established.

It is imperative that pharmacists continually update their skills and knowledge about HHC products and services. They should never attempt any service or sell any product unless they are knowledgeable and competent. All appropriate quality assurance procedures, documentation and adherence to established polices should be followed.

LIABILITY INSURANCE POLICIES

Just as with traditional pharmacy practice, pharmacists should maintain liability insurance to cover HHC products and services. Since many liability policies cover only traditional dispensing functions, pharmacists should examine their policies to determine if HHC functions are included. For example, the preparation of parenterals should be covered, as well as professional services provided at sites outside the pharmacy.

Employee pharmacists should also examine the pharmacy's liability policy to ascertain if they are covered. Although the employer is liable for the acts of its employees, the employer would have a right of subrogation against the employee if it is sued. Moreover, the plaintiff could always choose to sue the employee independently or jointly with the employer.

LIABILITY FOR THE ACTS OF EMPLOYEES

As a general rule an employer is liable for the negligent acts of its employees. This rule is called respondeat superior and applies when the employee is functioning within the scope of his or her employment. Several reasons are often advanced for respondeat superior including: (1) employers have the authority to direct and control employees and therefore should be responsible for their activities, their supervision and their proper selection; (2) employers should be at risk since they benefit from the acts of the employees; (3) the employer is more likely to be able to pay for the plaintiff's loss than the employee (called the deep pocket theory); and (4) the employer can be insured.

A pharmacy in the HHC business may employ several persons besides pharmacists including nurses and various types of technicians. These individuals have expertise different than the pharmacist owner or manager, making it more difficult for him or her to evaluate their performance and competence. Nonetheless, the pharmacy must take every precaution that employees are competent to perform the tasks assigned and that they are properly trained. The pharmacy should supervise and monitor its employees regularly to insure this.

A significant issue might arise whether a person is actually an employee or an independent contractor. Generally an employer is not liable for the acts of an independent contractor. In situations such as when a pharmacy contracts with a HHC nurse to make patient visits and administer drugs, the issue might become murky. Often the most important determinant is how much control the employer has over the time, manner and method of the work performed. The more control the pharmacy has over the nurse's services, the more likely that the nurse would be viewed as an employee.

Even if it is determined that an independent contractor relationship exists, it may not shield the pharmacy from liability. If a patient reasonably believes that because of the conduct of the pharmacy, that the independent contractor is acting on behalf of the pharmacy, liability could result under the doctrine of apparent or ostensible agency. Several factors might enter into this determination besides employer control including whether the patient had any input in choosing the contractor; the nature of the contract between the pharmacy and contractor; and whether the pharmacy supplies any equipment, space or support to the contractor.

Because of the foregoing discussion, the contract between the pharmacy and the contractor is very important. The contract should specify the scope of each parties' duties and responsibilities and the nature of the relationship between the parties. Although such provisions will not always be valid, the contract should include provisions holding one party harmless in the event of a negligent act by the other.

MEDICARE/MEDICAID ANTI-FRAUD & ABUSE LAW

Since the enactment of the Medicare and Medicaid programs in 1965, some health care providers have exploited the programs for personal financial gain. Most notably this exploitation has occurred by physicians who refer patients to health care facilities in which they either have an ownership interest, or from which they receive kickbacks or other types of incentives. Often these situations have resulted in substandard and unnecessary treatment for the patient and added expense for the federal government.

Pharmacists who market their HHC products and services frequently encounter situations where a physician or other health care provider will ask: "What's in it for me if I refer patients to your business?" From the other perspective, pharmacists have been known to offer discounts, rebates or other inducements to providers to obtain patients. These practices would be illegal for Medicare or Medicaid patients as described below.

The Anti-fraud And Abuse Statute

In an effort to curb fraudulent and abusive practices by health care providers, Congress enacted anti-kickback provisions in 1972, which made it a criminal offense to solicit, offer or receive kickbacks, bribes or rebates for referrals.[10] Nonetheless, fraud and abuse continued, prompting Congress to toughen the law even further in subsequent years. The current law, as amended in 1991, prohibits anyone from knowingly and willfully soliciting, receiving, offering or paying any remuneration in exchange for inducing referrals, or for the furnishing of any goods or services which Medicare or Medicaid pays. Violation of this law is a felony punishable by a maximum fine of $25,000 and/or five years imprisonment. Violators will also be expelled from the Medicare and Medicaid programs. The Office of Inspector General (OIG) is charged with the responsibility of investigating and identifying instances of fraud and abuse; while the Department of Justice prosecutes offenders.

The federal courts have construed the anti-kickback statute very liberally in favor of the government. In United States v. Greber, physicians ordered Holter-monitor tests to be performed and interpreted at the defendant cardiologist's lab.[11] The lab billed Medicare for the test and the interpretation by the defendant. After receiving the payment the defendant remitted 40% of it to the referring physician. The government charged the defendant with intentionally inducing referrals in violation of the anti-kickback statute. The defendant contended that the payments to the referring physicians were simply to compensate them for their initial consultations and explanation to the patient of lab results. The defendant also admitted, though, that if he did not pay the physicians the fee they would not use his lab. The court concluded that even if the payment was for compensation for actual services, if one purpose of the payment was also to induce referrals, then the payment violated the statute.

A subsequent federal case supported the Greber decision,[12] while another case held that the payment would not be illegal unless it was for the primary purpose of inducing referrals.[13] Despite this controversy, providers would best be served to follow the holding of Greber and avoid making or receiving any payment, even for a legitimate purpose, if it might be construed as inducing a referral.

Safe Harbor Regulations

In 1991, after considerable public controversy and commentary, the Department of Health and Human Services (DHHS) promulgated final regulations for the purpose of giving health care providers better guidance as to the types of investments and business arrangements which would be safe from the anti-fraud statute.[14] These regulations are commonly called the safe harbor regulations and are summarized below.

Large Entity Investments

Under the regulations, investors capable of making or influencing referrals to a health care entity may invest in the entity so long as the dividends they receive are actually dividends and not kickbacks disguised as dividends. To assure this, the investment must meet six conditions: (1) the entity must hold more than $50 million in net undepreciated tangible assets; (2) if the investment is in corporate stock, the entity must be registered with the Securities and Exchange Commission; (3) if the investor is in a position to generate business or referrals to the entity, the investor's interest must be obtained on terms equally available to the public through a registered national securities exchange; (4) the entity may not market products or services that favor passive investors (e.g., stockholders, limited partners) over non-investors; (5) the entity may not provide or guarantee a loan to an investor who is in a position to generate business for the entity; and (6) the investor's return on investment must be directly proportional to the investor's capital investment.

Small Entity Investments

Entities such as joint ventures, partnerships and corporations with less than $50 million in net assets must meet the following seven requirements: (1) no more than 40% of the investment interests of the entity can be obtained from investors in a position to refer or generate business for the entity; (2) no more than 40% of the entity's gross revenue for the previous year is generated from business from investors; (3) the terms for investment are offered equally to all investors in order to prevent illegal payments disguised as higher profit returns; (4) investment opportunities offered to potential referral sources must not be based upon previous or anticipated business from the investor; (4) an investor cannot be required to be a referral source; (5) there can be no cross-referral arrangements between entities or their investors; (6) the entity must not loan or guarantee investment capital to potential referral sources; and (7) returns to an investor must be directly proportional to the investor's capital investment.

Space and Equipment Rentals; Personal Services and Contracts

Rental payments between providers, as well as personal services and management contracts between providers are safe from violation if: (1) the agreement is in writing, signed and for one year; (2) the agreement specifies the premises, equipment or service covered; (3) the terms of a periodic lease must specify the schedule length, and exact charge for each period; and (4) the aggregate rental charge or compensation must be established in advance based upon fair market value without regard to the potential for referral value. This requirement aims at precluding commission agreements with independent contractors. For space and equipment leases, fair market value cannot be adjusted based upon proximity or convenience to referral sources.

Sale of a Practice

A contract by one practitioner to sell a practice to another practitioner is legal so long as the sale is completed within one year and the seller does not make referrals or generate business for the purchaser for one year.

Referral Services

Referral services are businesses which refer patients to certain providers which pay to be listed with the service. These referral services are legal provided: (1) the payment by the provider is based upon a flat fee, not upon a commission for the number of referrals; (2) the service discloses its relationship with the providers and the criteria used to select providers; and (3) the service applied criteria for membership equally to all participants.

Warranties

Manufacturers and suppliers may make payment to a purchaser for a faulty product or replace the product pursuant to a written warranty provided (1) the purchaser and seller report the warranty and the resulting price reduction; (2) the seller does not pay a provider for medical expenses incurred by a beneficiary other than for the cost of the item; (3) the seller documents the terms of the warranty when the sale is made before the price reduction is known and informs the buyer when the amount is known; and (4) the buyer discloses the information to the DHHS upon request.

Discounts

If a provider gives a discount for a product or service to another provider in exchange for patient referrals and the full price is billed to Medicare or Medicaid, the discount is illegal. The safe harbor regulations allow discounts if (1) they are obtained at the time of purchase in an "arm's length" transaction; (2) the discount is in the form of a rebate check, credit or coupon directly redeemable from the seller, but not as cash, warranties or the furnishing of one product or service free or at a lower cost in exchange for the purchase of another product or service; (3) if the discounts are applicable to any other payer, they must be applicable to Medicare and Medicaid; and (4) the discount buyer must disclose the discount and upon request of DHHS or the state provide the information obtained by the seller. Waivers of the patient's deductible or copayment does not constitute a discount for the purposes of the safe harbor regulation.

In 1992 the OIG challenged a program in which the manufacturer offered $75 rebates to individuals who purchased home blood glucose meters from pharmacists. The pharmacists submitted the claims to Medicare for the patient and as a result the claims often did not reflect the rebate given to the individual. Since the discount was not disclosed it did not fall within the safe harbor regulation. The program was thus restructured such that the rebate was paid to the pharmacist, who reflected the discount on the claim. As part of this same program the manufacturer also offered discount airline vouchers worth up to $110 off airline tickets. Since this type of rebate is not reportable it would not fall under the protection of the safe harbor and the manufacturer was forced to eliminate it.

Pharmacists should avoid bundling services or products, such as providing nursing and consulting services at a discount in exchange for receiving prescription drug business. The OIG has specifically stated that Congress did not intend for these types of arrangements to be included under the safe harbor for discounts.

Payments to Employees

Payments by an employer to a bona fide employee even for the purpose of making referrals is protected by the safe harbor.

Group Purchasing Organizations

Payment of a fee by a vendor to a group purchasing organization which serves as a purchasing agent for providers is protected so long as (1) there is a written agreement between the organization and the provider members; (2) the written agreement includes the vendor's fee, if it is not fixed at 3% or less of the purchase price; (3) the organization is not owned by a participating provider; and (4) the organization makes an annual disclosure to the member providers of the amount received from each vendor.

Waiver of Coinsurance and Deductibles

Providers may legally attempt to attract inpatients by waiving Part A coinsurance and deductible charges. The provider is then prohibited from reporting this as a bad debt to Medicare. Moreover, the waiver must be made available to all Medicare inpatients. This safe harbor does not apply to outpatient Medicare (Part B) recipients, but does apply to outpatient Medicaid patients.

Safe Harbors as Guidance

The OIG stated that the purpose of the safe harbors is to define innocuous arrangements that should not be prosecuted, even though all of the activities would be illegal under the anti-kickback statute if not protected. The safe harbors are quite narrow in scope and exclude many common business practices. If a particular business practice does not fall into a safe harbor it could mean that the practice is either (1) clearly legal since it does not intend to induce referrals; (2) clearly illegal in violation of the anti-kickback statute; or (3) unclear, but containing risk as it may violate the statute in a nonobvious or less serious manner. Pharmacists should be aware of the nature of their business practices and be aware of activities which fall outside of the safe harbors and which could be construed as inducing referrals.

ANTITRUST LAWS

HHC business practices can present antitrust legal problems ranging from restraint of trade or monopolization to price discrimination. Although several state and federal laws could be applied to various business practices, the primary laws encountered include the Sherman Antitrust Act and the Robinson-Patman Price Discrimination Act.

Restraints Of Trade And Monopolization: The Sherman Act

The Sherman Antitrust Act includes two sections. Section 1 prohibits contracts, combinations and conspiracies in restraint of trade.[15] Section 2 prohibits monopolization, attempts to monopolize and conspiracies to monopolize.[16] Although a literal interpretation of the Act would essentially prohibit every contract or combination in restraint of trade, the Supreme Court has established that only contracts which unreasonably restrain trade are unlawful. A violation of Section 1 can occur only if there is an agreement, formal or informal, between competitors. Absent any concerted activity, the behavior will be judged under Section 2. The plaintiff must also establish that he or she suffered injury and the extent of that injury.

In addition to proving unreasonable conduct, concerted behavior and injury, a section 1 plaintiff must also often prove that the defendant possessed sufficient market power to cause actionable harm. Market power is usually defined as the ability of a defendant to raise prices or exclude competition and is dependent upon the defendant's percentage of the available market. In Section 2 cases, the degree of market power must rise to the level of monopolization. The percentage of the market necessary to constitute market power or monopolization is very specific to the facts of each case. Some courts have found sufficient market power exists in some cases when the defendant has captured as little as 10% of the market and have found monopoly power to exist when the defendant has owned 30% of the market.

Although it is sometimes difficult for competitors to understand, the purpose of the antitrust laws is to protect free competition, not a particular competitor or group of competitors. Economic injury to competitors is not in itself a violation of the antitrust laws. "In an openly competitive market the inefficient fail; in a noncompetitive system the efficient are precluded from competing."[17]

Rule of Reason and Per Se test

In analyzing whether a particular activity violates the Act, courts will apply either a rule of reason or a per se test to the activity. Under a rule of reason analysis a court will examine whether the activity is reasonable based on a balancing of the pro-competitive and anti-competitive effects. Factors considered in the balancing include the purpose, nature and effects of the restraint, the duration of the restraint, the justification for the restraint, the market power of the entities involved, the number of entities, the nature of the industry, the relevant market, etc. The bottom line is "whether the restraint imposed is such as merely regulates and perhaps thereby promotes competition or whether it is such as may suppress or even destroy competition."[18]

Certain activities are usually anti-competitive. With respect to these activities courts will generally not examine the competitive effects, but rather consider such activities per se unlawful, regardless of any justification. Per se rules are applicable only to "Agreements or practices which because of their pernicious effect on competition and lack of any redeeming virtue are conclusively presumed to be unreasonable and therefore illegal without elaborate inquiry as to precise harm they have caused or the business excuse for their use."[19]

Some examples of activities generally held to be per se unlawful include price fixing among competitors (horizontal price fixing); price fixing between suppliers and their customers (resale price maintenance or vertical price fixing); group boycotts; and tying arrangements. The type of analysis which the court applies, rule of reason or per se test, could be crucial to the determination of the case. Application of the per se test is greatly advantageous to the plaintiff, obviating the necessity of introducing extensive economic proofs. HHC providers engaged in activities which could potentiate an antitrust lawsuit must seek to avoid actions which could lead to a per se classification.

Several types of general business activities by health care providers have been scrutinized by the courts and many of these are discussed below.

Price Fixing

Explicit or implicit agreements among competitors which affect the price or the allocation of services may constitute a per se violation of the Act.[20] However, novel, procompetitive structures in the health care system will likely be subject to a rule of reason analysis despite ancillary price fixing ramifications of the structure. Prohibited activities include not only setting specific prices but also setting maximum or minimum prices, and attempting to stabilize prices among competitors. Pharmacists must resist any temptation to conspire with competitors to establish prices or fees to patients or third party payors. Similarly, HHC providers must submit bids for contracts unilaterally.

Group Boycotts

A group boycott is an agreement among competitors not to deal with a third party payor. Boycott issues may also occur when a provider contends he or she as been excluded by other providers. As a general rule a boycott is a per se violation of the Act, however, novel situations in the health care industry where competition was not intentionally affected may warrant a rule of reason approach.[21] Pharmacists must not agree among themselves to reject a third party plan; and must exercise extreme caution when collectively rejecting a particular buyer or seller.

Purchasing Cooperatives

Since a purchasing cooperative represents an association of competitors, Sherman Act questions can arise. The Supreme Court, however, has viewed purchasing cooperatives quite favorably. In Northwest Wholesale Stationers, Inc., v. Pacific Stationery and Printing Co., a wholesale purchasing cooperative expelled a member without any explanation, notice or hearing.[22] The member alleged that the expulsion without procedural protection was a group boycott and constituted a per se violation of the Sherman Act.

Reversing the court of appeals decision and remanding the case, the Court held that the absence of procedural safeguards cannot determine the antitrust analysis. Rather the case must be decided based upon whether the decision to expel the member can properly be viewed as a group boycott mandating per se invalidation. Reviewing previous decisions where the per se rule had been applied, the court found that these involved situations where the boycott disadvantaged competitors by denying them suppliers, facilities, or markets necessary to compete. The Court found that the purchasing cooperative in question was "...not a form of concerted activity characteristically likely to result in predominantly anti-competitive effects."[23] Recognizing the value of cooperative purchasing arrangements to small retailers, the court found that such cooperatives might actually increase economic efficiency rather than decrease competition.

Preferred Provider Organizations (PPOs)

Since PPOs are usually composed of competitors, concerted behavior raises Section 1 concerns. Properly structured PPOs, however, are procompetitive and regarded favorably by both the FTC and the Justice Department. This does not mean, however, that any exceptions to the Sherman Act will be allowed. Any activity which can be characterized as a group boycott or price fixing may be considered as a per se violation of the Act, regardless of any economic benefits to the consumer which might result from the activity.

For example, in Arizona v. Maricopa County Medical Society, the Supreme Court applied the per se rule to a medical care foundation's maximum fee schedule.[24] The physician members agreed to accept certain fixed fees as full payment for service performed for patients insured under plans accepted by the foundation. The fees were established by the medical care foundation and were generally lower than those normally charged by its member physicians. In its decision the Court stated, "The anti-competitive potential inherent in all price-fixing agreements justifies their facial invalidation even if procompetitive justifications are offered for some."[25] Despite the Maricopa decision, competitive entrants into the health care market will likely be accorded a rule of reason analysis by the courts, rather than per se invalidation.

Joint Ventures

Of particular recent concern to many HHC providers is the issue of joint venturing, especially when a hospital integrates in some manner with a community HHC provider. Joint ventures arise when entities contract to carry out a single business venture and in the process combine their efforts, property, money, knowledge, or other assets. These joint ventures raise antitrust concerns when the hospital has market power in the geographic market of HHC patients and "steers" these patients to its "downstream" affiliate to the exclusion of other community providers. A court would likely apply a rule of reason approach to the joint venture, examining whether the purpose of the venture was for a legitimate business reason to enhance competition; or, to injure or destroy competition.

In Key Enterprises of Delaware, Inc., v. Venice Hospital, the defendant Venice Hospital purchased a one-half interest in the codefendant's home medical equipment (HME) supply business, Medicare Patient Aid Centers (MPAC).[26] The plaintiff, Venice Convalescent Aids Medical Supply (VCA), witnessed its percentage share of the HME market dwindle from 72.8% prior to the joint venture to 30% two years after the joint venture. Meanwhile the hospital affiliate's market share increased from 9.2% to 61%. VCA charged the defendants with violating Sections 1 and 2 of the Sherman Act by "coercing or unduly influencing" the home health agencies to refer patients to MPAC; and by unreasonably restricting and excluding competition. At trial the jury found for VCA and awarded it $2,282,949. The district court overturned the jury's decision and the court of appeals reversed the district court's decision and reinstated the jury verdict.

The court of appeals found that the defendants' behavior supported the charge of anti-competitive behavior for the following reasons: home health agency nurses were allowed access to the hospital's patients only if they recommended MPAC; the hospital changed its no solicitation policy prior to the joint venture to allow an employee of MPAC to make recommendations to patients; the joint venture appeared to be created expressly for the purpose of eliminating a potential competitor; the hospital allowed home health nurses to have access to patients, but not HME providers; the hospital followed a default rule, automatically selecting MPAC if a patient did not choose a HME provider.

The district court held that even this behavior would not be anti-competitive since the patients retained their freedom of choice to pursue any HME vendor. The court of appeals, however, found that the actions of the defendants were unnecessarily restrictive and that patient freedom of choice was illusory: "Patients rarely have a preference for an HME vendor. The patients know very little about the equipment or the companies that rent the equipment. Thus, they are very susceptible to recommendations made by anyone who appears to be knowledgeable on the subject."[27]

The Venice decision is currently being appealed, but as it stands it is a warning to hospitals and other providers with market power that they must exercise caution in their referral practices to affiliates.

Tying Arrangements and Exclusive Contracts

A court might conclude that a joint venture arrangement between a hospital and community home health entity constitutes an illegal tying arrangement. Tying arrangements exist when the seller, in this case the hospital, conditions the purchase of one product or service (hospitalization) with the purchase of another product or service (HHC).[28] Similarly an exclusive contract between the hospital and its affiliate, whereby the hospital agrees to steer all its patients to the affiliate might be viewed as anti-competitive. Exclusive contracts are normally legal, but not when they freeze out a significant portion of the market. Hospitals would be wise not to expressly enter into either a tying arrangement or exclusive contract with an affiliate.

Monopolization

A hospital which diversifies into HHC or HME as the owner cannot be held accountable under Section 1, but is susceptible to section 2 claims.[29] Simply being a monopoly is not illegal, but exploiting monopoly power unfairly for the purpose of injuring competition, as opposed to having a legitimate business purpose, is illegal. The distinction between engaging in tough, honest competition and engaging in anti-competitive conduct can be very difficult for a court to make. As a result, courts require that the plaintiff prove that the defendant's conduct was a willful acquisition or maintenance of monopoly power, as distinguished from growth or development through better products, services or good business practices.

In Venice Hospital, the court found that the defendant hospital willfully intended to injure competitors by using its monopoly power to foreclose competition and thus gain an unfair competitive advantage. This is termed monopoly leveraging and could occur when a hospital exploits its monopoly power in one market (inpatients) to obtain a monopoly or competitive advantage in another market (e.g., HHC).

Another monopolization theory under which a hospital could be found liable is called the essential facilities doctrine. This doctrine might apply when access to the hospital's patients is crucial in order for competing home health agencies to compete with the hospital's HHC business. Two important factors must be determined under this theory. Firstly, is the plaintiff really precluded from competing without access to patients in the hospital, or are alternative routes of marketing available to capture patients? As part of this question, a court would have to confront the issue of how much of the market should be available to the plaintiff. Secondly, does the hospital have a valid business reason for excluding competitors, such as for patient care and efficiency issues? A valid business reason would likely validate the exclusionary practice of the hospital.

Attempt to Monopolize

Section 2 not only prohibits monopolization but attempts to monopolize. Under this action the plaintiff need not establish that the hospital is a monopoly, but rather that the defendant specifically intended to acquire monopoly power; and that there is a dangerous probability that the defendant will succeed in obtaining a monopoly. In Venice Hospital, the court of appeals judged that the defendants attempted to monopolize the home health market since they had an intent to monopolize and had a dangerous probability of succeeding. The court reached this conclusion based upon the following facts: MPAC captured 39% of the HME market through referrals, and the hospital owned 46% of the total HME market; MPAC had only 9.2% of the market before the joint venture, but 61% of the market two years later; the joint venture devastated HME competitors by running one out of business, leaving another likely to go out of business, and leaving the others with a small market share to divide; finally, the joint venture created a barrier to entry making it highly unlikely that any new HME competitor could survive.

Price Discrimination: The Robinson-Patman Act

The Robinson-Patman Act (R-P Act) makes

it unlawful for a seller in interstate commerce to discriminate in price between different purchasers of like goods when the effect of the discrimination may be to injure competition, unless the discriminatory prices can be cost justified because of differences in the cost of manufacture, sale or delivery of the products.[30] Hospitals should be cautious of the R-P Act when they purchase pharmaceuticals and medical products at reduced prices and then resell those products to an affiliate home health business or to patients in competition with community home health operations.

NonProfit Institutions Act

An important exemption to the R-P Act is created by the NonProfit Institutions Act.[31] This law exempts from the application of the R-P Act sales to nonprofit schools, colleges, universities, etc "for their own use." A landmark U.S. Supreme Court decision in 1976, Portland Retail Druggists Assn., Inc. v. Abbott Laboratories, et. al., established the scope of the "own use" doctrine when nonprofit hospitals sell prescription drugs in competition with retail pharmacies.[32] In its decision the Supreme Court concluded that not all purchases by hospitals are exempt from the Act. "Own use," stated the Court, "is what reasonably may be regarded as use by the hospital in the sense that such use is a part of and promotes the hospital's intended institutional operation in the care of persons who are its patients."[33] Pursuant to this definition the Court established classifications of permissible and impermissible uses for drugs purchased at preferential prices.

Permissible activities constituting "own use" include the sale of drugs to an inpatient for use in the patient's treatment in the hospital; to an emergency room patient for use in the patient's treatment there; to an outpatient for personal use on the hospital premises; to an inpatient or emergency room patient, upon discharge and to outpatients for personal use away from the premises (take home medications); to the hospital's employee or student for personal use or for the use of a dependent; or to a staff physician who is not an employee, for personal use or for the use of a dependent.

Impermissible activities, or those not included under "own use" include sales of refills to former patients, emergency room patients or outpatients; sales to physicians for dispensation by the physician in his or her private office practice; or sales to the walk-in customer who is not a patient of the hospital.[34] It is very important to note that if a hospital engages in any of these impermissible activities, it does not necessarily mean that the hospital has violated the R-P Act. It simply means that the activity is not exempt and may be legally scrutinized under the R-P Act.

In a later decision, De Modena v. Kaiser Foundation Health Plan, Inc. the Ninth Circuit Court of Appeals found that HMOs selling prescriptions to enrollees were exempt from the Act under the Nonprofit Institutions Act.[35] The Court considered HMOs to be charitable institutions within the meaning of the Nonprofit Act and the purchases to be for the HMO's "own use" if sold to its members.

Application of "Own Use" to HHC

The Portland decision leaves several unanswered questions as applied to HHC. Two related questions of particular interest to many HHC providers include: (1) for how long a period of time can a discharge medication be supplied, and, (2) at what point in time is the patient no longer a patient of the hospital? In its analysis, the Court stated that take-home medications are part of the continuous treatment of the patient as he transcends from an inpatient to a home patient. However the court also emphasized that the take home prescription must be intended for a "...limited and reasonable time, as a continuation of, or supplement to, the treatment that was administered at the hospital...."[36]

It would not seem that therapies which must continue indefinitely, such as parenteral nutrition, would qualify under the "own use" doctrine. Whether, home IV antibiotic and chemotherapy started at the hospital which continues for several months would be included under "own use" is unclear. One could make the argument that after a few days, the patient would have had time to select a competing HHC provider and at that point in time, all competitors are obliged to play on a level-priced playing field. The limited and reasonable time issue also raises the issue of when is the drug therapy continuous and when is it a refill. Is it a refill when the admixture is prepared or at the end of the course of therapy? Similarly, although a hospital might view a patient for HHC purposes as an outpatient and eligible for continuous treatment, competing providers will argue that the patient is no longer exclusively the domain of the hospital's, since they can provide comparable treatment. All of the these questions remain unanswered as yet by the courts.

Establishing a Robinson-Patman Act Violation

Regardless of whether the hospital is a nonprofit hospital engaging in an impermissible activity, or a proprietary hospital, a plaintiff must establish competitive injury. This requires a plaintiff initially to establish that the hospital or its home health affiliate is selling differentially priced products to its HHC patients. Courts will likely require the plaintiff to provide documentation of the actual extent of the competitive injury suffered because of the discriminatory pricing and the amount of damages attributable to that injury. A causal connection must be established between any decline in market share or profits and the discriminatory pricing practices of the manufacturer. Evidence must be presented documenting diverted sales from the plaintiff to the defendants through witnesses and profit and loss statements.

One of the intriguing legal issues which must be decided ultimately by the courts is whether competitive injury can be established if the defendant does not undersell its rival retail competitors. One could certainly argue that competitive injury can still be inferred, since a substantial price advantage can enlarge the favored buyer's profit margin and enable it to offer more services, thus drawing more customers.

Defenses to the R-P Act

Assuming that the plaintiffs establish competitive injury they still must contend with various defenses to the Act which are available to the seller and favored purchaser. The most important of these are the cost justification and meeting competition defenses. Under the cost justification defense, a seller may sell its goods at a lower price if that price is cost justified through economies of manufacture, sale or delivery. This defense would not appear to be applicable to situations involving discriminatory pricing where the drug prices available to the defendant are much lower than those available to the plaintiff.

The meeting competition defense provides that a price discrimination is justified if the price is made in good faith so as to meet the equally low price of a competitor. The meeting competition defense is most often applicable to situations where the plaintiff purchases drugs pursuant to bid. Under this defense, if a manufacturer sold drugs to the defendant, at a lower price than that offered to the plaintiff, in good faith believing another manufacturer would offer those prices, the manufacturer would be protected under the meeting competition defense, as would the purchaser. This defense would be applicable even though the purchaser competes with plaintiffs who had to pay a higher price and regardless of the resultant economic injury to the plaintiff. Needless to say, it is not easy for a plaintiff to prevail in a R-P Act case, having to prove competitive injury, as well as rebut the defenses.

PRESCRIPTION DRUG MARKETING ACT

Hospitals and affiliate health care entities (HCE) must be cautious of the Prescription Drug Marketing Act.[37] Passed in 1987, this law prohibits hospitals and HCE from reselling, purchasing or trading prescription drugs which it has purchased. A HCE is any organization that provides diagnostic, medical, surgical, or dental treatment, but does not include a retail pharmacy. The law is intended to prohibit black-market drug diversion schemes whereby a hospital purchases drugs at very low prices as if for its own use, and then resells to someone else, who then in turn resells the products. These schemes create inequitable pricing problems for competitors, and result in the sale of misbranded, adulterated and counterfeited drugs.

Exceptions to the law include purchases from the hospital's group purchasing organization or from other member hospitals for the hospital's own use; sales or purchases to nonprofit affiliates; sales or purchases among hospitals or HCE under common control; sales or purchases for emergency medical reasons; and selling or dispensing prescription drugs pursuant to prescriptions. Thus, this law would not seem to apply if the hospital's joint venture affiliate was nonprofit, or if the hospital owned the HHC business. Apart from these relationships, the reach of the law becomes murky depending upon how the issue of common control is determined.

PHARMACY COMPOUNDING VERSUS MANUFACTURING

No one denies that compounding is an historic right of pharmacy. Certain activities by some HHC pharmacists, however, may cross the line from compounding into manufacturing. Section 510(g) of the Act provides in part that pharmacies are exempt from registering as manufacturers under the Federal Food Drug and Cosmetic Act (FFDCA) if they: "...do not manufacture, prepare, propagate, compound or process drugs or devices for sale other than in the regular course of their business of dispensing or selling drugs or devices at retail."[38] The exemption provided by Section 510 is important since if a pharmacy is deemed a manufacturer, it must then be licensed as such by the FDA and conform to the Code of Good Manufacturing Practices (CGMP) regulations.

The distinction, however, between compounding and manufacturing is not always clear. In Cedars North Towers Pharmacy, Inc. v. U.S., a Florida pharmacy compounded bulk quantities of a physician's dermatological medication.[39] This medication was then dispensed to other physicians pursuant to prescriptions by these physicians written "For Office Use Only," rather than for individual patients. In finding that the pharmacy was not exempt under §510(g), the court established the following factors as important in whether a pharmacy is exempt from the Act: (1) whether particular drugs are being compounded on a regular basis as opposed to periodic compounding of different drugs; (2) whether drugs are being compounded primarily for individual patient prescriptions as opposed to orders contemplating larger amounts for office use; (3) the geographic area of distribution; (4) whether any form of advertising or promotion is being utilized; (5) the percentage of gross income received from sales of particular compounded drugs; and (6) whether particular compounded drugs are being offered at wholesale prices.

The FDA had been quite concerned about compounding by pharmacists for some time, but two events in 1989 prompted the Agency into action. In one incident, a Pittsburgh pharmacist prepared indomethacin eye drops which resulted in eye infections in twelve patients. Two of these patients had to have an eye surgically removed. In the second incident, patients died because a hospital pharmacy in Lincoln, Nebraska prepared surgical solutions which became microbially infected. As a result, the FDA published an "Alert Letter" on Compounding in November of 1990, which was subsequently published in the October 1991 edition of American Pharmacy. The Alert Letter states in part: "Deaths and eyesight loss stemming from microbially contaminated drug products purporting to be sterile have occurred recently. The Food and Drug Administration (FDA) has determined that [some] pharmacies are using incorrect procedures and controls for the batch production of drug products intended to be sterile. The unacceptable packaging of nonpreserved sterile solutions in multiple dose containers is also occurring in pharmacies. These are matters of serious concern to the FDA. In the interest of patient safety, pharmacists preparing batches of sterile drug products are responsible for providing adequate sterility assurance through adherence to principles of good manufacturing practices and for using safe packaging to ensure continued sterility during use...."

The Letter continued by warning pharmacists to weigh their need to prepare batches of sterile products with their capacity for doing so. The FDA concluded that it did not wish to discourage pharmacists from compounding, but hoped that the Letter would serve as a "strong reminder" to pharmacists of the seriousness of batch producing sterile drugs.

FDA 1992 Compliance Policy Guide

Prompted by the two tragic incidents involving the batch preparation of contaminated sterile drugs and intense interest by pharmacists that the FDA not interfere with pharmacists' right to compound, the FDA published a compliance policy guide in 1992.[40] The Policy Guide emphasized that the FDA has no intention of regulating pharmacy's historic exemption to extemporaneously compound drugs in reasonable quantities pursuant to prescription. Pharmacies may also prepare "very limited quantities" of drugs before receiving valid prescriptions, provided these anticipated quantities can be documented historically with prescriptions on file. However, the FDA stated: "FDA believes that an increasing number of establishments with retail pharmacy licenses are engaged in manufacturing, distributing, and promoting unapproved new drugs for human use in a manner that is clearly outside the bounds of traditional pharmacy practice and that constitute violations of the Act."[41]

The Policy Guide emphasized that pharmacies may not compound, provide or dispense drugs to third parties for resale to individual patients, and then listed nine factors it would consider in whether to bring enforcement action against a pharmacy.

1. Soliciting business (e.g., promoting, advertising, or using sales persons) to compound specific drug products, product classes, or therapeutic classes of drug products.
2. Compounding, regularly, or in inordinate amounts, drug products that are commercially available in the marketplace and that are

essentially generic copies of commercially available, FDA-approved drug products.
3. Receiving, storing, or using drug substances without first obtaining written assurance from the supplier that each lot of the drug substance has been made in an FDA approved facility.
4. Receiving, storing, or using drug components not guaranteed or otherwise determined to meet official compendia requirements.
5. Using commercial scale manufacturing or testing equipment for compounding drug products.
6. Compounding inordinate amounts of drugs in anticipation of receiving prescriptions in relation to the amounts of drugs compounded after receiving valid prescriptions.
7. Offering compounded drug products at wholesale to other state licensed persons or commercial entities for resale.
8. Distributing inordinate amounts of compounded products out of state.
9. Failing to operate in conformance with applicable state law regulating the practice of pharmacy.

New Drug Issue

An inherent issue of compounding is whether the compounded product becomes a new drug for the purposes of the Act. Pharmacies are not exempt from the new drug provisions of the Act. In United States v. Baxter Healthcare Corp., the court held that reconstituting, repackaging, freezing and distributing approved antibiotic drugs made them new drugs.[42] In United States v. Sene X Eleemosynary Corp., Inc., the court considered whether the compounding and promotion of a product containing procaine hydrochloride by a pharmacy resulted in a new drug.[43] The court found that unlike in the normal practice of pharmacy, the defendants received a large volume of out-of-state prescriptions, compounded and dispensed a single product on a routine basis from the purchase of bulk chemicals and advertised and promoted its product, soliciting prescriptions. These activities resulted in the court holding that the product was a new drug, and thus illegally marketed. In contrast, a HHC pharmacy compounding a chemotherapeutic drug pursuant to prescription for a particular patient would not violate the new drug provision of the law, even through the pharmacy has in essence dispensed a new drug.

STATE GOVERNMENT REGULATION

Many states have laws and regulations governing the provision of HHC of which the pharmacist must be aware. In particular to pharmaceutical services, these laws and regulations are usually contained within the state's pharmacy practice act. California regulations, for example, prescribe specifications, standards and equipment for the area in which the preparation of parenterals occur.[44] The regulations also detail such issues as recordkeeping requirements; the training of staff; quality assurance; and necessary policy and procedures.

CONCLUSION

Although a pharmacist who expands the scope of his or her practice to include HHC will incur added liability exposure, this should never be a reason not to expand. Pharmacists who are competent, knowledgeable and diligent will seldom experience professional liability actions. Although product liability actions could exist regardless of the degree of care exercised by a pharmacist, the incidence of these actions can be mitigated by selling and leasing quality products made by reputable manufacturers who warrant their products. Medicare/Medicaid fraud and abuse situations can be avoided with the knowledge of what the statute is attempting to forbid and by knowing the safe harbors. Antitrust problems can be avoided by understanding what the laws are designed to prevent and by analyzing whether the business is unfairly competing with or harming competitors. A pharmacy can avoid being deemed a manufacturer by following the policy guidelines of the FDA. In addition, pharmacies should make every effort to follow all accreditation standards and the conditions for participation established under Medicare/Medicaid.

SUGGESTED READINGS

Abood RR. Antitrust Implications when Hospitals Diversity into HHC. Pharmacy Law Annual. 1990; 3:3-28.

Abood RR. Differential Pricing of Pharmaceuticals and Retail Competition Under the Robinsion-Patman Act. Am. J. of Law & Med. 1986; 11:293-317.

Carder EB. The Safe Harbor Regulations: An Overview. NARD J. 1992; 114:65-72.

Fink JL, Ed. Pharmacy Law Digest. Facts and Comparisons. 1993.

Lasky PC. Principles of Hospital Liability. Hospital Law Manual, Administrator's Volume IB. Germantown MD, Health Law Center, Aspen Systems Corp.

Pozgar GD. Legal Aspects of Health Care Administration. 4th ed. Rockville MD. Aspen Systems Corp. 1990.

Prosser WL. Law of Torts. 4th E. St. Paul. West Publishing Co. 1971.

Southwick AF. The Law of Hospital and Health Care Administration. 2nd ed. University of Michigan. Health Administration Press. 1988.

Tedrick S. Legal Issues in Physician Self-Referral and Other Health Care Business Relationships. J. of Legal Med. 1992; 13:521-561.

REFERENCES

1. See Ingram v. Hooks, 476 N.E.2d 881 (Ind. 1985); McKee v. American Home Products, Corp., 782 P.2d 1045 (Wash. 1989).
2. Omnibus Budget Reconciliation Act of 1990, Public Law 101-508.
3. Darlington v. Charleston Community Memorial Hospital, 211 N.E.2d 253 (1963).
4. Bichler v. Willing, 397 N.Y.S.2d 56 (1977).
5. Uniform Commercial Cod §2-313 (1972).
6. Id. §§2-314, 2-315.
7. Restatement Second Tors §402A. American Law Inst. 1965.
8. Abood R. Pharmacist Dispensing: Service or Sale? Applicability of Strict Liability. American Pharmacy. 1980; 20:25-29.
9. Magrine v. Krasnica, 227 A.2d 539 (1967), aff'd sub nom. Magrine v. Spector, 241 A.2d 637 (1968).
10. Pub. L. No. 92-603, 242(b)-(c).
11. 760 F.2d 68 (3d Cir.), cert. denied, 474 U.S. 988 (1985).
12. United States v. Kats, 871 F.2d 105 (9th Cir. 1989).
13. United States v. Bay State Ambulance and Hospital Rental Service, Inc. 874 F.2d 20 (1st Cir. 1989).
14. 42 C.F.R. §1001.952 (1991).
15. 15 U.S.C. §1 (1982).
16. 15 U.S.C. §2 (1982).
17. Klamath-Lake Pharmaceutical Assn. v. Klamath Medical Service Bureau, 701 F.2d 1276, 1292 (9th Cir. 1983)
18. Chicago Board of Trade v. United States, 246 U.S. 231, 238 (1918).
19. Northern Pacific Railway Company v. United States, 356 U.S. 1,5 (1958).
20. Northern California Pharmaceutical Ass'n v. United States 306 F.2d 379 (9th Cir. 1962), cert. den. 83 S.Ct. 119 (1962).
21. See Note 17 supra. Everhart v. Jane C. Stormont Hospital, 1982-1 Trade Cas. ¶64,703 (D. Kan. 1982).
22. 472 U.S 284 (1985).
23. Id. at 287.
24. 457 U.S. 332 (1982).
25. Id. at 351.
26. 703 F. Supp 1513 (MD Fla 1989); rev'd and remanded, 919 F.2d 1550 (11th Cir. 1990).
27. 919 F.2d 1557.
28. Jefferson Parish Hospital District No. 2 v. Hyde, 466 U.S. 2 (1984).
29. Section 1 claims cannot be brought since there can be no conspiracy as the hospital and home health operation would be one. Section 2 claims can be brought, as well as section 1 claims when there is concerted action, as well as monopolization such as in Venice Hospital.)
30. 15 U.S.C. §13(a) (1982).
31. 15 U.S.C. §13(c) (1982).
32. 422 U.S. 1 (1975).
33. Id. at 14.
34. The court applied a similar analysis to state and local government hospitals which are not included under the Nonprofit Institutions Act. In Jefferson County Pharmaceutical Assn., Inc. v. Abbott Laboratories, 455 U.S. 999 (1982), the Supreme Court determined that the sale of pharmaceutical products to state and local government hospitals for resale in competition with private retail pharmacies is not exempt from the Act.)
35. 743 F.2d 1388 (9th Cir. 1984).
36. Portland Retail Druggists at 15.
37. Public Law 100-293 (Apr. 22, 1988).
38. Federal Food Drug and Cosmetic Act, §510(g).
39. 1978-1980 FDLI Jud. Rec. 668 (S.D. Fla. 1978)
40. Compliance Policy Guide 7132.16, March 16, 1992.
41. Id.
42. 901 F.2d 1401 (1990).
43. 479 F. Supp. 970 (1979).
44. Ca. Code of Regulations, Chpt. 17, Title 16, §§1751-1751.10.

3 Home Health Care Reimbursement

Virginia Tobiason, R.N., M.B.A.

The use of home health care (HHC) has increased dramatically over the past decade. A recent Bureau of the Census Report estimated that home health revenues grew slightly over 19% between 1990 and 1991, almost double the rate of hospital care.[1] The key factors contributing to this increase include the introduction in 1983 of a fixed per case reimbursement methodology for inpatient hospital services, which shifted patient care to higher reimbursed outpatient services; the development of new technologies specifically targeted for the home market; and a growing acceptance of home therapies by patients, physicians and payers.

The escalating pressure for health care reform will continue to encourage the use of HHC services as providers will be encouraged to treat patients in the lowest cost setting. In the past, HHC has been able to demonstrate significant cost savings over inpatient care. If this continues, HHC has the potential to benefit greatly from the changing health care paradigm shift towards less costly health care delivery.

HHC is comprised of three major market segments: home health nursing, home medical equipment and home infusion therapies. This chapter will review the current reimbursement for home therapies by major payer and identify future trends and payer initiatives impacting the HHC industry.

MEDICARE

Home Health Nursing

In 1991, Medicare expenditures for HHC were $5.6 billion, up 26 percent from 1990. Actual visits totaled approximately 78 million with an average of 45.7 visits per patient.[2] Medicare nursing services must be provided by Medicare certified home health agencies (HHA) that meet government mandated conditions of participation, as well as applicable state and local regulations. Home health services are covered under both Part A and Part B and include:

- Part-time or intermittent nursing care provided by or under the supervision of a registered professional nurse.
- Physical, occupational or speech therapy.
- Medical social services.
- Part-time or intermittent services of a home health aid.
- Durable medical equipment and medical supplies.[3]

To qualify for care, a number of conditions must be met, namely, the services must be furnished under a physician's plan of care and updated periodically, the patient must be confined at home, and the nursing services must be provided only on an intermittent or part-time basis.[4] As a result of these restrictive guidelines, most beneficiaries are able to receive only some limited post-acute nursing care. The average duration of therapy is 35 hours a week for a total of two to three weeks.[5]

In 1989, the Medicare Home Health Agency Coverage Manual (HIM-11) was rewritten as a result of a lawsuit brought by Congressman Staggers and others against the government for illegally denying home health claims as a result of restrictive coverage policies. The favorable ruling expanded the definition of intermittent services and clarified the medical necessity criteria used to adjudicate claims. As expected, there has been a dramatic increase in HHA visits over the last two years.

Payment by Medicare for home health nursing services is based on a reasonable cost payment methodology subject to limits. It is anticipated that within the next few years, a prospective payment system will be implemented for home health nursing services. Actual demonstration projects have already been initiated by the Health Care Financing Administration to test reimbursement mechanisms based on a fixed reimbursement per visit or episode of care.

Home Medical Equipment

The Home Medical Equipment (HME) industry is comprised of durable medical equipment, orthotics and prosthetics, respiratory equipment and medical supplies. The next section will provide an overview of Medicare coverage and payment by product type.

Durable medical equipment is defined as those items which 1) can withstand repeated use, 2) are primarily and customarily used to serve a medical purpose, 3) generally not useful to a patient in the absence of illness or injury, and 4) appropriate for use in the home.[6] Some examples of durable medical equipment are hospital beds, wheelchairs, and walkers. HME providers include home medical supply companies, HHA, outpatient clinics, pharmacies, physicians and home infusion companies. Payment for HME is made under Medicare Part B. Durable medical equipment is classified into six categories. The six categories are:

1) Inexpensive or other routinely purchased equipment. This includes items with a purchase price less than $150 and items that are routinely purchased at least 75% of the time.
2) Items requiring frequent and substantial servicing. Examples of these items include ventilators, nebulizers and intermittent positive pressure breathing (IPPB) machines.
3) Customized items. This category is very limited and include only those items which are highly customized for an individual, such as a customized wheelchair.
4) Oxygen and oxygen equipment. This category is divided into oxygen, stationary oxygen equipment and portable oxygen equipment.
5) Other equipment or the "capped rental" category. This category includes items that are not included in one of the other categories and are usually rented. Items included in this category are wheelchairs and hospital beds.
6) Items other than durable medical equipment. This category includes prosthetic devices, orthotics and prosthetics. Examples of these products are braces, artificial limbs and ostomy supplies.[6]

Beginning January 1, 1989, Congress changed the reimbursement methodology for durable medical equipment. The payment is now based on the lesser of the actual charge or a fee schedule amount. Known as the "six-point" plan, this fee schedule was established with 1986 to 1987 data (subject to caps) and is to be updated yearly by the consumer price update. Unfortunately, durable medical equipment has been subject to the same cost pressures that other Medicare providers have experienced and expected payment increases have either been eliminated or cut back due to federal budget pressures As a result, the six-point plan reimbursement methodology has effectively been dismantled. Recent changes to the fee schedule under OBRA 1990 include:[6]

1) Replacing the regional pricing system for capped rental items with a national fee screen.
2) Establishing a separate fee screen for each prosthetic and orthotic item.[6]

These cutbacks have resulted in lower profit margins for providers of these services, particularly those companies with large numbers of Medicare patients.

In addition to payment pressures, the home medical industry has been the focus of government fraud and abuse investigations. While the majority of providers offer reputable and legitimate services, there have been instances of abusive practices, including carrier shopping and falsification of claims. Concerned with the lack of industry regulation, the government and Congress have initiated a number of reform proposals. In 1992, the Health Care Financing Administration proposed consolidating the current Medicare carriers.[7] Starting October 1, 1993, all claims for durable medical equipment, prosthetics, orthotics and supplies must be submitted to one of four regional carriers, down from the current 34 carriers. The four regional carriers are listed in Table 3-1. As part of this consolidation, claims will no longer be based on the point of sale, which is the location where the transaction for the sale occurred, but on the state where the beneficiary resides. This is called "zip-code" jurisdiction. Medicare also intends to establish uniform and consistent coverage policies between all four carriers. These changes should eliminate carrier shopping, where providers falsely bill those carriers where the reimbursement and coverage is more favorable. Suppliers will also need to obtain new billing numbers requiring disclosure of the identity of the ownership interest, the managing employees of the entity and any employees with a history of criminal convictions and/or Medicare/ Medicaid sanctions. In addition, the supplier must meet established standards which include:

Table 3-1 Medicare Regional Carriers

Region A	Connecticut, Delaware, Maine, Massachusetts, New Jersey, New York, New Hampshire, Pennsylvania, Rhode Island, and Vermont	The Travelers Insurance Company, Hartford, Conn.
Region B	District of Columbia, Illinois, Indiana, Maryland, Michigan, Minnesota, Ohio, Virginia, West Virginia, and Wisconsin	Associated Insurance Co., Inc. Indianapolis, Ind. (doing business as Blue Cross and Blue Shield of Indiana)
Region C	Alabama, Arkansas, Colorado, Florida, Georgia, Kentucky, Louisiana, Mississippi, North Carolina, Oklahoma, Puerto Rico (Virgin Islands,) South Carolina, Tennessee, and Texas	Blue Cross and Blue Shield of South Carolina, Columbia, S.C.
Region D	Alaska, Arizona, California, Hawaii (Guam), Idaho, Iowa, Kansas, Missouri, Montana, Nebraska, Nevada, North Dakota, Oregon, South Dakota, Utah, Washington, and Wyoming	Cigna Corporation Hartford, Conn.

1) The supplier must fill orders from its own inventory of companies with which it has a contractual arrangement to fill orders.
2) The supplier must be responsible for delivery of Medicare-covered items to Medicare beneficiaries.
3) The supplier must honor any warranties, answer any questions and complaints a beneficiary might have.
4) The supplier must maintain and repair items rented to beneficiaries and accept returns of substandard or unsuitable items from beneficiaries.[7]

The current local Part B carriers will continue to handle claims by physicians.

Home Infusion Therapy

The past few years have seen a tremendous growth in the use of home infusion therapies. These therapies include home parenteral nutrition, intravenous antibiotics, pain management as well as the administration of drug therapy for cardiac support and the prevention of premature labor. Unlike other HHC services, Medicare is not a major payer for home infusion therapy since Medicare generally excludes self-administered drugs from coverage, except for certain limited diagnosis.

Parenteral and Enteral Nutrition (PEN). Coverage for PEN therapy is covered under the Part B prosthetic device benefit. In order to be covered the patient must have a permanent impairment of the gastrointestinal tract prohibiting digestion of nutrients. Nutritional supplementation is not covered. Payment for PEN is currently based on a national fee schedule which covers the nutrients, supplies, pump, pharmacy and delivery services. This fee schedule is updated yearly.

Part B Durable Medical Equipment. The Medicare Part B program includes coverage for some drugs and related supplies when infused by an external infusion pump. The Medicare Carriers Manual instructs carriers to cover the following limited therapies: deferoxamine for the treatment of acute iron poisoning and iron overload;
morphine used for the treatment of intractable cancer pain; and cancer drugs used to treat primary

unresectable liver or colorectal cancer.[8]

Medicare also allows the local carrier's discretion to expand coverage for other diseases as long as an external infusion pump is required. Therefore, some local carriers have modified coverage to include intravenous antibiotics, dobutamine, and additional pain management drugs such as hydromorphone and demerol. While most carriers still have very limited reimbursement coverage for home infusion therapy, more and more carriers are in the process of expanding coverage. The payment methodology for these therapies is based on reasonable charges established by the local carrier. Payment for the drugs and supplies under this benefit is considered very limited and in most cases is usually based on the average wholesale price of the drug and supplies. Payment for pharmacy compounding, delivery to the patient's home, and other necessary services are usually not paid for.

PRIVATE INSURANCE

Private insurers, such as Blue Cross/Blue Shield plans, and commercial insurers are a major payer source for HHC services. Private payers have long recognized the cost-effectiveness of HHC as compared to the higher cost of inpatient hospitalization. In the past, providers were often reimbursed at close to full charges since payers were saving the higher cost of hospitalization. However, these payers have recently initiated a number of cost-containment measures, including the use of case managers to negotiate lower rates for services on a case-by-case basis and fixed "per-diem" or per item fee contracts. Additionally, as the government and other payer sources seek to reduce health care costs, there will be a continued increase in managed care plans as subscribers are shifted from the standard indemnity plans into managed care programs such as health maintenance organizations and preferred provider organizations. According to the Group Health Association of America in 1992 there were 550 health maintenance organizations in the U.S. with 38.6 million members, or approximately 15% of the U.S. population.[9]

The two major types of managed care organizations are defined below:

1. Health Maintenance Organizations (HMO). An HMO is a health plan which offers prepaid (capitated) health coverage for both hospital and physician services. Members are limited to receiving care by participating providers. HMO include specific model types such as staff, group and independent practice associations (IPA). In response to concerns over limited provider choice, the fastest growing type of HMO is the point of service (POS) plan. This plan allows the member to receive services out of network in return for a higher out of pocket cost.
2. Preferred Provider Organizations (PPO). PPO are networks of providers who agree to provide services at a discounted rate. Subscribers can elect to go outside of the network for a higher co-pay. Exclusive Provider Organizations (EPO) require the member to use a network provider. PPO are becoming increasingly more like HMO as they adopt the more stringent HMO utilization control mechanisms.

The continued emphasis on reducing health care costs will further the growth of HMO and PPO. The current incentives to treat patients in a higher reimbursed site of care will disappear as the provider will have an incentive to manage a patient's whole episode of illness for the lowest cost irregardless of the site of service. The adoption of capitated mechanisms which shift the financial risk onto the provider will also encourage this trend. It is anticipated that HHC will continue to expand under this scenario as providers will recognize the home as the lowest cost setting and shift patients where possible to home therapies. Currently, the most successful managed care programs are those that have been most effective in using ancillary services. According to a recent Interstudy report on managed care, 97.1% of managed care programs consider HHC as one of five key cost control measures.[10]

Managed care programs are able to reduce cost by either providing pharmacy and nursing services directly through their own health care system or setting up limited provider panels through contracts with other providers which guarantee patient referrals for a discounted rate. Other cost-containment measures include utilization review, establishment of usual and customary rates and the use of professional case managers. Case management services employ registered nurses or other health care professionals which arrange for a patient's therapy for a discounted price. In the last two years, it is estimated that utilization of these services for HHC grew from around 5% to 35% of all referrals. It is expected that this trend will continue growing rapidly over the next few years with the majority of HHC patients being subject to cost and service utilization controls.

MEDICAID

Medicaid is a state-administered program that provides health care coverage to low-income and medically needy people. Most state programs cover HHC services and can vary from state-to-state. Federal mandates require coverage for durable medical equipment and home health nursing services. While prescription drugs are optional, all states routinely cover them. However, providers may be required to obtain prior approval through a labor intensive process before initiating therapy. Reimbursement is generally poor since Medicaid does not, in many cases, cover the actual costs of providing nursing and drug therapies. Additionally, as many states are increasingly having severe budget shortages, payments can be substantially delayed or not paid at all.

REIMBURSEMENT OUTLOOK

Health Care Reform

The United States currently spends approximately 14% of our Gross National Product on health care. President Clinton, in response to the public concern over rising health care costs and lack of coverage for all Americans, has made health care reform one of the major priorities of his administration. While his proposal has not yet been finalized or enacted by Congress, there are a number of options being explored and publicized.

The anticipated approach is a system based on the managed competition type of model. Key options include 1) the establishment of purchasing cooperatives called Health Alliances, which would cover small employees and individuals; and 2) a mandated basic benefit package modeled on the federal HMO benefits plan. Other issues still undecided include universal coverage, tax deductibility of insurance benefits, and the use of price controls and rate-setting mechanisms.

While HHC services should have a significant role in the health care debate, there are a number of critical issues confronting HHC providers. First, it is essential that HHC services be included in the basic benefit package as a separately defined benefit in order to ensure adequate coverage and payment. Secondly, the growth of managed care will force providers to negotiate discounted managed care contracts. This will accelerate already eroding prices. Providers will also be expected to demonstrate quality through the use of patient outcome measurements. Payers will continue to reduce the number of providers they are willing to contract with to those who can provide quality services at an acceptable price. To be successful, a provider must develop the necessary tools to compete in this environment and be able to demonstrate the ability to provide quality services.

COST CONTAINMENT

While it is anticipated that HHC services will continue to grow, particularly under health care reform, prices will continue to erode as insurers explore ways to cut costs. Recent initiatives include establishment of preferred provider rates, case manager negotiations to obtain the best price, and capitated contracts with HMO and PPO. It is also likely there will be more financial risk-shifting to providers as the use of capitated fees grow. Providers will also be expected to "bundle" services and negotiate the patient's entire episode-of-care with the insurer at one cost effective price.

According to Cabin,[11] managed care organizations are shifting their reimbursement for home infusion therapy to an all-inclusive per diem fee. This method is also becoming increasingly popular among commercial insurers. Pharmacists may use a variety of strategies in response to reimbursement contract proposals of the per diem type. Negotiating strategies include devising per diem rates for each type of therapy; establishing a per diem fee schedule based upon dosage level, number of drugs, and frequency of administration; stating limits on nursing care that is included in the per diem, with all other nursing care listed under the HHA fee.[11]

EXPANDED MEDICARE COVERAGE

The Office of Technology Assessment (OTA) recently completed a comprehensive study of home infusion drug therapy at the request of Congress. Ever since the repeal of the ill-fated Medicare Catastrophic Act of 1989, Congress has explored ways to legislate home infusion benefits. The study is generally favorable on the benefits of home infusion drug therapy and recommends initiating a number of demonstration projects. However, any legislation is unlikely in the near future due to Medicare budget concerns.[5]

PHYSICIAN REFERRAL

Opposition to physician self-referral arrangements is growing as many states and the federal government are proposing legislation to prohibit physician ownership of health care facilities. In 1991, the Office of the Inspector General published a list of regulations defining safe harbor payment practices that exempt health care entities from prosecution under federal fraud and abuse laws. These regulations provide an exemption for physicians with investment interests in large publicly-traded entities with assets greater than $50 million. It also provides an exemption for smaller entities requiring that no more than 40% of the value of the investment interests be held by investors who are in a position to make or influence referrals, and no more than 40% of the gross revenue be generated by referrals from investors. (See also Chapter 2.)

Current legislation in Congress proposes to extend the current prohibition against physician self-referral, originally enacted as part of OBRA in 1989, to additional health care entities, including durable medical equipment, parenteral and enteral equipment suppliers, home infusion providers and other home health services.

Many states, including New York, New Jersey, Florida and Illinois, have either enacted or are in the process of enacting laws banning physician self-referral. It is clear that this trend will continue.

OFFICE OF INSPECTOR GENERAL (OIG) INVESTIGATIONS

As a result of concern over fraud and abuse in the home care industry, the OIG has initiated a number of investigations in this area. Included are the following:

1. Durable Medical Equipment Payment Reforms: Audit to determine the effectiveness of the new reforms over Medicare payment for medical equipment.
2. Home Oxygen: Inspection to determine the existing level of service provided to beneficiaries by oxygen suppliers. Also, inspection will determine if Medicare should encourage lease-purchase arrangements for oxygen concentrators.
3. Validation of Claims for Infusion Therapy: Inspection to determine the accuracy of coverage determinations and claims processing for outpatient infusion therapy.
4. Financial Arrangements for Infusion Therapy: Inspection to determine the type and extent of financial arrangements between physicians and home infusion therapy suppliers.
5. Total Parenteral Nutrition: Inspection to examine payment data and certificate of medical necessity for Medicare beneficiaries receiving total parenteral nutrition on an outpatient basis.[12]

These investigations are part of the growing concern over the lack of regulation from home health services. While HHA are subject to state and federal conditions of participation under Medicare Part A, Medicare Part B suppliers, such as durable medical equipment and home infusion providers are not. These industries are primarily regulated through the Joint Commission on the Accreditation of Health Care Organization (JCAHO) voluntary accreditation program. Continuing concern over quality issues, pricing practices and fragmentation of services will likely lead to increasing federal and state regulations being enacted.

In summary, HHC as a health care alternative will continue to expand during this decade as additional treatment sites, product innovations and drug therapy regimen are identified. The underlying question is to what extent will cost-containment efforts by payers have in controlling availability as well as coverage of future home health programs.

REFERENCES

1. Bureau of the Census 1991 Service Annual Survey. BNA Health Care Policy Report 1993; Volume 1, Number 6, 274.
2. Prospective Payment Assessment Commission. Medicare and the American Health Care System Report to Congress June 1992; Part 2, p. 111.
3. CCH Medicare and Medicaid Guide; § 1404.
4. CCH Medicare and Medicaid Guide; § 1411, 1414, 1448.
5. Prospective Payment Assessment Commission. Medicare and the American Health Care System Report to Congress June 1992; Part 2, p. 111.
6. CCH Medicare and Medicaid Guide; § 3144.
7. Medicare Program Criteria and Standards for Evaluating Regional Durable Medical Equipment, Prosthetics, Orthotics and Supplies (DMEPOS), Final Rule and Request for Comments. Federal Register; Vol. 57, No. 118, pp. 27296-27298.
8. Medicare Carriers Manual § 60-14.
9. Anonymous Managed Care: Where Will Your Hospital Fit In? Hospitals. 1992; 67:18.
10. Burns J. Interstudy, a division of Decision Resources, Inc. St. Paul MN, 1992.
11. Cabin WD. Home Infusion Per Diem Reimbursement. Home Health Consult. 1993; 5:1.
12. CCH Medicare and Medicaid Guide; § 40917.

4 Establishing Quality in Home Health Care

Jeff A. Keimach, Pharm. D.

The goal of this chapter is to introduce the reader to the established management theories of Total Quality Management (TQM) and Continuous Quality Improvement (CQI), and how these theories apply to the home health care (HHC) accreditation process. For the purposes of this chapter, programs such as TQM and CQI, and the familiar sounding Quality Assurance, will be called, "Quality Programs". Many HHC organizations have been utilizing these concepts for years in order to manage and improve the quality of their services and products.

HHC organizations have had the opportunity to seek accreditation since 1988, when the Joint Commission for the Accreditation of Healthcare Organizations, (JCAHO) began its Home Care accreditation process. In contrast, the JCAHO has been providing accreditation services to American hospitals for decades. Without accreditation, hospitals and home health agencies have difficulty participating in federal programs such as Medicare, as the Medicare program "deems" that JCAHO accreditation is a sufficient replacement for a full scale Medicare survey. Currently, JCAHO has deemed status for hospitals and HHC organizations. The effect of this new deemed status may affect HHC organizations which primarily provide home health services (i.e., home care nursing visits) to a much greater extent than less Medicare dependent organizations such as pharmacies. The full extent of these changes may only become evident in the years ahead. JCAHO is not a government agency, but rather an independent organization geared to improve the quality of health care provided to the public. JCAHO develops standards of quality in collaboration with health professionals and others and stimulates health care organizations to meet or exceed the standards through accreditation and the teaching of quality improvement concepts.[1,2]

The types of organizations eligible to apply for JCAHO accreditation include those that provide one or more of the following: home health services (home nursing); personal care or support services (e.g., home nursing aides); pharmaceutical services (home infusion services); and home medical equipment.[3] JCAHO regularly publishes its standards, which are developed in collaboration with input from industry representatives. Much of the content of the HHC standards is similar to the published JCAHO hospital standards. The home care standards have been published for 1988, 1991, and 1993 and are expected to be revised and published again in 1995. There are eleven chapters of standards, and in addition to the four listed above they include: rights and responsibilities, patient care, safety management, infection control, home care record. The standards address pharmaceutical care (clinical monitoring), home health services, durable medical equipment (e.g., intravenous infusion devices), drug dispensing, drug compounding, and drug information. The standards are not rules, laws, or regulations (although the JCAHO may have as a standard that an organization follows applicable rules, regulations, and/or laws). There are various ways to meet the intent of the standards.

Some of the most challenging of the JCAHO standards are those related to Quality Assessment and Improvement. Successfully meeting these standards sets the superior patient-oriented provider of health care apart from the average organization. In the simplest terms, quality programs are designed to help organizations do the right thing, the right way, all the time. Quality programs help organizations meet the customer's needs utilizing cost effective and cost efficient processes. When successfully implemented, quality programs include top to bottom changes in culture, management, and support processes. A quality program facilitates efficient work patterns, so that the staff will work more efficiently, not harder.

There are many acceptable methods of implementing quality programs such as TQM and CQI. Some methods focus on process refinement, systems development, statistical process control, and "zero defects," whereas others focus on outcome.

WHY IMPLEMENT A QUALITY PROGRAM?

Appropriate reasons or goals of a quality program are to decrease costs associated with poor quality; continually improve the processes that provide for a positive outcome of patient care; and decrease the risk inherent in providing health care services (risk management). Although accreditation for HHC organizations is strictly voluntary, confirmation of having a well implemented quality program is usually established through accreditation by JCAHO or The Community Health Accreditation Program (CHAP).[3] Because the majority of HHC organizations, especially those offering pharmaceutical, HME, or respiratory care services, seek JCAHO accreditation, that process will be the focus of the chapter.

The rationale for establishing a quality program includes:

- to qualify for reimbursement by many insurance company programs;
- to maintain accreditation with JCAHO;
- to receive referrals from certain sources;
- a method of decreasing the costs of doing business;
- to decrease the risk associated with the provision of HHC;
- to meet state regulations and laws; and,
- to focus on outcomes of services as a method to position one's organization for the future of health care.

In order to decrease the costs associated with poor quality, it is necessary to understand the processes that are involved in reaching any outcome. Most quality programs focus on process management. The process leading to an outcome is defined, developed, executed, analyzed, and monitored. In HHC, practical examples of avoidable costs include redelivery of poorly managed patient supplies or a faulty infusion device, hospitalization in order to re-establish the patency of a poorly managed central venous catheter, or the denial of insurance reimbursement due to inadequate qualification of the patient for admission to service. Each one of these services have several processes which can be independently assessed and improved. With such a process orientation, it is understandable why the next industry buzzwords may be "Process" or "Performance" Improvement.[4]

Some states require pharmacies that provide home parenteral services to have a quality assurance program. However, quality assurance is interpreted by some to mean "quality control" which is a method of statistical process control such as the random testing of compounded parenterals for the presence of precipitation or contamination. Tennessee, for example, has proposed a pharmacy law which requires that pharmacies engaged in the provision of home IV therapy "...shall be responsible for ... the ... establishment of a quality assurance program"[5] and California state pharmacy law has a stipulation requiring that licensed pharmacies involved in the provision of parenteral services have policies and procedures for their quality assurance component.[6]

Another reason for implementing a quality program includes the increasing focus on outcomes of various health care delivery systems as a means to compare organizations (this comparison is also known as "bench-marking"). Although the traditional measures of quality evaluated structures and processes, ideally quality programs measure the outcomes of those processes. In HHC, this may call for the comparison, for example, between Company A and Company B in terms of which provider of home IV antibiotic therapy was more successful in both meeting the goals of therapy and providing for a higher level of patient (customer) satisfaction. Both of these aspects, goals and satisfaction, are identifiable and quantifiable. The current challenge is to develop universal techniques for outcomes data analysis. A familiar health care example is the annual publication of statistics comparing hospitals on mortality rates by the Health Care Financing Administration (HCFA).[7] Examples of home infusion therapy indicators that may be used to compare HHC organizations are listed in Table 4-1.

An illustration of the role of a quality program in improving the processes that provide patient care may be found in HHC organizations that manage a patient's central venous catheters. If less than desirable results are noted, an organization could categorize the management of the central venous catheter into several processes. Some of the procedures involved include patient or caregiver

Table 4-1 Home Infusion Therapy Indicators

- Unscheduled inpatient admission by type of therapy
- Discontinued infusion therapy
- Interruption in infusion therapy by type of therapy
- Prevention and surveillance of infection by type of therapy
- Reporting adverse drug reactions (ADRs)
- Patient/client monitoring and appropriate intervention

education, return demonstration by the patient or caregiver, and monitoring of routine compliance with the procedures. Using common statistical tools, a study may be undertaken which will focus on these processes. Once quantified, it may be found that although education and return demonstration are adequate, routine compliance with catheter maintenance techniques is not being carried out. Analyzing the data, it could be decided to develop and implement a formal method of monitoring compliance. With the new processes in place, the organization could, after a period of time, again perform an evaluation of the changes that were implemented.

According to Zitter, "As customers increasingly use outcomes data to select and reimburse providers, the ability to determine outcomes accurately and to improve results measurably will become a competitive necessity."[7] It is possible that in the not too distant future, the HHC patient will be referred to the organization with the best statistical outcomes. In addition, although it is not mandatory to achieve accreditation as proof that an organization espouses quality, accreditation may act as a "stamp of approval" of an organization's quality program.

QUALITY, AN HISTORICAL PERSPECTIVE

Discussion of the methods of establishing quality in any industry, including HHC, necessitates the presentation of an historical perspective of the quality movement in the modern industrialized world. The concepts of TQM, CQI, and Zero-Defects were based on theories espoused in American academia, developed and perfected by the Japanese, and then finally, but only recently, introduced on a wide scale to American industry and service organizations. Major players in the quality revolution include Deming, Juran, and Crosby. Any person or organization desiring to implement a successful quality program should become familiar with the teachings of these three leaders in quality programs. A thorough understanding of the historical perspective will provide a basis for understanding how the current JCAHO standards for "Quality Assessment and Improvement" were developed.

W. Edwards Deming

W. Edwards Deming is an internationally renowned consultant whose work led Japanese industry into new principles of quality management and revolutionized their quality and productivity. He is often credited with introducing the concepts of quality management to industry. A statistician by background, his work with the Japanese began in the 1950's, but it was not for another 30 years that American industry responded to his advice. The American health care industry is a relative late comer to quality management, only establishing quality management programs as recently as the 1980's.[8]

Deming espoused fourteen points of quality management, and taught his fourteen points as, "the basis for transformation of American industry." The fourteen points apply anywhere, to small organizations as well as to large ones.
(See Table 4-2.)

Joseph M. Juran

Joseph M. Juran is an administrator, lecturer, writer, and consultant. Along with Deming, he had a major impact on the Japanese quality renaissance and continues to contribute internationally. Juran defines quality as product performance that results in customer satisfaction and freedom from product deficiencies, which avoids customer dissatisfaction.[10] He believes that users of a product or service should be able to count on it for what they needed or wanted to do with it, a concept commonly referred to as "fitness for use".[11]

In his definition of poor quality, Juran included various problems, such as customer complaints, product liability lawsuits, defective work, and scrapped products. He was concerned that poor quality costs companies 20 to 40 percent of sales. Or, about 20 to 40 percent of the companies' efforts are spent in redoing things that went wrong because of poor quality.[12] He felt that the goal of quality programs is to keep improving quality until there is no longer a positive economic return.

Table 4-2 Deming's Fourteen Points of Quality Management[9]

1. Create constancy of purpose toward improvement of product and service, with the aim to become competitive and to stay in business, and to provide jobs.
2. Adopt the new philosophy.
3. Cease dependence on inspection to achieve quality.
4. End the practice of awarding business on the basis of price tag. Instead, minimize total cost. Move toward a single supplier for any one item, on a long-term relationship of loyalty and trust.
5. Improve constantly and forever the system of production and service, to improve quality and productivity, and thus constantly decrease costs.
6. Institute training on the job.
7. Adopt and institute leadership.
8. Drive out fear, so that everyone may work effectively for the company.
9. Break down barriers between departments (staff areas).
10. Eliminate slogans, exhortations, and targets for the work.
11. Eliminate numerical quotas for the work force and numerical goals for people in management.
12. Remove barriers that rob people of pride of workmanship.
13. Institute a vigorous program of education and self-improvement.
14. Take action to accomplish the transformation.

Juran proposed that attention to quality should be made a priority similar to attention to financial management. This attention includes the establishment of policies and goals for quality; plans for meeting those quality goals; providing the resources needed to carry out the plans; establishing controls to evaluate progress against goals and to take appropriate action; and, providing motivation to stimulate the personnel to meet the quality goals.[13-16]

Juran's strategy included quality planning, quality control, and quality improvement.[17] Quality planning is the activity of developing the products and processes required to meet customers' needs, and involves establishing quality goals. Quality control consists of evaluating performance. Finally, quality improvement is the process of raising quality performance to unprecedented levels, termed "breakthrough." (See Table 4-3.)

Table 4-3 Juran's Breakthrough Sequence [14]

- Breakthrough in attitudes
  Managers must create a climate conducive to change. To demonstrate need, data must be collected to show the extent of the problem; the data must be convincing. To get the resources required for improvement, expected benefits can be monetized and presented in terms of return on investment.
- Identify the vital few projects
- Organize for breakthrough knowledge
  Steering group (a multidisciplinary quality committee); diagnostic group of professionals to analyze problems
- Conduct the analysis:
  Operator or management controllable
- Determine how to overcome resistance to change
- Institute the change
  Corrective action
- Institute controls
  Monitor the solution

Philip B. Crosby

Philip B. Crosby, also one of the leaders of the modern quality revolution, popularized the "Zero-Defect" movement which relied on management establishing the highest standards of performance. According to Crosby,[15] management really has three basic tasks to perform: establish the requirements that employees are to meet; supply the resources employees need in order to meet those requirements; and, encourage and help employees to meet those requirements. Like Deming, Crosby established a fourteen step approach to Quality Improvement. (See Table 4-4.)

Crosby also described the Four Absolutes of Quality Management.[15] The First Absolute answers the question: What is quality? Crosby[15] defined quality as conformance to requirements, and suggested that improvement occurs when management and staff are committed to conformance. "Do it right the first time" (DIRFT) is one of his mottos that exemplifies this concept. The Second Absolute answers the question: What system is needed to cause quality? Crosby suggested that if systems and

Table 4-4 Crosby's Approach to Quality Improvement[15]

1. Management Commitment
2. Quality Improvement Team
3. Measurement
5. Quality Awareness
6. Corrective Action
7. Zero Defect Planning
8. Employee Education
9. Zero-defect Day
10. Goal Setting
11. Error-cause Removal
12. Recognition
13. Quality Councils
14. Do It Over Again

requirements are in place and well communicated, then quality will be caused by the prevention of deviation from those requirements. Crosby's Third Absolute asks, What performance standard should be used? Crosby endorses the "Zero Defects" concept, that was described previously.

The Fourth Absolute asks: What measurement system is required? Crosby measured quality as a price, either as conformance or nonconformance to the requirements. In HHC, this may be translated as the risk exposure relative to professional and clinical competence, or incompetence.[15] In presenting arguments as to why any organization should have a quality program, Crosby, like Juran, described the financial cost of having poor quality. His two cost centers were the "price of nonconformance" and the "price of conformance." The price of nonconformance consists of all the expenses involved in doing things wrong. The price of conformance consists of what must be spent to make things right.[15]

Comparing Quality Programs

In HHC, the demonstration of quality may be established by meeting the standards of JCAHO. Although there is no current equivalent of the Baldrige Award[16] for quality HHC organizations, the awarding of accreditation assists in validating that a quality program exists and is making progress toward achieving its goals. JCAHO states that quality of care is the extent to which care provided is expected to achieve the most favorable balance of risks and benefits.[18]

In surveying the literature, common themes reappear in all quality programs (e.g., TQM, CQI, Deming, Juran, Crosby), namely

- Top management embraces and providing resources and leadership for implementation of a quality program.
- There is a planned and methodical process, involving all aspects of the organization; organized by committee.
- There is objective data collection, analysis, monitoring.
- There is extensive education and training; attitude changes.
- There is collaboration between departments, and with suppliers.
- There is continuous improvement that is goal-oriented.
- There is a customer (patient) focus.
- It is a positive, rather than negative, experience.
- Value and cost effectiveness are promoted.

JCAHO ACCREDITATION

The JCAHO evaluates a HHC organization for accreditation based on compliance with applicable standards.[19] The standards are organized within the following categories or chapters: Patient/Client Care, Safety Management, Infection Control, Home Care Record, Quality Assessment and Improvement, Governance and Management, Home Health Services, Pharmaceutical Services, Personnel Care and Support Services, Equipment Management, and Clinical Respiratory Services.

HHC organizations, offering various kinds of services, have been awarded accreditation, since JCAHO established their HHC accreditation process in 1988. Many different types of HHC facilities may be evaluated for accreditation. For example, a pharmacy that provides infusion therapy only will be evaluated against standards in all the above chapters, except, typically, Personnel Care and Support Services and Clinical Respiratory Services. A provider of DME/HME may be evaluated against all of the above standards except Home Health Services, Pharmaceutical Services, and Personnel Care and Support Services. A HHC nursing agency will typically not be evaluated against the standards for Pharmaceutical Services, Equipment Management, or Clinical Respiratory Services. Finally, a hospital based pharmacy (inpatient) providing IV pharmaceuticals to patients at home (outpatient), may be evaluated against the Home Care Standards in addition to standards from the Accreditation Manual for Hospitals.

The best preparation for a survey is an ongoing, day to day quality improvement program.[19] The JCAHO's mission ("to improve the quality of health care provided to the public")[19] is well reflected in its standards. The following are selected standards for Quality Assessment and Improvement as reprinted with permission from the JCAHO publication, Accreditation Manual for Home Care, Volume I, Standards. 1993. Chicago, Illinois. JCAHO:[2]

STANDARD

QA.1 The organization's leaders set expectations, develop plans, and implement procedures to assess and improve the quality of the organization's governance, management, clinical, and support processes.

QA.1.1 The leaders undertake education concerning the approaches and methods of quality improvement.

QA.1.2 The leaders set priorities for organization wide quality improvement activities that are designed to improve patient/client outcomes.

QA.1.3 The leaders allocate adequate resources for assessment and improvement of the organization's governance, managerial, clinical, and support processes.

QA.1.4 The leaders assure that organization staff are trained in assessing and improving the processes that contribute to improved patient/client outcomes.

QA.1.5 The leaders individually and jointly develop and participate in mechanisms to foster communication among individuals and among components of the organization, and to coordinate internal activities.

QA.1.6 Quality assurance activities are defined in a written plan.

QA.1.7 The quality assessment and improvement program addresses all home care services, whether provided directly or through a written contract.

QA.1.8 Relevant results from the quality assessment activities listed in QA.1.6. through QA.1.7.1.6

QA.1.9 There is a planned, systematic, and ongoing process for monitoring, evaluating, and improving the quality of care and improving key governance, managerial, and support activities that has the characteristics described in QA.1.9.1 through QA.1.9.10.2.

QA.1.9.1 Those aspects of care that are most important to the health and safety of the patients/clients served are identified.

QA.1.9.2 Indicators are identified to monitor the quality of important aspects or care.

QA.1.9.3 Data are collected for each indicator.

QA.1.9.4 The data collected for each indicator are organized so that situations in which an evaluation of the quality of care is indicated are readily identified.

QA.1.9.10 The finding, conclusions, recommendations, actions taken, and results of actions are

QA.1.9.10.1 documented, and

QA.1.9.10.2 reported through established channels.

QA.1.10 The governing body receives reports at least annually on the quality of patient/client care and the allocation of resources.

The Monitoring and Assessment Process for JCAHO accreditation is patterned after existing Quality Programs. Although defined as a quality assurance approach, a JCAHO ten step process expands upon the theories of Deming, Juran and Crosby (See Table 4-5.)

INSURING SUCCESS

A common theme of Deming, Juran, Crosby, and the JCAHO, is that management must embrace the quality program. For any quality program to be successful, it must be embraced by everyone in the organization, from upper level management to the per diem employee. Rather than assigning the quality program to a particular staff member or committee only, management should develop teams that become highly involved in the day to day quality process. Administrative support should also be provided even though extra resources must be provided for staff members to carry out their quality program duties. Incentive programs, salary increases, employee evaluations, and even an annual bonus could be based upon individual participation or performance in the quality program.

As seen in the above JCAHO standard QA.1.1, leaders of the organization, i.e., management, must educate itself in the principles of quality management. The education then must filter down through the organization, and include all staff members. Without the participation of all staff, most well intentioned quality programs will be difficult to perform on a daily basis.

Table 4-5 Ten Step Monitoring and Evaluation Process[18,19]

Summary of the Ten-Step Monitoring and Evaluation Process:
• Assign responsibility • Delineate the scope of care • Identify important aspects of care • Identify indicators • Establish thresholds for evaluation • Collect and organize data • Evaluate care • Take actions to solve problems or improve care • Assess the effectiveness of the actions, • Communicate findings to the quality assurance program.

REFERENCES

1. Joint Commission, Department of Home Care Accreditation Services, One Renaissance Blvd., Oakbrook Terrace, IL 60181.
2. Reprinted with permission from Accreditation Manual for Home Care (Vol I: Standards; Vol II: Scoring Guidelines). Copyright 1992 by the Joint Commission for Accreditation of Healthcare Organizations, Oakbrook Terrace, Illinois
3. Community Health Accreditation Program, Inc., A subsidiary of the National League of Nursing, 350 Hudson St., New York, NY 10014.
4. The Measurement Mandate. On the Road to Performance Improvement in Health Care. JCAHO. Oakbrook Terrace, Illinois. 1993.
5. Tennessee Pharmacist. Proposed IV Regulations Presented to Board. Chapter 1140-7: Sterile Product Preparation in Pharmacy Practice. [1140-7-.03(1)(f)] Feb 1993. pp 5-6.
6. California Pharmacy Law, California State Board of Pharmacy, Sacramento, CA 1991.
7. Zitter M. Outcomes Assessment: True Customer Focus Comes to Health Care. Medical Interface. 1992; 5:32-37.
8. Gabor Andrea. The Man Who Discovered Quality. New York. Penguin. 1990.
9. Deming WE. Out of the Crisis. M.I.T. Cambridge, MA. 1986.
10. Juran JM. Juran on Planning for Quality. New York. The Free Press. 1989.
11. Juran JM, Gryna FM Jr. Quality Planning and Analysis. New York. McGraw-Hill, 1980.
12. Juran JM. Juran on Planning for Quality. New York. The Free Press. 1989.
13. Juran JM. Juran on Quality by Design. New York. The Free Press. 1992.
14. Juran JM and Gryna FM Jr. Quality Planning and Analysis. New York. The Free Press. 1980.
15. Crosby PB. Quality Without Tears. New York. Plume. 1984.
16. Gabor Andrea. The Man Who Discovered Quality. New York. Penguin. 1990.
17. Quality Assessment in Home Infusion Therapy. First Ed. JCAHO. Oakbrook Terrace, Illinois. 1993.
18. Hearst MR, Ed. Quality Assurance in Home Care and Hospice Organizations. Chicago. Ill. JCAHO. 1990.
19. JCAHO Accreditation Manual for Home Care, Vol II: Scoring Guidelines. 1992.

5 Drug Information in Home Health Care Practice

Julio R. Lopez, Pharm.D.

A body of knowledge associated with home health care (HHC) pharmacy practice is evolving in this relatively new field. However, HHC is neither extensively nor routinely taught to all students at schools of pharmacy in the United States. HHC practice-specific knowledge is frequently acquired with experience on the job. Furthermore, many pharmacists practicing in HHC graduated before HHC in its present format was born. Consequently, the information base of pharmacists may vary widely. Pharmacists working in HHC may have different backgrounds, with some individuals originating from traditional community pharmacy practice while others having hospital background. Indeed, HHC pharmacy practice contains elements found in both traditional pharmacy practice settings. In order to bridge this gap, a greater reliance on sound drug information skills is needed.

The provision of pharmaceutical care to patients at home presents potential logistical problems to accessing drug information when questions arise at the patient's home. In addition, the home setting itself may generate unique questions. Consequently, a good understanding of information sources is needed for effective home care pharmacy practice.

The types of questions facing pharmacists in HHC may include traditional drug information as well as unique questions associated with the use of drugs at home. Furthermore, these questions may arise from other health care practitioners, the patient, or from the pharmacist himself. Traditional drug information questions are those related to adverse effects, drugs of choice, pharmacology, drug interactions, or pharmacokinetics, to name just a few. Since the pharmacist may routinely come in contact with the patient and his family, many of these questions may arise from them. In addition, questions related to technical operation of the pumps used in home IV therapy, drug compatibilities and stability at home, waste disposal regulations, and many other unique questions may arise from the fact that patients are receiving drugs traditionally administered in the hospital setting.

A sound approach to handling drug information questions is also needed to ensure that the information is correctly applied to patient care. This includes obtaining sufficient background into the patient or situation that originated the question. Clarifying the question is essential. Consideration of drug dosing according to indication and clinical characteristics of the patient (e.g., renal function) is an example of how drug information needs to be understood in the context of the HHC patient to make it useful information. When combined with the pharmacist's training in pharmacology and clinical therapeutics, expertly retrieved and evaluated drug information can provide the elements needed for resolution of many patient-oriented problems.

This chapter is designed to highlight useful drug information resources and to list some key references for HHC pharmacy practice. In addition to serving as a guide for building a HHC pharmacy library, this chapter also gives some tips and techniques for accessing off-site information such as electronic on-line information services.

INFORMATION SOURCES

A brief description of books, information systems, and key journal articles is given. This list was not designed to be complete, but rather reflects the author's choice of references that have proven most useful in drug information practice.

General References

As their name states, these references contain general and varied information on drugs. Typically, general references are used as the starting point for answering most questions. A general reference will be able to handle most drug information questions.

Martindale, The Extra Pharmacopoeia (30th edition, JEF Reynolds, editor. The Pharmaceutical Press, London:1993). Considered by many as the best overall drug information book, Martindale's contains drug monographs listing physico-chemical drug properties, toxicology information, extensive adverse reaction and indications information, pharmacokinetic data, and international drug availability. References are provided throughout the text. The book is published approximately every 4 years and tends to get outdated. However, there is an electronic version accessible through on-line information vendors such as Data-Star and in CD-ROM from the Micromedex Company.

Handbook of Clinical Drug Data (Seventh Edition. JE Knoben and PO Anderson. Drug Intelligence Publication, Vancouver, WA:1993). This is an excellent compilation of useful data on drugs either by brief monograph or tables. Specialized sections deal with nutrition, drug interactions, pharmacokinetics and drug-induced disorders, among others. Perhaps the greatest strength of this book is that it is small enough to be carried in a coat pocket.

Facts and Comparisons (Olin BR, Hebel SK, Dombek CE, Eds. Facts and Comparisons, Inc. St Louis, MO, updated monthly). An excellent general information source that provides summarized drug data and many tables comparing drugs by pharmacological class. Facts and Comparisons is notable for its extensive inclusion of over-the counter, prescription, and diagnostic products. A loose-leaf and microfiche version are updated monthly making Facts and Comparisons one of the best sources for new product information. A hardbound book version is published annually and is best suited for nursing unit use. Several surveys indicate that Facts and Comparisons is the most widely used information resource in American pharmacies.

AHFS Drug Information (McEvoy GK, Litvak K, Eds. American Society of Hospital Pharmacists, Bethesda, MD:1992). An annual publication from ASHP with quarterly updates provides complete drug monographs for products commonly used in the hospital setting. While the information provided is very extensive, not all drugs are included in AHFS. Furthermore, the quarterly updates frequently do not reflect recently introduced drugs. Comprehensive monographs make AHFS a useful reference particularly in the institutional setting.

USP DI (United States Pharmacopeial Convention, Inc, Rockville, MD:1992). A three volume annual publication with quarterly updates. The first volume covers drug information for the health provider. This volume contains complete drug monographs presented in a very nice outline format that makes location of information very easy. The second volume is information for the patient and is discussed below. The third volume contains a reproduction of the FDA's list of approved drug products with therapeutic equivalencies (the FDA Orange Book) which is useful in locating drug manufacturers and, most importantly, for generic equivalency ratings.

Handbook of Nonprescription Drugs (Tenth Edition, American Pharmaceutical Association, Washington, DC:1993). A textbook that specializes in over-the-counter products. Each chapter contains both a thorough description of therapeutic considerations as well as a listing of most products available in the United States. Of particular interest for the HHC pharmacist will be chapters discussing in-home diagnostic products, diabetes care products, and ostomy care products.

Physicians' Desk Reference (PDR) (Forty-seventh edition, Medical Economics Company, Montvale, NJ: 1993). A book that compiles the package inserts for most brand-name products in the United States. While the therapeutic information presented in these monographs is non-comparative and of limited value, the package inserts commonly list official FDA-approved indications, inert ingredients in product formulations, and some compatibility and preparation data for parenteral products. Some of the information in the PDR may not be listed in other general references and therefore can be very useful. The PDR is published annually and is widely available to most physicians and pharmacists in the country.

Drugdex (Micromedex, Inc, Denver, CO:updated quarterly). Although a microfiche version of this drug information compilation is still available, Drugdex is commonly used in its CD-ROM (Compact Disc) electronic version. Drugdex is made up of three parts: the complete drug evaluations database, an index to side effects that points to the complete drug evaluations, and the drug consults database. The complete drug evaluations offer excellent comprehensive and fully referenced drug reviews. Within the drug evaluations, the section on therapeutic uses approaches being an abstracting service as it describes in detail most clinical trials with the drug. The drug consults are cross-referenced from the drug evaluations database. The drug consults database consists of answered drug information questions that are supplied by pharmacy practitioners throughout the United States. A limitation of these drug consults is that they can become obsolete since they are not routinely updated. It is necessary to check the author's section to find the date the consult was written. Furthermore, since the consults are supplied by many people, errors in transcription and data interpretation are possible. Overall, Drugdex is an excellent source of information. It is fast and very complete. Some drawbacks are the requirement for computer hardware and a high annual subscription cost of several thousand dollars which varies depending on the number of users at one location, configuration, and access to related databases. A new CD is mailed quarterly updating the entire system.

Indexing/Abstracting Services

Whenever information is not located in a textbook or when one needs the most current information available, it will be necessary to access the published literature. Indexing and abstracting sources exist to facilitate access to the primary literature. Computer technology now makes all of these indexing services available electronically. On-line access is described in a separate section below.

International Pharmaceutical Abstracts (IPA) (American Society of Hospital Pharmacists, Bethesda, MD). Billed as the only pharmacy-specific indexing and abstracting source, IPA is produced by the ASHP and indexes approximately 700 journals, newsletters, and trade magazines. Many of these are pharmacy journals not indexed anywhere else. A strength of IPA is its key-word thesaurus that includes not only drugs and diseases but also pharmacy topics. This includes topics such as "nutrition, parenteral" and "health care, home" that can be used to search for published practice models and administrative issues related to HHC delivery. IPA is published in print twice a month with a cumulative index every 6 months. An on-line and a CD-ROM version that enable electronic searching are also available from third party information vendors.

IDIS (Iowa Drug Information Service, Iowa City, IA). The Iowa Drug Information Service (IDIS) is a microfiche indexing service for drug articles found in major medical and pharmacy journals. Approximately 300 journals are indexed. In addition, the articles are available as full text copies in microfiche. The IDIS can be used as an alternate medical library source focusing on drug information, albeit there is some lag time between the publication of an article and its inclusion in IDIS. Monthly updates are shipped. A new CD-ROM version is now also available that allows fast searching of the index covering articles from 1985 to the current month. The article copies are not on the CD-ROM, however. One limitation of IDIS is the somewhat difficult and restrictive key word thesaurus used to index the articles. On the other hand, major advantages are that indexing is done by pharmacists and that the full article is in microfiche. The system requires, at a minimum, a microfiche reader.

Inpharma (Adis International, Inc, Langhorne, PA): This is a weekly publication that selectively provides abstracts to key drug therapy articles. Inpharma is very current and is most useful to keep up with advances in clinical pharmacology and therapeutics. The abstracts are very complete. An on-line Inpharma is also available through some third party information vendors. A shortcoming of Inpharma is its very high cost, currently $1,550 per year, making it one of the most expensive alternatives.

Therapeutics

Applied Therapeutics. The Clinical Use of Drugs. MA Koda-Kimble and LY Young, Editors. (Fifth Edition, Applied Therapeutics, Inc, Vancouver, WA:1992). An excellent textbook that presents information on disease states and therapeutics in a case-oriented fashion. In addition to being a complete therapeutic reference, this textbook also teaches clinical problem-solving skills.

Pharmacotherapy. A Pathophysiologic Approach. JT DiPiro, Talbert RL, Hayes PE, Yee GC, Posey LM, Editors. (Elsevier Science Publishing Co., New York, NY: 1989). Another excellent therapeutics text that includes summaries of landmark studies supporting the therapeutic approaches to diseases. It also provides extensive background into the disease including pathophysiologic and diagnostic discussions.

Infectious Diseases

Principles and Practice of Infectious Diseases. (Third Edition. Mandell GL, Douglas RG, Bennett JE, Editors. Churchill Livingstone, New York, NY:1990). One of the best infectious diseases textbooks, Mandell's describes diagnostic principles, classic syndromes, drugs, and pathogens in major sections of the textbook.

Manual of Antibiotics and Infectious Diseases. (Seventh Edition. JE Conte and SL Barriere. Lea and Febiger, Philadelphia, PA:1992). This book contains summarized practical information on the use of antimicrobials. In addition, it is small enough to be portable.

The Medical Letter Handbook of Antimicrobial Therapy. (The Medical letter, New Rochelle, NY: 1992). Another small practical guide to the use of antimicrobials. It contains the standard antibiotic regimens used to treat various infections as well as other useful information such as tables on how to adjust drug dosing in renal failure.

Cancer Chemotherapy

Handbook of Cancer Chemotherapy, (Third Edition. Skeel RT. Little Brown and Company, NY:1991). The field of oncology therapeutics has undergone a small revolution with the introduction of biologic response modifiers and new antineoplastic drugs. There is no textbook that is entirely current. This Little-Brown manual is one of the most recently published.

Geriatrics

Prescribing for the Elderly. PP Lamy. (John Wright PSG, Inc, Boston, MA:1980). Although old, this classic textbook thoroughly describes considerations for the use of medications in the elderly patient.

Geriatric Clinical Pharmacology. WG Wood and R Strong. (Raven Press, New York, NY:1987). This textbook has detailed descriptions of infectious diseases in elderly persons as well as the factors that affect drug response in the elderly.

The Merck Manual of Geriatrics. (WB Abrams and R Berkow. Merck and Co., Inc, Rahway, NJ:1990). Concise yet complete coverage of diseases of the elderly arranged by organ system.

Pharmacokinetics

Basic Clinical Pharmacokinetics, (Second Edition. ME Winter. Applied Therapeutics, Vancouver, WA:1988). This is an excellent book that explains the practical considerations that must be taken when evaluating serum drug levels. It includes cases as examples.

Dosing

Handbook of Drug Therapy in Liver and Kidney Disease. (RW Schrier and JG Gambertoglio. Little Brown and Co, Boston, MA:1991). Whenever drug elimination is compromised in patients, questions arise on how to modify the dose. This reference provides dosing adjustment information in renal and liver disease. In addition, other guidelines and discussion focus on how to use drugs safely in these patients.

Parenteral Therapy/Compatibilities

Guide to Parenteral Admixtures. JC King. (Pacemarq, Inc, San Francisco 1993). An excellent reference for locating compatibility and stability information for parenteral products, especially those given intravenously. This 3-volume loose-leaf publication is updated on a quarterly basis.

Handbook on Injectable Drugs, (Seventh Edition. LA Trissel. American Society of Hospital Pharmacists, Bethesda, MD:1992). One of the most extensively used references for compatibility and stability information. New editions are published every two or three years.

Nutrition Support

Training Manual for Total Parenteral Nutrition, (Second Edition. RE Dean. Precept Press, Chicago, IL:1990). This is a practical textbook on how to determine nutritional needs as well as how to manage care of the patient with catheters. For example, it illustrates how to change catheter dressings.

Total Parenteral Nutrition. (Second Edition. JE Fischer. Little, Brown and Company, Inc, Boston, MA:1991). A comprehensive textbook on parenteral nutrition, including chapters on the use of total parenteral nutrition in specific disease states.

Pain Management

The pathophysiology and therapeutic approaches to pain management are usually included as part of other textbooks. For example, the therapeutics texts listed above contain chapters on this topic. However, pain management crosses many medical disciplines. An effort has been made to sensibly organize pain management strategies through the publication of guidelines. The following guidelines and review articles are widely used:

Analgesic Therapy in the Terminally Ill Cancer Patient. A supplement to the American Journal of Hospital Pharmacy, August 1990.

American Pain Society. Principles of Analgesic Use in the Treatment of Acute Pain and Chronic Cancer Pain. Second Edition. Clin Pharm 1990; 9:601-11.

Agency for Health Care Policy and Research. Acute Pain Management. Operative or medical procedures and trauma. Part 1 in Clin Pharm 1992;11:309-31. Part 2 in Clin Pharm 1992;11:391-414.

Drug Interactions

Drug Interactions Facts. (Facts and Comparisons, St. Louis, MO: updated quarterly). Drug Interaction Facts presents information listing the significance of an interaction, its management, and a summary of the supporting documentation. In addition to the printed loose-leaf updated version, hardbound and electronic editions are available. The electronic edition can be loaded into a personal computer or the system can be accessed on-line through modem.

Drug Interactions and Updates. PD Hansten and JR Horn. (Applied Therapeutics, Inc, Vancouver, WA: updated quarterly). Another excellent reference on the clinical significance of drug interactions. The database in Drug Interactions has been sold separately for use in microcomputer.

In addition, various pharmacy computer systems integrate drug interaction databases. These systems typically check for interactions as part of routine medication order processing.

Adverse Drug Reactions

Most common adverse drug reactions will be listed in general references such as Facts and Comparisons. In some cases, incidence rates are provided on the basis of pre-marketing data. Specialized textbooks for certain kinds of adverse reactions also exist. For a detailed general coverage of adverse drug reaction information, the Textbook of Adverse Drug Reactions, fourth edition by DM Davies is a good source. Available from Oxford University Press, New York, NY:1992.

Patient Education

Several good patient education textbooks are available. They all have monographs on drugs or drug classes written in plain language for ease of patient understanding. The most commonly used ones are:

Medication Teaching Manual, (Fourth Edition. American Society of Hospital Pharmacists, Bethesda, MD:1987).

Patient Drug Facts. Olin BR, Hebel SK, Covington TR, Eds. (Facts and Comparisons, St. Louis, MO: updated quarterly).

USP DI, Volume II: Advice for the Patient. (United States Pharmacopeial Convention, Rockville, MD: 1992). The USP patient information is also supplied in an electronic version, for example in the Micromedex CD, that can print patient information in a low english literacy mode and in spanish.

ON LINE INFORMATION

Access to on-line information systems is made possible due to the growth of personal computer use with modem capabilities. On-line systems are traditionally bibliographic. Namely, they include citations to published articles. The databases can be searched for words in various parts of the citation. In addition, these citations are classified according to key-words so that the articles can also be searched by key words. A few full-text on-line electronic databases also exist. For example, full text versions of major medical journals are available from some third party information vendors. Searching databases on-line has the advantage of speed and currency of information. Searching has been made easier by advances in user interface and tutorials.

Typically a local number is dialed connecting to a telecommunications network. Consequently, even though the vendors may be located far away (sometimes in other countries), no long distance telephone charges are incurred. Once the connection is established, the right database is accessed and the search is input. Charges vary depending on connect times, citations printed and, in some cases, according to the database that is searched.

While many databases exist that may be interesting to HHC pharmacists, the most widely used is the Medline database, with backfiles dating to 1966, produced by the National Library of Medicine. This is the same database that is used to produce Index Medicus. Medline is accessed through various third party vendors, such as PaperChase, DataStar, Dialog, and BRS Colleague. Many of the third party vendors reformat the information in order to make searching easier. Third party vendors also provide access to many other medical databases such as International Pharmaceutical Abstracts and Excerpta Medica. Many pharmacists will select third party vendors because of the variety of databases that can be searched. Some vendors have minimum monthly fees that are applied to search charges while other do not. When selecting a third party information vendor, one should check the types of databases available, ease of use, customer support, and costs.

It is not necessary to use a third party vendor to access Medline, however. Direct access to Medline can be established by setting up an account with the National Library of Medicine. In addition, a "front-end" program called Grateful Med makes searching very easy. This program allows entry of the search before connecting on-line, then automatically runs and downloads the search results. Grateful Med has a glossary of the Medical Subject Terms (MeSH) used to index the Medline database. Versions of Grateful Med are available for PC and Macintosh at $29.95 each with free upgrades. Connect charges will vary on the length of the search and average between $2 to $5 per search. For information on Grateful Med contact the MEDLARS Management Service Desk at 1-800-638-8480. Grateful Med may be ordered from the U.S. Department of Commerce, National Technical Information Service, 5285 Port Royal Road, Springfield, VA 22161.

Another good source of on-line information is the Food and Drug Administration. Notices on new drug approvals, recalls, and regulatory actions are posted in a toll-free BBS. To access set up your modem to 7 bits, even parity, full duplex, and 1 stop bit. Dial 1-800-222-0185 (301-227-6849 in Maryland). At the prompt "login" respond with "bbs" in lower case letters and then follow the instructions.

MANUFACTURERS

Manufacturers of medical equipment, supplies, and drug products will often have information that is not published in journals or textbooks. As an example, questions about drug stability for many of the automatic infusion pumps will need to be directed to the manufacturer of the equipment rather than the company that produces the drug. Salespersons for the various equipment and supplies companies can be a good source of practical information.

Whenever calling a drug company for information, the pharmacist must understand that delays in getting the information can exist. Frequently drug companies call back an answer after their files are searched. Patient-specific questions on adverse effects may also trigger a medical event report to the company as this is required by FDA regulations. Phone numbers to contact pharmaceutical companies are located in most general textbooks, including Facts and Comparisons.

INFORMATION FILES

The practice of HHC pharmacy involves more than therapeutic knowledge. Information on drug delivery systems and equipment, medical supplies, and other types of specialized knowledge are also needed. Since this information is not routinely collected in textbooks, pharmacists will need to set up information files. These files should include equipment brochures, medical supplies descriptions, and other company information in addition to the standard reprinted articles from journals.

Systems for organizing this information are diverse and depend on personal preference. Typically an alphabetical filing system is created with topic headings according to disease, drug, or other information category. However, if more than one individual will use the filing system, it is best to have consistent organization of the materials so that they are readily accessible to all. One could go as far as cataloging the information and setting up an index to the files. Although it may be time consuming to set up, computer database programs may ease retrieval of information. A specialized PC software program called Cite Search is available from ASHP for this purpose. Information files should be periodically purged to delete obsolete materials.

PEERS

Even with the best printed or electronic information resources available, there will be questions for which no apparent answer exists. In some of these cases it may be possible to call upon colleagues to see if a similar question has arisen in their practice. In some cases, other health practitioners may be practically familiar with how to solve a particular problem. For example, a nurse may have practical experience on managing ostomy care so that she can provide information on the benefits of one product versus another. The development of a network of consultants is thus important. Yet, the limitations of using consultants must also be recognized. Consultants may have limited experience with certain products or their area of practice may be somewhat different. In developing a network with outside consultants, it is imperative to understand their area of practice and credentials.

The advent of electronic communications also allows wider access to peers for advice. Bulletin board systems now operate within certain professional organizations such as ASHP and the American College of Clinical Pharmacy, and in the Department of Veterans Affairs' Clinical Pharmacy Forum. At least one commercial system exists, the F.I.X. or formulary information exchange, available from The Formulary Company. Questions may be placed in these bulletin board systems and satisfactory answers are frequently received. To access many of these systems a personal computer with a modem is used. Standard communications software is all that is needed.

DRUG INFORMATION CENTERS

Drug Information Centers serve most areas of the United States. They maintain extensive drug information libraries and often have access to on-line information sources. Drug Information Centers often provide services at no charge to the caller. They should be used as a source of information after local resources are exhausted. Drug Information Centers are an excellent and often overlooked source of information for HHC practice.

USEFUL HOME HEALTH CARE REFERENCES

Solomon DK, Holt JM. Home Health Care - 1991. Hosp Pharm 1991;26:261. A basic bibliography.

Monk MR. Home Intravenous Therapy Bibliography for Pharmacists (1970-1989). Hosp Pharm 1991;26:203-233. A comprehensive listing of references covering all aspects of the provision of home IV therapy.

PERIODICALS

American Journal of Hospital Pharmacy. American Society of Hospital Pharmacists, Bethesda, MD. A monthly journal that frequently presents research on IV drug compatibilities and stability as well as descriptions of parenteral therapy techniques and pharmacy practice research.

Home Health Care Business. Cassak Publications, Union, NJ. It includes an annual buyers guide listing products and vendors.

Hospital Pharmacy. J. Lippincott Company, Philadelphia, PA. A monthly journal that has an abstracting section on parenteral therapy techniques, with some issues also containing information on new devices.

JPEN. Journal of Parenteral and Enteral Nutrition, Silver Spring, MD. A multidisciplinary journal that contains articles related to enteral and parenteral nutritional support.

Pharmacy Practice News. The McMahon Group, New York, NY. A monthly periodical that, among many other topics, describes new devices and supplies used in IV therapy.

Rx Homecare. Barrington Publications, Los Angeles, CA. A monthly journal describing issues related to home health care. It includes an annual buyers guide listing manufacturers of durable medical equipment.

6 The Needs of the Elderly Patient

Peter P. Lamy, Ph.D., Sc.D.

Substantial and dramatic changes in the geriatric long term care sector have taken place in the past decade—and the changes continue. Home-based community care is a major part of the long-term care sector now. A greater proportion of the elderly with complex health problems and consequent complex care needs now remain in the community rather than entering some form of institutional care. The levels of dependency, as measured by activity of daily living scores, are increasing in the home care sector, and this suggests that there is now a greater degree of overlap in the characteristics of people cared for in the various segments of long term care. The blurring of boundaries may be of little consequence to the people receiving the various forms of longterm care, but it does have consequences and implications for the type of care they receive. In home care, the family plays an important, vital, and substantial part in the delivery of it.

A woman living in the United States now can expect to spend 17 years caring for children and 18 years helping an aging parent, likely at a high economic, physical and emotional price. Nearly four of every ten women will care for a disabled adult.[1] Eighty percent of family caregivers to the elderly provide care seven days a week, and it has been estimated that caregivers to the elderly provide over 27 million days of unpaid care every week. One of every five caregivers to the elderly has been providing care for five years or more.[2] Perhaps based on these findings, there is strong national support for longterm care programs. One survey found that 84 percent of the American public supports the idea of new programs.

THE ELDERLY

Life expectancy has increased across all age groups. A 68 year old woman, living today, has a life expectancy of another 20 years, while a man of equal age can expect to live another 12 years. The projected median age of the US population, now 31.8 years, will rise to 36 years by the year 2000 and to 42 years by the year 2040.

Two facts are thought to be responsible for these dramatic, projected increases. The first of these is the "aging" of the population. Life expectancy at age 85 years has increased 24 percent since 1960 and is projected to increase another 44 percent by the year 2040.[3] At that time, or shortly thereafter, at least 50 percent of Americans will survive to their 85th birthday and those 85 years old and over will constitute at least 15 million people.[4] This part of the population is expected to be seven times as large in 2050 as in 1980. This particular age cohort will have increased in number from 123,000 in 1900 and 2.2 million in 1980 to more than 18 million in the year 2080. It has been estimated that there were 15,000 centenarians in 1980 and 25,000 in 1986, a number likely to increase to more than 100,000 by the year 2000.

The other factor is the dramatic shift in the age distribution of the US population, a shift that will change the well-known age pyramid to a near rectangle. Table 6-1 depicts the average remaining lifetime in years at specified ages[5,6] and Table 6-2 shows the projected and actual population changes in the United States.[7]

The elderly are the population segment most in need of long-term care, perhaps because they are stricken most often with chronic diseases and, importantly, with a multiplicity of chronic diseases.

A chronic disease is a sickness (e.g., diabetes, arthritis) or limitation of function that lasts a long time (more than two to three weeks). The condition will likely require adjustment of an individual's lifestyle and provision of medical, nursing, and social services.[8] Indeed, the conditions may mandate long-term care. Longterm care is the range of medical and

Table 6-1 Average Remaining Lifetime in Years at Specified Ages: 1900 to 1991[6]

AGE	1900-02	1939-41	1949-51	1959-61	1969-71	1979-81	1989-91 (est)
birth	49.2	63.6	68.1	69.9	70.8	73.7	75.4
60	14.8	15.9	7.0	17.7	18.5	19.9	20.8
65	11.9	12.8	13.8	14.4	15.0	16.4	17.3
70	9.3	10.0	10.9	11.4	12.1	13.3	13.9
75	7.1	7.6	8.4	8.7	9.5	10.4	10.9
80	5.3	5.7	6.3	6.4	7.2	7.9	8.3
85	4.0	4.3	4.7	4.6	5.3	5.9	6.2
Median Age at Death	58.4			74.3	74.9	77.4	79.1

Table 6-2 Population Changes in the United States[7]

	55+		65+		(% total pop.)		75+	
1900	7.1M(a)	-	3.1(a)	-	(4.1%)(a)	-	0.89M(a)	-
1920	11.5	-	4.9	-	(4.6%)	-	1.5	-
1940	19.7	-	9.0	-	(6.8%)	-	2.6	-
1960	32.3	-	16.7	-	(9.2%)	-	5.6	-
1980	45.6	47.2(b)	24.5	25.5(b)	(11.0%)%	(11.3%)(b)	9.1	10.0(b)
1990	-	52.8	-	31.7	-	(12.7%)	-	13.7
2000	53.5	58.7	30.6	34.9	(11.7%)	(13.0%)	13.5	17.2
2010	65.7	74.0	33.2	39.2	(12.0%)	(13.8%)	13.9	18.9
2020	79.5	91.7	42.8	51.4	(14.6%)	(17.3%)	15.4	21.6

(a) 1976 data[7]
(b) 1988 data[7]

social care for individuals having chronic functional impairment in activities of daily living, and it may be provided by formal or informal support systems.[8] Long term care is also defined as the sustained and prolonged health, social, and personal care given to individuals who are chronically ill and/or disabled. It is the type of care given to those (older) persons whose chronic conditions (physical and cognitive impairments) and accompanying problems (inability to carry out a range of tasks, deal with isolation, depression, etc.) have affected their daily functioning. It is interesting to note, though, that there are many elderly with chronic conditions, even multiple chronic conditions, who are not restricted in their activities of daily living.[9]

On the other hand, there are increasing numbers of "homebound" elderly. Homebound status may predict the need for more intensive and costly services. A patient who needs skilled services must be considered homebound and certified as such by a physician. Persons are homebound if leaving home requires a "taxing" effort and necessitates the assistance of another person or supportive device.[10] Once somebody becomes homebound, there is, in general, a unidirectional path of decline. Rarely does somebody, living in the community, return to non-homebound status.[11]

THE ELDERLY AND CHRONIC ILLNESS

About 80 percent of the elderly have at least one chronic illness. Certain diseases and problems are largely age-dependent, such as dementia, coronary heart disease and most cancers.[12] Even a single chronic disease, such as Alzheimer's can produce an ever-increasing burden of illness and progressively deteriorating physical dysfunction.[13] Being overweight is a serious health problem for older people, especially for those with long-standing weight problems.[14] Urinary incontinence, from which a large proportion of elderly women suffer, is one of the most overlooked problems.[15] Arthritic diseases are common, as are cardiovascular problems. The prevalence of elevated isolated systolic blood pressure may range from 10 percent in men aged 60 and over to 37 percent in women aged 70 and over. The prevalence of elevated diastolic pressure ranges between 43 percent of men aged 60 and 38 percent of women aged 70 years.[16] Occult significant coronary artery disease is present in the majority of elderly.[17] Ischemic heart disease or hypertension or a combination of both is found in more than one-third of the elderly.[18] Functional bowel distress and peptic ulcer disease may be present in more than 40 percent of community-living elderly.[19] Cognitive impairment is a major problem.[20] Among the potentially severely disabling non-lethal conditions, one might list arthritis, visual impairment, and dementia. Those that can be variably disabling and lethal would include stroke, heart disease, and circulatory disorders, cancer, and chronic lung disease. Those that are potentially less disabling and less lethal include diabetes, depression, and high blood pressure.[21] Unfortunately, more than 40% of those elderly suffering from one chronic disease also suffer from multiple chronic diseases, as shown in Table 6-3.

Table 6-3 The Most Common Medical Problems Coexisting in Elderly

1. Hypertension
2. Congestive heart failure
3. Depression
4. Dementia
5. Chronic renal failure
6. Angina pectoris (atherosclerotic heart disease)
7. Degenerative joint disease (osteoarthritis)
8. Gait disturbance
9. Urinary dysfunction
10. Constipation
11. Peripheral vascular disease
12. Diabetes mellitus
13. Chronic pain
14. Sleep disturbances

Often, in an elderly hypertensive patient one should expect to find conditions related to hypertension, such as generalized, coronary, or cerebrovascular atherosclerotic cardiovascular disease, renal dysfunction, left ventricular hypertrophy and heart failure. It is also likely that the patient may present with a coincidental disease process, such as diabetes mellitus, chronic obstructive lung disease, or arthritis. Finally, the patient may also suffer from conditions related to adverse effects of the treatment of hypertension, such as hypovolemia, hypo- or hyperkalemia, hyponatremia, and/or orthostatic hypotension.[23]

With increasing age, the number of chronic

illnesses increases (Table 6 - 4). Long term care recipients usually suffer from multiple and often interrelated chronic problems. Chronic disease in the elderly presents more frequently with functional impairment than in younger people. For example, the ratio of chronic disease in patients over 65 years of age versus that of patients below 45 years of age is 9.74 for arthritis, 6.98 for hypertension, and 9.69 for diabetes.

Table 6-4 Illness Conditions for Elderly Medicare Beneficiaries by Selected Characteristics[26]

Characteristic	Elderly Population (in Millions)	Number of Illness Conditions Percentage Distrubution					Average Number of Conditions
		None	1-2	3-4	5-6	7 or more	
AGE							
65 - 69 years	9.1	8	30	27	16	20	4.0
70 - 74 years	6.8	8	25	25	21	22	4.4
75 - 79 years	4.3	7	20	25	19	30	5.1
80 years & over	3.5	6	22	30	19	24	4.9
SEX							
Male	9.8	9	28	29	16	18	3.9
Female	13.9	6	23	24	20	26	4.8

As pointed out, many elderly suffer from multiple medical problems that need ongoing attention and from functional impairments that prevent independence. In short, impairments, disabilities and handicaps (Table 6-5) abound, often overlaid by cognitive impairment (Table 6-6). The number of old-old so afflicted may triple in the years ahead.[24,25]

Table 6-5 Definitions of Functional Problems[24]

Impairment: Disturbances at organ level. Abnormalities of body structure

Disability: Consequences of impairments in terms of functional performance and activities of an individual (Also defined as primarily a medical problem, a health-related inability to work, physical limitation).

Handicap: Disadvantage to an individual as a result of impairments and disabilities (Also defined as inability to perform certain social functions).

Table 6-6 Indicators of Cognitive Deficits

TYPE OF DEFICIT	INDICATOR
Disorientation	Unable to give information related to living arrangements, age, family, others.
General Confusion	Unable to follow instructions and procedures Incoherent speech.
Memory Deficit	Unable to list medications. Unable to give correct recent medical history.

Activity limitations data are presented in Table 6-7. The number of community-living elderly 65 years old and over with functional dependencies increase from 12.6% for those 65 to 74, to 25.0% for those 75 to 84, and 45.8% for those 85 years and over. Dependency data are presented in Table 6-8.

Disability has been classified into eight different levels by the Veterans Administration.[26]

Level O (no disability): Individuals at this level are essentially well and need no services. They should have access to and take advantage of periodic examinations to rule out and treat nascent and otherwise unrecognized disorders, particularly those with serious potential. Older individuals, just as the very young, should receive appropriate immunizations.

Level 1 (minimal disability): These are patients with established diagnoses which require periodic services, especially visits to the physician's office or the clinic, but are otherwise able to maintain an independent life style.

Level 2 (mild disability): These are patients who require a greater level of support because of disability, but only on an intermittent basis. Additional requirements may include transportation, assistance in shopping or housekeeping, or the availability of oxygen in the household.

Level 3 (moderate disability): At this level the patient requires someone in the household daily,

Table 6-7 Activity Limitation of Non-institutionalized Elderly Medicare Beneficiaries by Selected Characteristics[26]

Characteristic	Elderly Population (in Millions)	Percent with Some Activity	Percent with Limitation
Age			
65 - 69 years	9.1	31	69
70 - 74 years	6.8	39	61
75 - 79 years	4.3	47	53
80 years and over	3.5	52	48
Sex			
Male	9.8	52	48
Female	13.9	31	69
Total	23.7	40	60

Table 6-8 Numbers of Non-institutionalized Dependent Persons and Rates of Dependency by Age Groups[26]

	Personal Care		Mobility		Household Activities		Health Services		Total Dependency
Age	**Number**	%	**Number**	%	**Number**	%	**Number**	%	**Number**
0-64	898,000	0.5	268,300	0.1	966,300	0.5	659,000	0.3	1,791,000
65-74	370,000	2.5	206,700	1.4	431,500	2.9	90,000	0.6	1,098,200
75 +	710,000	8.5	336,300	4.0	708,200	8.4	107,500	1.3	1,862,800
Total	1,978,800	0.9	811,300	0.4	2,106,000	1.0	856,500	0.4	5,752,600
65 +	1,080,800	4.6	543,100	2.3	1,139,700	4.9	197,500	0.8	2,962,000

In this scheme, the categories are mutually exclusive - individuals were classified by their most severe dependency.

but not necessarily continuously. Examples include patients with arthritis or significant residuals of a stroke, as well as many psychiatric patients in remission.

Level 4 (moderately severe disability): These patients require the constant availability of support and supervision, but relatively little actual performance of services. Examples include certain types of cardiac patients, such as those convalescing from a myocardial infarction, or patients with severe brain damage who cannot be alone.

Level 5 (severe, chronic, stable disability): Includes those patients who require intensive non-professional nursing care. A typical and frequent example is the stable, but totally incapacitated, aphasic patient with the residuals of a stroke. Usually, this is the highest level for a skilled nursing facility.

Level 6 (severe, chronic, unstable disability): These are patients who require frequent, even daily medical supervision, extensive skilled nursing care, and many of the services generally available only in the hospital. Most of these patients are unstable, and can be expected to improve or get worse over a period of months. Examples include patients recovering from severe accidents or complex surgical problems, patients with severe respiratory diseases, patients in the terminal phases of cancer, and patients with severe neurological disorders, such as traumatic paralysis of all four extremities.

Level 7 (acute disability or diagnosis): This level represents traditional acute hospital care. The hospital provides specialized facilities for diagnosis and treatment not readily available in an alternative setting, and the utilization of specialized services is high. Nursing care can vary from minimal to intense. The duration of stay at this level is usually relatively short.

Level 8 (severe acute disability): Patients in this category are critically ill, with need for intense use of all hospital services and facilities. The typical setting includes the intensive care, coronary care, respiratory care and surgical intensive care units. The general ward also continues to serve many of these patients. The duration of stay tends to be brief, with early transfer to a less intense status.

The Health Interview Survey of the National Center for Health Statistics estimated that about 12% of elderly are either confined to their home or need help in getting around. That, though, may be an underestimate. It is reasonable to assume that the impaired elderly population ranges between 12% and 17% and that 20% to 33% of the elderly need in-home services of varying kinds. Others[27] have reported that among both males and females, the greatest increase in Medicare recipients is among those 95 years and over, with females showing a greater increase than males. About one in 20 of institutionalized or community-living elderly between 65 and 74 needs assistance in walking, but 75% of institutionalized and 25% of community-living elderly 85 years and older need that kind of assistance. Indeed, 70% of those 85 years and over need assistance in performing normal daily activities. Hospitalization is always a danger to the elderly, and among those 65 to 74, there are 306 hospital stays per 1000 population, increasing to 507 per 1000 for those 85 years and over.

Various parameters are employed to measure assistance need (Table 6-9), impairment (Table 6-10) and disability. There are no recent studies which can be used to estimate the level of impairment and disability among the elderly, particularly those 85 years old and over. Two studies, which did not look at persons over the age of 84, found disability levels of up to 50%, depending on the category studied.[28,29]

An evaluation of the Survey of Income and Education (SIE) of the Census Bureau reported 28 million people at that time in physical, emotional, or mental problems that limited their ability to pursue activities or daily living (ADL) consistent with their age. There were 2.3 million severely dependent persons in that group who were very restricted in ADL and in need of help to leave their home. Of those, 18% lived alone which was more than double the number of unimpaired people living alone at that time.[30]

The severely dependent persons represented 1.1% of the total U.S. population and their families represented 3.4% of all families. Among the severely dependent, the disability prevalence rate for persons 65 years and over is ten times that of those 18 to 64, and 25 times more than that of those under 18. Females over 65 constitute one-third of all severely dependent people, compared with older men who made up only one-sixth of the total. The leading causes of dependency among elderly are

Table 6-9 Methods of Measuring Assistance Need[26]

Scales & Measures to Help Needs	Indicators
Katz Activities of Daily Living (ADL) Scale	• Eating; Continence; Transferring; Toileting; Dressing; Bathing
Mobility	• Assistance in Walking • Help in Going Outside
Instrumental Household Activities of Daily Living (IADL)	• Meal Preparation • Managing Money • Household Chores (e.g., yard work) • Shopping
Health Services Administration	• Administering Medications • Changing Bandages • Administering Physical Therapy

Table 6-10 Impairment Scale

IMPAIRMENT LEVEL	SOCIAL, ECONOMIC, MENTAL, PHYSICAL AND ACTIVITIES OF DAILY LIVING
Unimpaired	Good to excellent in all 5 areas
Slightly Impaired	Good to excellent in 4 areas
Mildly Impaired	Mildly impaired in 1 and severely or completely impaired in another.
Moderately Impaired	Mildly or moderately in 3, or mildly or moderately impaired in 2 and severely or completely impaired in another.
Generally Impaired	Mildly or moderately impaired in 4.
Greatly Impaired	Mildly to moderately impaired in 3 and severely or completely in another.
Very greatly Impaired	Mildly to moderately impaired in 4 and severely or completely in the other; or severely or completely in 2 or more.

Adapted from Older Americans Rating Scale, Duke University Center for the Study of Aging & Human Development and Administration on Aging heart problems, arthritis, respiratory disorders, vision problems and hearing disorders.[31] Mental retardation and speech impairment are significant among those under 25, and orthopedic handicaps peak in the 18 to 24 year old group. Dependency increases with age for persons reporting hearing impairments, blindness, spine or back problems, and, particularly, cardiac problems. Thirty-seven percent of males over 65 and 42% of females in that age group were unable to work.

The Veterans Administration has estimated that about 2.7% of the non-institutionalized population is dependent, compared to 7.4% of those 65 to 74 and 22.1% of those 75 and over.[25,26] About 8.5% of those 75 and over have reported a dependency in their personal care needs, which is the most important indicator of probable institutionalization. Still others[32] have estimated that approximately 4.6 million community-living persons 65 and over are limited in activities of daily living (ADL) or instrumental household activities of daily living (IADL). The National Long Term Care Survey predicts that between now and the year 2040, this number may double, triple or even quadruple, depending on the category (unmarried, male, female, etc.). The largest absolute and relative increases are seen and will continue to be seen for unmarried females over the age of 85.

Current data suggest that disability increases in the same proportion as aging.[33] Furthermore, diseases that decrease function in the elderly will probably increase in the future.[34] Growing dependency of elderly patients has already been observed. Yet, disability does not seem to be the determinant for nursing home placement, since there are twice as many equally disabled elderly living in the community with only informal assistance from their families as there are residing in nursing homes.[35] The elderly impaired are depicted in Table 6-11, and the primary care sites of elderly are listed in Table 6-12.

National data on the utilization of home health services reveal a substantial growth. Visits per user, total number of visits, and visits per 1,000 Medicare enrollees rose from 17 per 1,000 in 1974 to 46 per 1,000 enrolles in 1983.[37] During the 20 year period between 1967 and 1987, the number of Medicare certified home health agencies rose from 1,753 to 5,877.[38] Expenditures by Medicare on home health care doubled between 1980 and 1983, from $ 772 million to $1.5 billion, growing at an annual rate of approximately 34 percent.[35] By 1985, it had already become a $9 billion industry.[40]

It is estimated that about 5 million chronically ill community living elderly, 20 percent of all aged living in the United States, are in need of at least minimal assistance to perform their activities of daily living.[41] By the year 2000, over 15 million older persons will suffer at least one chronic illness that will limit their functioning, a 50 percent increase over 1980 estimates.[42] The demand for more formal home care services is bound to intensify. This is confirmed by the fact that in fiscal year 1985, Medicare paid about $ 1.7 billion for HHC services, more than six times the amount spent in 1976.[41] Medicare's prospective payment system of DRGs requiring hospitals to discharge patients at an earlier stage of convalescence places additional stress on post-hospital services.[43]

ADDITIONAL FACTS ON HOME HEALTH CARE

Eighty percent of the 7.1 million elderly needing long term care and assistance with activities of daily living reside in the community, either at home or some other segment of the long term care system.[44] Almost 75% of elderly unable to pursue one or more activities of daily living rely almost

Table 6-11 The Impaired Elderly[36]

	Percent	Number (million)
Impaired elderly	19	5
Of those, severely impaired	20	1.6
Impaired elderly living alone	33	1.7
Of those, severely impaired	19	0.32
Impaired needing equipment	36	1.8
Incontinence problems	24	1.2

Table 6-12 Long Term Care Sites[36]

Place of Care	Number of Elderly
Nursing Home	1.3*
Assisted Living	0.75
Home Care	
- High Tech	0.25
- Low Tech	4-6

*Estimates in million

exclusively on families and volunteers for support, which enables them to remain at home.[45,46] Others are cared for via home health agencies (HHA).

HHC includes preventive, supportive, therapeutic or rehabilitative services, supportive social services, respite care and adult day care.[47] These definitions apply mostly to "organized and structured" HHC services, which, incidentally may be extended in 1993 to elderly Medicaid patients under OBRA 1990 at each individual state's discretion. This would mean that OBRA regulations, including those that demand much more intensive pharmacy services, would be applicable to this sector. The need for HHC is increasing, as the number of elderly increases and, proportionally, the number of nursing home beds decreases. Importantly, elderly want to stay at home. There are currently over 9,000 HHC agencies, certified by Medicare to provide services, including medications, parenterals nutritional supplements, HHC products such as durable medical equipment, incontinence and ostomy supplies. It is a market that will soon reach approximately $2 billion/year.[48] If the HHC agency is accredited by JCAHO, standards demand that pharmacists must assume responsibility for the continual monitoring of home care patients.[52] The total expenditures for HHC are shown in Table 6-13.

One must realize, though, that these numbers apply to a relatively small number of HHC patients, likely those qualifying for 90-day post-hospital skilled care. For those, some records may be available, but as has been shown repeatedly, records on drug use are poor and for non-prescription drug use are often non-existent. The vast majority of elderly is cared for at home by family caregivers, not by personnel from HHC agencies. No structure has been developed for this system, where elderly receive their drugs most likely from a community pharmacy.

Average patient visits/week are on the rise. Not-for-profit (VNA) agencies still make the most visits/week, at an average of 527 visits/week per agency. The average for all agencies was 380, up 1.6% from 1991, a very significant slowing of the rate of increase demonstrated in prior years. Home health aides made the most visits, followed by registered nurses, physical therapists, and licenses practical nurses. Others making home visits included occupational therapists, speech pathologists, respiratory therapists, social workers, dietitians, and still others. Most patients required two or three visits per week and only 3.7% required 24-hr care. Almost three-quarter of all patients received care for more than 30 days.

In 1992, the gender ratio of HHC patients was 61:39, female:male.[80] The demographics of HHC patients based upon age in 1992 were pediatric, 5%, adults, 26%, and geriatric, 69%. Over half (53%) of all home care patients in 1992 were chronically ill, 20.5% were recovering from major surgery, 23% were incontinent, 8.6% were Alzheimer's patients, and 15.4% suffered from another type of dementia. Over 12% of all home care patients were within the last six months of their life.[80]

Major changes were seen in ancillary services offered in 1992. Slightly more than one-third of all home care agencies provided medications, a decrease of 44% from the year before. This is cause for concern, since among the most often used drugs for the elderly in the community (Table 6-14)

Table 6-13 Total National Health Expenditures for Home Health Care[47]

Year	Total ($)	Facility based HHA ($)	Non-Facility based HHA ($)
1970	154	11	143
1975	446	46	404
1980	1,494	147	1,347
1985	4,401	561	3,841
1986	4,719	859	4,182
1988	5,439	1,012	4,427

are those most often cited by the Food and Drug Administration as being the cause of adverse drug reactions, and monitoring of drug outcome is one of the principal means of detecting and overcoming adverse drug reactions. Major reductions were also seen in the provision of IV pumps and sets, medical supplies and hospital beds, which was especially true for proprietary agencies.

The most prevalent services offered were skilled nursing services (90.1%), personal care (83.6%) and home infusion therapy (70.5%), all of which have been the leading services since 1988. Government-owned agencies were more likely than other agencies to offer skilled nursing, personal, and home maintenance services. Hospital-owned agencies were less likely to offer unskilled nursing, cooking, or housekeeping services as well as home renal dialysis.

As has been the case, Medicare Part A covers home care services deemed medically necessary by a physician for Medicare patients who are confined to home (in Medicare terms) and require skilled or intermittent care. Medical equipment and supplies may be included in this coverage.[49]

Outpatient IV antibiotic therapy is a cost-effective modality to shorten hospital stay (or prevent hospitalization) and provide continued care to patients with infections. Tamper-proof pumps can deliver multiple antibiotics of independently timed regimens.[50] The development of computerized ambulatory infusion drug delivery pumps has enabled providers to treat patients previously considered ineligible for home IV antibiotic therapy.[51]

Still, home IV antibiotic therapy requires selection of patients who are medically and psychologically stable, are capable of being trained to administer IV medications, will not abuse the IV system, and have insurance coverage. Patients with conditions such as osteomyelitis, septic arthritis, pelvic inflammatory disease, endocarditis, and skin and soft tissue infections are appropriate candidates. Individual patients have received IV therapy at home for as long as three years and more.[52]

Table 6-14 The 20 Most Often Prescribed Drug Classes for Elderly

Rank	Therapeutic Class	Percent of Total Drug Used
1	Calcium Blockers	4.8
2	Digitalis preparations	4.2
3	Antiarthritics, systemic	4.1
4	Diuretics, other	4.0
5	ACE Inhibitors	3.3
6	Nitrites/Nitrates	3.0
7	Beta Blockers	2.9
8	Cephalosporins	2.8
9	Antispasmodics	2.6
10	Diabetes, Insulin	2.5
11	Diabetes, oral	2.4
12	K-Sparing Diuretics	2.3
13	Aspirin, APC, etc	2.1
14	Codeine & combinations	1.8
15	Antihypertensives	1.8
16	Xanthines	1.8
17	Potassium Supplements	1.6
18	Corticoids (oral)	1.5
19	Benzodiazepines	1.5
20	Diuretics, Thiazides	1.4

It is desirable to keep cancer patients at home whenever possible to maximize their physical comfort and well-being.[53] Indeed, changes in the health care system have made the patient's home the primary site of cancer care.[54,57] While it is possible to train family caregivers to administer IV chemotherapy,[55] it must be realized that there are multiple and complex needs of the patient that the family caregiver must address. The patient's pain and the management of that pain do impose a major burden on the caregiver: what to give, when to give, night duty, reminding, encouraging, keeping records, fear of addiction, and doing everything else.[54] There are also major caregiving roles not involved with drug interventions, including positioning/mobility, massage, use of ointments and lotions, cold and heat, being there (through touch), and talk and other distractions.[54]

The prevalence of congestive heart failure and its progressive degeneration course continue to generate pressure for alternative and more effective means of treatment. A confluence of factors (number of patients, costs, etc.) has lead to the development of an effective therapy that increases myocardial contractility and output and can be administered at home.[58]

Psychotropic drugs are often used for the patient at home and, often, people receiving these drugs do not have a diagnosed psychiatric disorder.[59] Home oxygen therapy is clearly beneficial for the chronically hypoxemic patient,[60] and severe pain due to malignancy can be treated at home with epidural morphine infusions.[61] Patients with psoriasis are also treated at home.[62] Recent reports indicated that malnourishment among elderly institutionalized and home care patient is common, despite the fact the total parenteral nutrition and enteral nutrition is often used.

Total parenteral nutrition (TPN) has been used for as long as 11 years for home care patients with Crohn's disease,[63] and its use demands experienced catheter insertion and management,[64] the need to address possible psychosocial problems of the patient [65] and, of course, the teaching of the patient and the family caregiver how to self-manage the administration of these agents.[66] Nevertheless, problems can and do arise. In patients receiving long-term home parenteral nutrition, superior vena caval obstruction may occur.[67] In one study, patients receiving home TPN for the short-bowel syndrome showed progressive bone loss, affecting mainly the cancellous bone.[68] Patients receiving home TPN can also develop a diffuse granulomatous interstitial pneumonitis secondary to calcium phosphate deposition.[69]

Home enteral nutrition can result in stabilization of nutritional indices[70] and is now used for malnourished patients, such as cancer patients[71] or when a TPN must be replaced because of problems.[67]

HOSPICE CARE FOR THE ELDERLY

As a specialized program of care, hospice care is characterized ideally by comprehensive, continuous 24-hr services by an interdisciplinary team of professionals, non-professionals and volunteers with central administration and physician direction for quality and supportive care of the dying and their families. Family caregivers spend most of their time giving emotional support tending to household tasks and provision of transportation. Giving emotional support is the most time-consuming and difficult task, imposing the highest burden.[73] Most hospices have focused primarily on terminal illness from malignant disease. They are intended to treat the physical, emotional, and mental symptoms of a hospice patient, rather than the terminal disease. The hospice concept promotes HHC so that patients can maintain their life at home. The interdisciplinary team, comprised of physicians, nurses, medical social workers, therapists, home health aides, nutritionists, pharmacists, clergy and volunteers, supervises and coordinates the plan of care of each individual patient and family. Continuity of care programs resemble hospice programs in philosophy. However, there are major differences in admission criteria: the program is not restricted to dying individuals; patients may live alone; they may receive active therapy with a focus on cure or remission; and they continue to receive their care, including pain management.[74] (See also Chapter 8.)

CONCLUSION

With the long-term care sector developing rapidly and the number of patients in need of long-term care increasing dramatically, accessibility to medical care at affordable prices is fast becoming impossible for many elderly.[75] Federal cost containment measure may heavily influence the number of elderly receiving long-term care in the community.

The elderly prefer not to be institutionalized at the onset of chronic disabilities[76] and the overwhelming preference of the elderly is to remain in their own home, above all, living independently.[77] There are increasing demands not necessarily for more services but for different ones such as HHC services. Questions are being raised about death and dying, mental competency and independent living, and the quality of life in the final years of life.[78] Different services such as HHC are called for because the use of health care services is a joint, interrelated function of need, predisposing (e.g., age-related) and enabling factors and the characteristics of an individual.

If a medical care model is to be applied to long-term care, then Donabedian's model for the medical care process might apply. This model utilizes assessments provided by the patient, the health care provider, and the nonprofessional caregivers (who now provide most of the personal care services in HHC).[79] Health status, determined by self-appraisal and physician appraisal of physical and mental well-being, differs from the "need" for health care services. The latter refers to the various regimens needed to restore the former. Community-based, alternate care systems could result in lower mortality rates, higher patient contentment, improved functioning and increased social activity.

REFERENCES

1. Bureau of Census Projections of the Population of the United States by Age, Sex, and Race: 1988 to 2080. Series P-25 Washington, DC, 1989.
2. Jackson S. Failing America's Caregivers: A Status Report on Women Who Care. Older Women's League, Washington, DC, 1989.
3. Soldo B, Manton KG. The graying of America: demographic challenges for socioeconomic planning. J Socio-Econ Planning Sci. 1985; 19:227.
4. Siegal JS, Taeuber CM. Demographic perspectives of the long-lived society. Daedalus. 1986; 115:72.
5. Spencer G. Projections of the Population of the United States by Age, Sex, and
6. Vital Statistics of the United States, 1987. Life Tables, Volume II, Section 6. National Center of Health Statistics, Washington, DC, 1988; and Statistical Bulletin, 1992, 73(3), Metropolitan Life Insurance Company, New York, NY.
7. Bureau of the Census. Current Population Reports, Special Studies, Series P-23, No. 59, May 1976; and Series P-25, No. 952, May 1984.
8. Selby P, Schechter M. Aging 2000. MTP Press Ltd, Boston, MA. 1982; 211-214 .
9. Hammerman J, Friedsam HH, Shore H. Management perspectives in long-term care facilities. In: Sherwood S,Ed. Long-term care: a handbook for researchers, planners, and providers. Spectrum Publications, Inc., New York. 1975; 179.
10. Social Security Administration Compilation of the Social Security Laws. Vol 1, Title 18, Section 1814 (1) (7) (c). Government Printing Office, Washington, DC, 1989.
11. Gilbert GH, Branch LG, Orav EJ. An operational definition of the homebound. HSR. 1992; 26(6):787-800.
12. Brody JA, Schneider EL. Diseases and disorders of aging: a hypothesis. J Chronic Dis. 1986; 11:871.
13. Krenz C, Larson EB, Buchner DM, et al. Characterizing patient dysfunction in Alzheimer's type dementia. Med Care. 1988; 26:453.
14. Harris T, Cook EF, Garrison R, et al. Body mass index and mortality among nonsmoking older persons: the Framingham heart study. J Am Med Assoc. 1988; 259:1520.
15. Thomas TN, Plymat KR, Blannin J, et al. Prevalence of urinary incontinence. Br Med J. 1980; 281:1243.
16. Meyers AR, Branch LG, Lederman RI. Temporary disability among independent living adults with major disabling conditions. Med Care. 1988; 26:499.
17. Caird FI, Kennedy RD. Epidemiology of heart disease in old age. In Caird FI, Dall LC, Kennedy RD, Eds. Cardiology in Old Age. Plenum Press, New York, 1976.
18. Elveback L, Lie JT. Combined high incidence of coronary artery disease and hypertension at autopsy in Olmstead County, Minnesota. 1950-1979; Circulation. 1984; 70:345.
19. Sklar M. Gastrointestinal diseases in aged. In Reichel W, Ed. Clinical Aspects of Aging. Williams & Wilkins, Baltimore, MD, 1983.
20. Gentry WD, Aronson MK, Blumenthal J, et al. Behavioral, cognitive and emotional considerations. J Am Coll Cardiol. 1987; 10 (Suppl A):38.
21. Ford AB, Folmar SJ, Salmon RB, et al. Health and function in the old and very old. J Am Geriatr Soc. 1988; 36:187.
22. Office of Technology Assessment. Technology and Aging in America. U.S. Government Printing Office, Washington, DC, 1985.
23. Fisher ML, Lamy PP. Special considerations in the use of antihypertensive agents in the elderly with coexisting disease. Geriatr Med Today. 1987; 6(11):47.
24. International Classification of Impairment, Disabilities and Handicap. A Manual of Classification Relating to the Consequence of Diseases. Geneva, World Health Organization, 1990.
25. US Congressional Budget Office. Long Term Care for the Elderly and Disabled. Washington, DC, Government Printing Office, 1977.
26. Veterans Administration. Caring for the Older Veteran, US Government Printing Office, Washington, DC, 1984.
27. Rosenwaike I. A demographic portrait of the oldest old. Milbank Memorial Fund Quarterly Health & Society, 1985; 63(2):187.
28. Branch LG, Jetter AM. The Framingham disability study: I. Social disability among the aging. Am J Publ Health. 1981; 71:1202.
29. Jetter AM, Branch, LG. The Framingham disability

study: II. Physical disability among the aging. Am J Publ Health. 1981; 71:1211.
30. Perlman R, Giele JZ. An unstable triad: Dependents' demands, family resources, community supports. In Family Home Care: Critical Issue for Services and Policies. Edited by Perlman, R. New York, The Haworth-Press, 1983.
31. Lamy PP. Prescribing for the Elderly. PSG Publ Co., Inc., Littleton, MA, 1980.
32. Menton KG, Saldo BJ. Dynamics of health changes in the oldest-old: new perspectives and evidence. Milbank Memorial Fund Quarterly/Health & Society. 1985; 63(2):206.
33. Menton KG, Hausner T. A multidimensional approach to case mix for home health services. Health Care Financing Rev. 1986; 7(4):33.
34. Schroeder SA. Clinical intensity versus cost containment: conflicting pressures on hospital care. Transactions & Studies of the College of Physicians of Philadelphia, Ser. 1990; 12(2):175.
35. Doty P. Dispelling some myths. A comparison of long-term care financing in the U.S. and other nations. Generations, 1990, (Spring):10.
36. Macken CI. A profile of functionally impaired elderly living in the community. Health Care Financing Rev, 1986, 7(4):33.
37. Leader S. AARP, Home Health Benefits under Medicare: a Working Paper. American Association of Retired Persons, Washington, DC, 1986.
38. National Association for Home Care. Basic Statistics on Home Care. National Association for Home Care, Washington, DC, 1987.
39. Doty P, Liu K, Weiner J. An overview of long term care. Health Care Financing Rev. 1985; 6:70.
40. Nassif JZ. There is still no place like home. Generations, 1986/87, 5:8.
41. U.S. Government Accounting Office . Medicare, Need to Strengthen Home Health Care Payment Controls and Address Unmet Needs. U.S. Government Printing Office, Washington, DC, 1986.
42. Spiegel A. Home Health Care, Second Edition. Rynd Communication, Owings Mills, MD, 1987.
43. U.S. Senate Special Committee on Aging. The Crisis of Home Health Care: Greater Need, Less Care. U.S. Government Printing Office, Washington, DC, 1986.
44. U.S. Senate Special Committee on Aging. Aging America: trends and Projections. LR 3377 (188), US Dept Health & Human Services, Washington, DC, 1988.
45. Lamy PP, Gondek K, Feinberg M, et al. The Family Caregiver: A report from the Maryland Caregiver Program. ElderCare News. 1991; 7(3):17.
46. Gondek K, Lamy PP. Boosting medication compliance: helping the caregiver take charge. Senior Patient. 1990; 2(5):52.
47. Office of National Cost Estimates. National health expenditures, 1988. Health Care Financing Rev. 1990; 11(4):1.
48. Lamy PP, Feinberg M. Why better pharmacy services are needed in residential care facilities. US Pharm. 1990; 15:72.
49. Balinsky W. Reimbursement for outpatient parenteral antibiotic therapy: update. Rev Infect Dis. 1991; 13 (Suppl 2):S193.
50. Brown RB, Sands M. Outpatient intravenous antibiotic therapy. Am Fam Physician. 1989; 40:157.
51. Williams DN, Gibson JA, Bosch D. Home intravenous therapy using a programmable infusion pump. Arch Intern Med. 1989; 149:1157.
52. Ryan D. High tech home care: a look at a success story. Military Med. 1992; 157:266.
53. Mahmood T, Rubin AD. Home-based intravenous therapy for oncology patients. New Jersey Med. 1992; 89(1):43.
54. Ferrell BR, Cohen MZ, Rhiner M, et al. Pain as a metaphor for illness. Part II. Family caregivers' management of pain. Oncol Nurs Form. 1991; 18:315.
55. Jayabose S, Escobedo V, Tugal O, et al. Home chemotherapy for children with cancer. Cancer. 1992; 69:574.
56. Colford JM Jr, Corelli RL, Ganz JW, et al. Home antibiotic therapy for streptococcal endocarditis: a call for a controlled trial. Am J Med. 1993; 14:111.
57. Beijnen JH. Home-based chemotherapy confronts pharmacists with stability and compatability problems. Phamaceut Weekbld. Sci Ed. 1992; 14:337.
58. Baptista RJ, Mitrano FP, Perri-LaFrancesca J. Home intermittent amrinone infusions in terminal congestive heart failure. DICP. 1989; 23:59.
59. Clarke DJ, Kelley S, Thinn K, et al. Psychotropic drugs an mental retardation: 1. Disabilities and the prescription of drugs for behavior and for epilepsy in three residential settings. J Ment Deficiency Res. 1990; 34 (Pt 5):385.
60. Herrick TW, Yeager H Jr. Home oxygen therapy. Am Fam Physician.1989; 39:157.
61. Ohlsson L, Rydberg T, Eden T, et al. Cancer pain relief by continuous administration of epidural morphine in a hospital setting an at home. Pain. 1992; 48:349.
62. Volden G, Bjornberg A, Tegner E, et al. Short-contact treatment at home with Micanol. Acta Dermato-Venereol. 1992; (Suppl) 172:20.
63. Galandiuk S, O'Neill M, McDonald P, et al. A century of home parenteral nutrition for Crohn's disease. Am J Surg. 1990; 159:540.
64. McIntyre AS, Gertner DJ, Wood S, et al. Long-term parenteral nutrition: problems with venous access. J Royal Soc Med. 1990; 83:371.
65. Hoffman KC. Psychosocial concerns of home nutrition therapy consumers. Nutr Clin Pract. 1989; 4(2):51.
66. Burnes JU. Preparing self-managing home parenteral consumers. Nutr Clin Pract. 1989; 4(2):67.
67. Beers TR, Burnes J, Fleming CR. Superior vena caval obstruction in patients with gut failure receiving home parenteral nutrition. J Parent Ent Nutr. 1990; 14:474.
68. Foldes J, Rimon B, Muggia-Sullam M, et al. Progressive bone loss during long-term home total parenteral nutrition. J Parent Ent Nutr. 1990; 14:139.
69. Knowles JB, Cusson G, Smith M, et al. Pulmonary disposition of calcium phosphate crystals as a complication of home total parenteral nutrition. J Parent Ent

Nutr. 1989; 13:209.
70. Campos AC, Butters M, Meguid MM. Home enteral nutrition via gastrostomy in advanced head and neck cancer patients. Head & Neck. 1990; 12(2):137.
71. Sami H, Saint-Aubert B, Szalowski AW, et al. Home enteral nutrition system: one patient, once daily ration of an "all-in-one" sterile and modular formula in a single container. J Parent Ent Nutr. 1990; 14:173.
72. McDonnell A. Quality hospice care, administration, organization, and models. National Health Publishing. Owings Mills, MD, 1984.
73. Carey PJ, Oberst MT, McCubbin MA, et al. Appraisal can caregiving burden in family members caring for patients receiving chemotherapy. Oncol Nurs Forum. 1991; 18:1341.
74. Coyle N. Continuity of care for the cancer patient with chronic pain. Cancer. 1989; 63(11 Suppl):2289.
75. Heinz J. The search for long term care solutions. Business & Health. 1984; 2(2):5.
76. Sussman MB. Social and Economic Supports and Family Environments for the Elderly. Final Report No. A-316103. Washington, DC, Administration on Aging, 1979.
77. Tissue T, McCoy JL. Incomes and living arrangements among poor and singles. Soc Security Bull. 1981; 44(4):3.
78. Moody HR. The complex choices of caring for the frail elderly. Business & Health. 1984; 2(2):17.
79. Soldo BJ, Manton KG. Health status and service needs of the oldest old: Current patterns and future trends. Milbank Memorial Fund Quarterly/Health & Society. 1985; 63(2):286.
80. Managed Care Digest, Long Term Care Edition, 1993, Marion Merrell Dow, Inc. Kansas City, MO. 1993.

7 Assisting Caregivers in Home Health Care Settings

Madeline Feinberg, Pharm.D.
Ilene H. Zuckerman, Pharm.D.

There are few, if any, reliable data available on drug use in home health care (HHC), even though drugs are the mainstay of disease management in community care settings. Drug use in HHC settings is probably similar to that found in skilled nursing facilities (SNF), as the HHC patient is similar to the SNF patient. However, the control of drugs in HHC is different and more difficult, since HHC does not use the drug distribution systems that are utilized in institutional settings. Because of the differences in drug distribution, additional measures for drug control and medication management are warranted. This chapter will focus on the chronic care patient in the home care setting. Possible pharmaceutical care interventions directed toward the formal caregiver system and the informal caregivers will be suggested.

THE HOME HEALTH CARE SETTING

Clinical pharmacy services in the HHC setting are underutilized due to a lack of clear cut reimbursement mechanisms, failure of health care providers to recognize the need for pharmacist expertise in drug therapy management, lack of established guidelines for provision of pharmacy-consulting services in the home care environment, and in many instances lack of awareness by pharmacists of HHC opportunities. Clinical pharmacy services include services separate from delivery of a drug product, medical equipment or supplies. The goal of clinical pharmacy services is to provide complete pharmaceutical care, with pharmacists assuming the responsibility for drug therapy outcomes. Services provided, for purposes of this chapter, will be considered analogous to consulting pharmacist responsibilities in the nursing home setting. Patients are found in a variety of HHC settings, e.g., living alone in their own home, living with family members, living in senior congregate housing units, or utilizing community services such as adult day care centers. Some of these patients receive structured skilled services through a licensed home health agency (HHA). Even more challenging will be the delivery of pharmaceutical care to the community-based, high risk patient not receiving structured medical supervision as in the HHC setting.

Whether the home environment can meet the needs of a given patient depends on a multitude of factors including the patient's ability to manage medications. Problems of medication management have been documented among patients seen by HHA, the most common problems being drug misuse, drug administration, unsupervised use of non-prescription medications, lack of understanding of the purpose and goal of drug therapy, and the use of multiple medications which may be contraindicated.[1,2,3] HHC patients obtain medications from community pharmacies and often there are a multitude of pharmacy providers. Patients or friends may select non-prescription medications, and a variety of "health-food" products which also may have pharmacological activity. The home environment may contain medications from other family members and for previous illnesses which may be administered to patients without the knowledge or consent of any health care provider. Inability to adhere to the prescribed regimen may go undetected by the formal caregiver systems (visiting nurse) or unreported by family caregivers.

The Patient

Patients may be classified into two major categories: the acute care patient and chronic care patient.[4,5] An acute care patient needs intensive support in the home following discharge from the hospital. Medications prescribed for the acute care patient might include parenteral antibiotics or chemotherapy, parenteral or enteral nutrition therapy, respiratory therapy or dialysis. Provision of therapies may include clinical pharmacy support services.

The chronic care patient is in need of careful drug monitoring services. It is the chronic care patient who requires long term supportive services at home. The majority of these chronic care patients are elderly with multiple diseases and reduced functional status. They probably will not require high technology support services, but will be maintained on multiple oral medications. Successful management of drug regimens may be the factor which enables these patients to remain in the community with a degree of independent function. It is particularly in this population that clinical pharmacy services must focus to maximize drug therapy and to decrease the opportunity for drug-related problems.

The Caregiver

More than 85% of care for disabled elderly is provided by families (or significant others) in the community. This care encompasses both medical and social services as well as assistance with activities of daily living (ADLs) and instrumental activities of daily living (IADLs).[6] (See also Chapter Six) Approximately 7 million frail elderly are cared for by families and friends[7] who provide an array of services and personal care.[8] In addition to families, informal care is also provided in the alternate care system (Table 7-1). Licensure in alternate care settings usually does not require personnel to be medically trained, although individual jurisdictions or facilities may offer a variety of health-related services supervised by a registered nurse in addition to residential and recreational services. In contrast, "formal" care describes those services provided by trained personnel which can be purchased by consumers from private or public agencies, such as a HHA.

Since informal caregivers provide the majority of care for impaired or frail adults, it is crucial that the health care providers translate and transmit information, skills and technology to the caregivers to assure that treatment interventions are successfully carried out.[9] In addition, it is crucial that the health care providers recognize that stresses of family caregiving may negatively impact on the physical and emotional well-being of caregivers, to the extent that the caregiver has been called "the hidden patient."[10] For example, caregivers of dementia patients have been shown to use more psychotropic drugs than non-caregiver controls,[11] have poorer physical health,[12] and resort to institutionalization when the burden of caring becomes too great.[8]

Table 7-1 Selected Alternate Care Systems[9]

Assisted living homes
Board and care homes
Foster care
Domiciliary care
Homes for adults
Sheltered housing

The Home Care Nurse

The most prevalent services offered by HHA are skilled nursing services. Medicare guidelines for agency certification delegate the drug monitoring function to nurses specifically. In addition to supervision of drug administration and patient educations, nurses are also required to "identify ineffective and contraindicated medications."[13]

"Politics" must be recognized as a potentially negative factor which may hamper the participation of pharmacists in medication management functions. Reluctance to utilize a consultant pharmacist to assist in this function may represent fear of loss of control or authority by the nurse. Or, it may represent lack of knowledge that this can be done and is allowed by existing regulation. Also, it may indicate a lack of awareness of the pharmacist's expertise in drug therapy management.

The Home Care Physician

Physician education should be a major focus of consulting pharmacist participation in medication management in the home. This occurs when pharmacists intervene to alter a drug regimen, or when nurses contact physicians to suggest a change in regimen. The interactions between pharmacists and physicians are critical in HHC, as patients frequently see multiple physicians. The pharmacist can serve as a key communication link between prescribers. In embracing the philosophy of pharmaceutical care the pharmacist assumes the responsibility for assuring that prescribers are aware of real and potential therapeutic problems.

A Case Study

Mrs. F. is a patient being followed by an urban, community-based HHA. She is a white, 81 year old, obese female receiving Medicaid-covered HHC services. Her problem list on admission to

HHC included toxic encephalopathy, old cerebral vascular accident, dysarthria, seizure disorder, disorientation/mental confusion, congestive heart failure, and indwelling urinary catheter. The patient had been discharged to HHC following hospitalization due to a phenobarbital overdose. Medications listed at the time of referral included phenytoin, phenobarbital, potassium and digoxin. The patient was described as ambulatory with assistance but unable to perform most activities of daily living. She resides with her daughter, and is cared for by a neighbor during the day while the daughter works. She is reportedly seen by two physicians.

Persistent questioning of the patient's daughter by the pharmacist revealed that in addition to medications noted on the admission record, the patient also takes sulfamethoxazole-trimethoprim, furosemide, chlordiazepoxide-amitriptyline, diazepam, levodopa-carbidopa, acetaminophen, chlorpheniramine, aluminum-magnesium antacid, several vitamin supplements purchased by the daughter "for mother's heart", products purchased in the health food store, and five topical preparations including two prescription corticosteroid creams, one non-prescription corticosteroid cream, an antifungal and an anti-infective cream. Medications are set out by the daughter in open vials arranged into morning, noon, evening, and night-time doses for the convenience of a neighbor-caregiver. Upon inspection, it was impossible to identify several tablets due to multiple manufacturers that were dispensed by multiple pharmacies frequented by the patient's daughter. At least one actual duplication of drug was noted in the morning bottle.

Mrs. F. is not atypical among the homebound elderly, although she represents a dramatic example of medication mismanagement and what can go wrong. If the regimen remains uncorrected, it is likely that a drug overdose will be administered again which may result in hospitalization. This case serves as a basis for the discussion of the scope of clinical pharmacy services which can be developed in the HHC setting.

PHARMACEUTICAL CARE IN THE HOME SETTING - THE LONG TERM CARE PRECEDENT

Since 1974, the federal government has required pharmacist-conducted drug regimen reviews of patients receiving skilled nursing services. In 1987, with the passage of nursing home reform legislation known as OBRA (Omnibus Budget Reconciliation Act) 1987, the emphasis of care has shifted to outcomes which focus on maintaining or improving the quality of life for residents living in nursing homes. Specifically, legislation mandates that residents only receive medications which are necessary to manage a specific medical problem, and that the nursing facility assures that each medication achieves the desired outcome.[13] This mandate has resulted in expanded responsibilities and opportunities for pharmacists in the long term care setting. Increased clinical duties and administrative functions include quality assurance and assessment activities, membership in multidisciplinary teams, research activities and educational roles.

Cost savings from the reduction in drug use in skilled nursing facilities have been estimated at $25 million annually. This does not include savings which might result from decreased hospitalization when drugs are used more appropriately, nor do these savings reflect the potential for improvement in quality of life achieved by optimization of drug therapy. Several studies have shown a decrease in hospitalizations due to identification of potentially adverse drug reactions by pharmacists and acceptance of pharmacists' recommendations by physicians in the skilled and intermediate care nursing facilities.[14,15] Since the passage of OBRA 1987, pharmacists continue to demonstrate significant reduction in the use of psychotropic drugs and documentation of positive patient outcomes.[16,17]

Among the population of HHC patients, it is believed that the prevalence of disease and drug use is similar to patterns seen in the long term care patient. Therefore, it is reasonable to extend the concepts and practice of clinical pharmacy services in the long term care institutional setting to the HHC setting and ultimately to the patient cared for at home by the family caregiver.

An Approach to Pharmaceutical Care

Appropriate drug utilization by HHC patients should be the responsibility of the pharmacist. Table 7-2 describes overall objectives of providing pharmaceutical care services in home care. Pharmacists who offer their expertise will assure positive outcomes to drug therapy in a variety of HHC settings, which include formal and informal caregiver systems. As an example of a formal caregiver system, pharmaceutical care services which may be provided to a HHA are described in this

Table 7-2 Objectives for Pharmaceutical Care in the HHC Setting

To increase patient compliance
To enhance effective and safe use of medications
To decrease drug related problems
To decrease admission or readmission to an institution

chapter. These services include tools and tasks that improve documentation of drug use and drug therapy outcomes, in-service education programs and drug information services. Pharmaceutical care interventions for informal caregivers are also discussed in Chapter 9.

INTERVENTIONS FOR FORMAL CAREGIVERS: THE HOME HEALTH AGENCY

Although home care services are coordinated through the HHA and approved by the patient's physician, the home remains mostly unsupervised and HHC patients have a high degree of independence with regard to medication management. Nursing visits are by definition "intermittent" and physician supervision may be less than once every 60 days, according to Medicare guidelines for patient eligibility for HHA services. Because patients and their family or neighbors have the major responsibility for patient care, problems with drug therapy may not be detected by agency providers.

Pharmacists can assist the HHA staff with documentation of drug therapy, drug regimen review and development of policies and procedures. Table 7-3 describes the scope of services that a pharmacist can provide to a HHA.

The Medication Record (Profile)

The pharmacist's professional domain includes accurate documentation of each patient's drug therapy and related information. In the case study above, on referral to the agency, the records of Mrs. F., were incomplete. Although the daughter carried a written record of her mother's medications, the list did not correlate with the patient's actual medication use. Such inaccuracies are the rule, rather than the exception in a home care referral. On admission to the HHA service, i.e., at the time of the initial home visit, a comprehensive medication record form should be completed. This form should serve as the patient's profile for inclusion in the patient's chart.

The medication record should include prescription and non-prescription medications being used, and all other "medications" in the home, including health food products which might have pharmacologic activity, and medications which might have been prescribed by other physicians or recommended by friends. Techniques for taking a drug history need to be learned by nurses and taught by the pharmacist.

In addition to medications and related products, the medication record form should indicate all physicians the patient may be seeing, all pharmacies where medications are purchased, and very importantly, the record form should indicate the patient's functional status such as physical impair-

Table 7-3 Scope of Pharmacist Services to a Home Care Agency

Provide drug information to staff, physicians, and patients
Review appropriateness of drug therapy
Monitor drug therapy
Make home visits
Maintain patient medication profiles
Identify drug-related problems
Participate in case conferences
Provide inservice education to nursing, home health aide staff, and other professional staff
Offer patient education to understand drug regimen, its purpose, recognize and report side effects to enhance compliance
Coordinate drug therapy, i.e., prescription and non-prescription drugs
Participate in the agency utilization review committee
Establish policy and procedures related to drugs and therapeutics

ment, mental status, sensory impairments and living arrangement. All factors which could impinge on the outcome of drug therapy need to be noted on the medication record form. Wherever possible, a check-off format is best for convenience of both nurse and pharmacist. A simplified medication record should be given to all patients for their own use.

Drug Regimen Reviews

Instead of a monthly or periodic regimen review, some pharmacists have found it more practical to perform an intensive medication review on all incoming patients following the initial home visit, and then limit their reviews to selected problems found by the nurse, physician, caregiver, or patient. The patient receiving drug therapy should be monitored using pharmacokinetic parameters. In an unpublished study of prescribing patterns of renally eliminated drugs in a HHC population, dosage recommendation changes were accepted more frequently when the pharmacist directly contacted the physician compared to instances when the pharmacist left the recommendation up to the HHC nurse to follow-up (73% versus 26%, Chi Square analysis, $p = 0.001$).[18]

Staff Education

Regularly scheduled inservice programs for agency staff should be initiated and tailored to meet needs of all agency providers, not just nursing staff. Nursing needs will differ from needs of home health aides, other consultant providers (speech therapists, occupational and physical therapists, social workers, nutritionists, clergymen), yet all staff should be notified of pharmacy inservices by pharmacist and invited to participate.

Suggested topics for inservice programs are listed in Table 7-4. Topics dealing with drug therapy may include assessment of therapeutic outcome of drug regimens, identification of side effects, drug/nutrient interactions and compliance. Prevention and wellness topics should not be overlooked since a goal of HHC is to assist patients in achieving independence within limits of disease or functional status. Topics on skin care, nutrition, home diagnostics, and selection of OTC products, for example, can be presented to nursing staff who must prepare for discharge from HHA care.

Policies and Procedures

Policy and procedure manuals should be carefully written with input by pharmacists, as this will represent the standard of practice for pharmacist consultants. Using the existing format of agency policy and procedures, the pharmacist should identify consultant's responsibilities and be certain to include how staff will interact to achieve outcomes.

Table 7-4 Suggested Inservice Topics in the Home Care Setting

- Drug therapy management
  - drug categories
  - drug protocols
  - guidelines for monitoring adverse effects
  - drug/drug, drug/food, drug/disease interactions
  - nutritional needs altered by drugs
- Dosage forms
- Drug administration techniques
- Medication histories
- Patient education techniques
- Medication compliance

Case Conferences

HHA staff may hold regularly scheduled case conferences. HHC pharmacists can and should use the case conference to present patients whose medication management problems require a well-coordinated team approach. In Mrs. F.'s case, a multidisciplinary approach was needed to support proper medication-taking behavior by the patient and proper supervision by caregivers.

Drug Information

Drug information should be a service which heads the list of clinical services, because it is a need most readily identified by HHA nurses. (See also Chapter 5.) Community public health nurses, responding to a survey regarding drug-related needs have indicated that questions regarding medications arise often during the course of their practice. Of these questions, the overwhelming majority relate to possible side effects of medications, indications for use of a drug, and cost of medications. The major information resource for nurses was reported to be the Physicians' Desk Reference. Nurses, recognizing the inadequacy of this resource, identified the need for solving individual patient medication problems as a priority need.[19]

Many hospitals offer drug information services which can be used by health care providers in the community. However, this is merely an informational service, and little assistance is given with regard to medication use in a particular patient. In addition to providing drug information to HHA staff, the consultant pharmacist needs to maintain up-to-date resource materials at the HHA office and should take responsibility for selecting materials to be kept on the pharmacy resource shelf.

Unique approaches can also be developed for the HHC setting to facilitate exchange of information. For example, pharmacists reviewing medication profiles have developed drug monitoring guidelines for most commonly prescribed medications. These guidelines, which may include indications for drug use, side effects and special precautions, are recorded on the profiles by pharmacists. In addition to drug-monitoring guidelines, other pharmacists have developed laboratory test recommendations and dietary precautions, all in the form of a notebook to be carried around by the visiting nurse. Patient information materials about specific drugs, such as the USP Dispensing Information leaflets for patients can be provided by nurses. They, in turn, can distribute these written materials in conjunction with verbal information to patients during home visits.

Reimbursement For Consultant Pharmacy Services To HHA

Although there is little precedent in the literature describing clinical consultative services to HHA by pharmacists, a few do exist.[2,20,21,22,23] There is a trend toward the use of consulting pharmacists by HHA. In 1992, HHA used an average of 3.1 consulting pharmacists per agency, up 35% from 1991.[24] Thus, the opportunity for development of practice sites is possible, and the creative, highly motivated pharmacist can offer expertise to HHA and will be paid for these services. The mechanism for reimbursement for consultative pharmacy services is in place. However, HHA administrators will need to be educated and pharmacists will need to demonstrate the advantages of their participation in the delivery of quality patient care.

Medicare-covered HHC services do not include direct payment for pharmacy services. However, Medicare will reimburse a HHA for pharmacist consultation services just as the agency is reimbursed for services of medical, nutritional and psychological consultants, as well as nursing specialists and members of the clergy.

Since the drug-monitoring function is considered a skilled nursing function, the consulting pharmacist may be in a unique position to assist the nurse to perform this mandated function. Expenses incurred by an agency for its consultants represents an indirect cost of furnishing a covered service; as such, the agency will receive reimbursement for these costs.

When calculating a fee for services, the pharmacist will need to consider time spent with HHA personnel and patients, time spent reviewing drug regimens, time spent on home visits, time spent preparing and delivering inservice programs, travel and administrative expenses. The scope of services provided and HHA caseload will be the major factors in establishing charges to the agency.

INTERVENTIONS FOR INFORMAL CAREGIVERS

Caregiver research has suggested several interventions which may reduce caregiver burden and facilitate the caregiving role. Table 7-5 lists educational and supportive services identified by caregivers[25] that can and should be offered by pharmacists to enable caregivers to meet both the needs of the patient and family caregivers. There is little research that documents specific needs of those working in the alternate care setting. However, at a conference of alternate care system providers in Maryland, critical issues identified by participants included the need for help with medication management, since the key to independent living may be appropriately managed drug therapy.[9] Specific problems in medication management for patients at home have been described (Table 7-6). One could readily

Table 7-5 Educational and Supportive Needs of the Informal Caregiver

Information about the disease state and medications
Skills for communicating with medical providers
Guidance in evaluating options for treatment or services
Information about drug therapy and referral to community support services

Table 7-6 Medication-Related Problems Identified Among HHC Patients

Problem	Examples and Consequences
Improper use/compliance	Discontinued medication. Changed dose. Altered medication schedule. Shared others' medication.
Inadequate information	Unable to name medication or dose or reason for use. Confusion about pre and post hospitalization medications.
Possible adverse effect	Patient perceived problem but no follow up
Unsupervised OTC use	OTC use not documented in patient's medical record.
Inability to swallow	Crushing, breaking, dissolving medication enteric coated or extended release dosage forms
Mixing incompatible drugs	Misuse of enteral feeding tubes for medication administration

speculate that a community pharmacist using patient profiles would easily identify Mrs. F.'s inappropriate use of medications, perhaps saving the pain and anguish involved in the hospitalization of this patient, in addition to the costs involved.

Home Visits

Pharmacists should anticipate an occasional need for a home visit and might establish those conditions when such a home visit would be indicated. Home visits allow the pharmacist to obtain a complete drug history, assess compliance and assess the home situation. With certain patients, such as Mrs. F., home visits are essential to improve medication management, as well as for patient and caregiver education.

Home visits are time-consuming and direct reimbursement for home visits by pharmacists is not easily obtainable through Medicare and other third party payers. However, pharmacists should charge their patients for at-home medication reviews, and should not provide the service "for free". Pharmacists have been successful at providing home visits.[26]

Compliance Packaging

The HHC setting may require innovative packaging to facilitate compliance, auditing, accountability, safety and ultimately serve as a source of patient information.[12] Traditional medication vials will not work for some patients and clearly Mrs. F. is one example. Once a vial is opened, patients may never close the vial again and caregivers report that they often find more medication on the floor than in prescription bottles. When pharmacists identify patients unable to properly self-administer medications from the prescription vial, they need to be prepared to suggest alternate systems. Occasionally patients can manipulate the reusable daily, weekly or monthly plastic dispensers, and for these patients, such a system may be more convenient than keeping track of multiple containers. These reusable containers are relatively inexpensive, represent a one-time purchase and are available in most pharmacies. But it is patients such as Mrs. F. who need a more structured, controllable dispensing system. Today's state of the art system includes the use of multiple dose medication cards, also called bingo cards which dispense a week or a month supply of medications. Cards are organized by the time of the day, and each blister is labeled with the name and strength of the medication, lot number and description of tablet or capsule. More sophisticated systems permit the patient or caregiver to detach the appropriate blister for convenience when leaving the home. The United States Pharmacopoeial guidelines for multiple dose packaging permits pharmacists to evaluate the variety of multiple fill packaging systems now available for the HHC market.[27] Pharmacists should check with their respective State Boards of Pharmacy to determine if there are regulations which apply to use of these systems. Multiple dose packages can be customized for the visually impaired patient.

Pharmacists who provide clinical services to HHC patients should be familiar with community pharmacies that specialize in compliance packaging systems. If none exist, the HHC pharmacist may identify a community practitioner who would be willing to invest in a compliance system.

The use of medication compliance systems is particularly helpful to caregivers who work in the alternate care system. Although most states prohibit medication administration by unlicensed personnel, staff assumes responsibility to "supervise" medications for their residents which led to the identification of multiple medication related problems by the U.S. Congress and the General Accounting Administration.[28] It is anticipated that the Department of Health and Human Services will develop regulations and set minimum standards for medication use in residential care facilities. Pharmacists, however, should not wait for executive mandate to deliver minimum standards, but rather should anticipate caregiver needs, not just for medication administration, but for medication monitoring.

In addition to the provision of dispensing systems to enhance compliance and the accompanying recordkeeping requirements (e.g., medication-administration records), pharmacists should develop methods to teach caregivers to observe and monitor medication effects and to report findings to other health care providers responsible for drug therapy outcome. These educational and training efforts should be combined with the provision of compliance packaging systems, and the commitment for ongoing education and training must be assumed, particularly since staff turnover is high in the residential care setting.

Community Outreach

Participation in community service programs heightens the visibility and enhances the credibility of professionals, in addition to showing a willingness to work with other health care providers in the community. Pharmacists should consider presenting information on medication usage through community programs such as Elder-Health[a] or Elder-Care.[b] These programs often lead to invitations to speak about medication management to provider groups such as HHA personnel, homemaker staff, physical therapy or recreational therapy associations. All providers including home health aides, homemakers and chore service personnel should be trained in techniques of observation, such as changes in patient status, proper storage of medications, compliance behaviors by caregiver and patients, and the need to train nonprofessionals to observe and to report their observations. Their recommendations or suggestions for improved management of medication problems should be solicited because they tend to see patients

[a] Elder-Health, University of Maryland School of Pharmacy, Baltimore, Maryland.

[b] Elder-Care® Parke-Davis, Division of Warner-Lambert Company, Morris Plains, New Jersey.

Table 7-7 Pharmacist Interventions to Assist Informal Caregivers

Medication Management Skills
- Treatment goals and desired outcomes
- When to expect results
- How to assess effect of drug therapy
- When to communicate with provider
- What information to bring to provider
- Techniques for medication administration

Community Resources
- Accessing aging, respite, and other social services
- Follow up by pharmacist to assure caregiver has accessed system

Community Education
- Disease management for caregivers and patient advocacy groups
- Accident and poison prevention programs

Caregiver Well-Being
- Warning signs of caregiver burnout (e.g., alcohol or substance abuse, insomnia, social isolation, verbal or physical abuse of patient, weight loss)
- Physician or social service agency referral

for longer periods as they give personal care.[2] Table 7 - 7 summarizes information that pharmacists can teach informal caregivers to improve drug therapy outcomes.

Community services for HHC patients, especially the elderly and handicapped, are extensive and likely to become more so. Adult day care centers, nutrition sites, senior centers, housing units, domiciliary care units, community health clinics and recreation programs are among the services offered where medication management can be a problem for the elderly.

Pharmacists are the most accessible health care resource in the community. As the need for effective medication management increases in HHC settings, pharmacists should retain the ability to dispense the pharmaceutical product and provide comprehensive pharmaceutical care services that accompany the delivery of that product for its most optimal outcome.

REFERENCES

1. Kitt D. Pharmaceutical services for a visiting nurse home health service. Am J Hosp Pharm. 1984; 40:1542-1544.
2. Zuckerman IH, Feinberg M, Kerr RA, Fedder DO, Lamy PP. Consultant pharmacy services to a home health care agency. The Consultant Pharmacist. 1986; 1:123-128.
3. Solomon DK, et. al. Pharmaceutical services to improve drug therapy for home health care patients. Am J Hosp Pharm. 1978; 35:55-557.
4. Burke GC, Doren MJ. Home care: an industry on the horizon. Business and Health. 1984; 12:8-12.
5. Anonymous. Toward a national home care policy. A blueprint for action. A report presented by the National Association for Home Care, Washington, DC., January 1985.
6. Brody EM. The family at risk. In: Light E and Lebowitz BD, eds. Alzheimer's Disease Treatment and Family Stress. Directions for Research. New York: Hemisphere Publishing Corp. 1990; 3.
7. Anonymous. A National Survey of Caregivers: Working Caregivers Report. Washington, DC., American Association of Retired Persons, 1989.
8. Council on Scientific Affairs, American Medical Association: Physicians and family caregivers. A model for partnership. J Am Med Assoc. 1993; 269:1282.
9. The Maryland Alternate Care System Working Group. The alternate care system: problems, needs and care of the elderly. Elder Care News. 1988; 4(4):25-32.
10. Fengler A, Goodrich N. Wives of elderly disabled men; the hidden patients. Gerontologist. 1979; 19:175.
11. Clipp EC, George LK. Psychotropic drug use among caregivers of patients with dementia. J Am Geriatr Soc. 1990; 38:227.
12. Kiecolt-Glaser KJ, Dura JR, Speicher CE, Trask OJ, et al. Spousal caregivers of dementia victims: longitudinal changes in immunity and health. Psychosomatic Med. 1991; 53:345.
13. Health Care Finance Administration, Department Health and Human Services: Medicare and Medicaid Programs; Final Rule 42 CFR Parts, 442 et al., September 26, 1991. Doc.#869-017-00159-7, Govt Printing Office, WashingtonDC.
14. Kidder SW. The cost benefit of drug reviews in long-term care facilities. Am Pharmacy 1982; 22:63.
15. Miller SW, Marshall LL, Preston MW. Impact of pharmacist-conducted drug regimen review on drug use in an intermediate care facility. Consult Pharm. 1991; 6:317.
16. Hirshfield JS. Positive patient outcomes from interdisciplinary assessments of psychoactive drug use. Consult Pharm. 1993; 8:532-4.
17. Neel AB, Pittman JC, Marasco RA, Trimmer BK. Psychoactive drug use in Georgia nursing homes: effects of aggressive intervention. Consult Pharm. 1993; 8:245.
18. Fields C, McPherson ML. personal communication, 1993.
19. White SJ, Goodwin HN. Pharmacist-nurse liaison services. Am J Hosp Pharm. 1974; 31:1063-1065.
20. Eastman PF. Pharmaceutical services for home health agencies. J Am Pharm Assoc. 1971; 11:391-394.
21. Barker D. Clinical pharmacy services in the hospital based home care program. Contemp Pharm Pract. 1980; 3:239-242.
22. Jinks MJ. Pharmacy consulting services to agencies serving elderly clients. Am J Hosp Pharm. 1983; 40:1542-1544.
23. Kitt D. Pharmaceutical services for a visiting nurse home health service. Am J Hosp Pharm. 1984; 41:728-730.
24. Anonymous. Home care pharmacy. Marion Merrell Dow Manage Care Digest - Long Term Care Edition. Kansas City, MO: Marion Merrell Dow, Inc., 1993; 41.
25. Matthis EJ. Family caregivers want education for their caregiving roles. Home Healthcare Nurse. 1992; 10:19.
26. Meade V. Conducting at-home medication reviews. Am Pharm. 1992; NS32:37-39.
27. Board of Trustees, Committee of Revision, United States Pharmacopoeial Convention: Customized patient medication packages. In United States Pharmacopoeia, XXII revision. Rockville, MD: United States Pharmacopoeial Convention, Inc., 1990;1574.
28. Gore, MJ. Knowing when to listen: how to intervene in residential-care settings. Consult Pharm. 1992; 7:711.
29. Cooper JW, Griffin DL, Francisco GE, Francis WR. Home health care: drug-related problems detected by consultant pharmacist participation. Hosp Formulary. 1985; 20-643.
30. McPherson ML. Medicating home health patients. Considerations for the caregiver. Caring. 1990; 9:38.

8 Hospice Pharmacy Practice

Mary Lynn McPherson, Pharm.D., BCPS

In medieval times, the word "hospice" designated a place of shelter for travelers on a difficult journey. In 1967, St. Christopher's Hospice was founded by Dame Cicely Saunders in Sydenham, England, to provide care for dying patients. St. Christopher's has become a model for modern hospice care throughout the world, demonstrating that patients can die pain-free and with dignity. The first hospice in the United States was established in 1974 in Connecticut. Today there are over 1700 hospices in the United States.[1]

The hospice concept of care encompasses several unique features designed to address the challenging and difficult needs of the patient with a life expectancy of six months or less. In hospice, both the patient and the family constitute the unit of care. In caring for the patient, the goal is enhanced quality of life. Therefore, when cure is no longer a reasonable goal, the goals of care are to make the patient as comfortable as possible and provide the patient and family members with the physical, social, psychological and spiritual support they need.[2]

While the first model of hospice care (in England) was an inpatient palliative care facility, this is not characteristic of hospice care in the United States. The vast majority of hospice care in this country is carried out in the patient's home. The hospice program itself may be hospital or community based, as a part of a home health care (HHC) program, or a stand-alone hospice program. Inpatient hospice facilities are also available, but they are usually reserved for patients with symptoms that have become unmanageable at home, or for patient care when the family or caregivers need a respite. When the symptom is controlled, or after a short respite period, the goal is to move the patient home, if possible.

PHILOSOPHY OF HOSPICE CARE

Hospice care provides compassionate care for those with life-limiting illnesses. Hospice care recognizes that dying is an integral part of living. In a hospice program the dying individual has rights that are respected, namely,

- The right to enjoy a maximum quality of life;
- The right to die with dignity, as he/she perceives dignity;
- The right to participate actively in the management of the remaining life span, dying, and the event of death; and
- The right to remain a viable family member in the environment of choice.

The needs of the patient and family members are considered on an individual basis. The supportive needs of the family do not end with the death of the individual; bereavement support continues for a year or more as needed.

The objectives of hospice care are to maintain maximal life function through provision of a interdisciplinary team approach to provide:

- Good general physical care and relief of pain without great mental or physical incapacitation;
- Ongoing emotional support of the individual and his/her family caregivers;
- Support of the patient's participation as an active family member by enabling them the opportunity to remain at home, and by offering services to accommodate family relationships;
- Assistance to the patient and the family in working through the grieving process, and other problems involved in serious illness and changes in lifestyle;
- Assistance to the family in a healthy resolution of bereavement after death of the patient; and
- Initiation and maintenance of an ongoing community education program regarding hospice philosophy and its implementation.

Levels of Care

There are four levels of hospice care.

- Routine Home Care. Care provided in the residential setting, usually a patient's home or a long term care facility. Hospice services are provided on an intermittent basis according to the needs identified in the plan of care. The interdisciplinary team determines the frequency and intensity of services.
- Short-term Acute Inpatient Care. Care provided in a hospital or skilled nursing facility when a patient's symptoms cannot be managed in the residential setting with the routine home care level of care. Hospice inpatient services are generally provided under a contractual arrangement with a hospital or skilled nursing facility.
- Respite Inpatient Care. Care provided to the patient in a hospital or skilled facility to relieve the patient's primary caregiver and family members for a short period, usually up to five days.
- Continuous Care. Care provided in a residential setting on a continuous basis when the patient is in a crisis, and symptoms cannot be managed with routine home care. This level of care is usually initiated during a crisis to prevent transfer to an inpatient setting.

PATIENT ACCEPTANCE CRITERIA

In general, there are several criteria that must be met in order for a patient to be accepted into hospice care. Firstly, all curative treatment options should have been exercised. Secondly, the patient should be aware of the diagnosis and prognosis and should elect non-curative medical and supportive care for the terminal illness. Thirdly, the referring physician should believe that the patient has a prognosis of less than six months.

Most referrals to hospice care are for terminally ill cancer patients. While there are other diagnoses that may have a terminal prognosis, cancer seems more clear cut in establishing that all practical modalities of treatment have been tried and failed, and that the patient has approximately six months to live.[3] Other diagnoses that are amenable to hospice care include patients with AIDS, Alzheimer's disease, end-stage renal disease, or end-stage chronic obstructive pulmonary disease.[3]

Medicare Eligibility Criteria

In 1983, hospice care became a reimbursable benefit under Medicare.[1] For patients to receive the Medicare hospice benefit, they must receive care from a Medicare-certified hospice program. In return they receive physician, nursing, psychosocial, and spiritual services, as well as medications, medical appliances, nutrition and bereavement counseling. Eligibility requirements and conditions of coverage require that:[1]

- a physician must certify a short prognosis (months not years);
- full reimbursement for inpatient care be limited to no more than 20% of all hospice patient days;
- when patients elect the hospice benefit, they waive rights to regular Medicare benefits; and
- a written care plan is established for the patient and is reviewed regularly.

THE HOSPICE TEAM

If the patient is receiving care under the Medicare hospice benefit from a Medicare-certified hospice program, the hospice team consists of a physician, nurse, social worker, volunteers and clergy. The hospice medical director may serve as a referral source for patients to the program, provide administrative services, and/or serve as a clinician on the team. The nurse functions as the case coordinator, and provides much of the direct patient care. The social worker assesses the patient and family's financial and social situation, and evaluates their understanding of the patient's illness and impending death. Volunteers may be involved in direct patient contact, such as reading or visiting with patients, or providing relief for the caregiver. Volunteers may run errands, participate in bereavement follow up, or provide a professional service (e.g., financial counseling, legal services). Members of the clergy provide spiritual support to the patient, family, and often the hospice team as well. In addition to these hospice team members, there are other disciplines that may contribute to the patient's care, such as nutritionists, physical and occupational therapists, respiratory therapists, home health aides, and pharmacists.

The role the pharmacist plays in hospice care, and the extent to which he or she is involved may vary from hospice to hospice. In some cases, the pharmacist may serve as a consultant, and primarily fulfill clinical responsibilities. In other situations, the hospice pharmacist may be a primary medication supplier, yet still be available for consultation. In this day of pharmaceutical care, it is difficult to distinguish separate roles for the pharmacist, therefore it is not possible to say that a hospice pharmacist is either clinical or distributive, since the roles may overlap. For purposes of this discussion, however, hospice pharmacist responsibilities have been divided into clinical, distributive, administrative, and research.

CLINICAL RESPONSIBILITIES

Participation on the Team

The interdisciplinary team approach is an important part of the philosophy of hospice care. The pharmacist is a natural addition to this team, because drug therapy plays a major role in the palliative management of these patients.

When a patient is first admitted to hospice, the pharmacist may review the patient's history and medications. As part of the pharmacist's workup of drug therapy, the goal is to simplify and optimize the patient's medication regimen. Questions to consider in this process include:

- Are the appropriate medications prescribed?
- Are the doses appropriate?
- Can any medications be discontinued?
- Are there any potential drug interactions?
- Are there any therapeutic duplications?
- Is the patient at risk for cumulative adverse drug effects?
- How will the patient's nonprescription medications impact his overall medication regimen?
- Does the patient have a history of allergies?

The team, and especially the pharmacist, should be vigilant in deciding when medications can be discontinued. Two examples of groups of medications that are affected by disease progression are antihypertensives and insulin or oral sulfonylurea agents. If attention is not paid to which medications may be discontinued, the patient may become hypotensive, hypoglycemic, or suffer from another drug toxicity.

As part of the hospice team, the pharmacist should participate in hospice rounds. During rounds notes are taken, such as on the form presented in Appendix 8-A. An example of ongoing documentation from rounds is shown in Appendix 8-B. This form becomes part of the pharmacist's file, and is used as a reference.

Using the chart and information gathered from rounds, the pharmacist can then initiate a pharmaceutical care plan (see Appendix 8-C). The pharmaceutical care plan presents the medical or drug related problem, the desired therapeutic outcome or goal, pharmacist intervention, and suggested monitoring. This dynamic document should be a part of the patient's permanent record. Complementing this document, the pharmacist should write progress notes (see Appendix 8-D), which would also become a part of the patient's permanent chart.

Impact of the Pharmacist

There are many aspects of hospice care in which the pharmacist may have an impact. One of the most obvious is consulting on pain and symptom management. The World Health Organization has advocated a three step "ladder" approach in the management of cancer pain relief, progressing from non-opioid therapy, to a mild and finally strong opioid, with adjuvant analgesics as needed.[5] (See also Chapter 22.) The pharmacist may offer suggestions to the hospice team and primary physician regarding analgesic selection. Many times, the pharmacist may point out situations where traditional analgesics are not the drug of choice. For example: Mrs. Jones is a 68 year old female with history of wide-spread cancer, primary site unknown. The patient was receiving maximum doses of Percocet and was still in pain. The primary physician decided that the patient should receive a morphine infusion, even though the patient could swallow. The nurse reported in afternoon rounds that the physician ordered 4 mg/hr morphine, and the dose could be increased up to 6 mg/hr per nursing discretion. At 5 am the next morning, the nurse contacted the pharmacist. The patient was currently receiving 16 mg/hr of morphine, and was still in pain. Upon talking with the pharmacist, it appeared that the patient's complaints were consistent with probable bone metastases, and she demanded that something be done for the pain. The pharmacist called the physician, and requested a nonsteroidal agent (patient had ibuprofen 200 mg at home). The physician was reluctant because the patient had an ulcer 15 years ago, but had not had problems since. The pharmacist persevered, and the physician agreed to prescribe ibuprofen 400 mg q4h x 2. Two hours after the first dose of ibuprofen, the patient was asleep for the first time in two days. The ibuprofen was continued, and the morphine was titrated back down to 4 mg/hr, with excellent pain relief.

Another area in which the pharmacist may help the hospice patient is the selection of alternate routes of medication administration when the patient can no longer swallow solid oral dosage forms. The pharmacist may recommend a commercially available liquid or rectal form of the same medication, or a therapeutic equivalent. The pharmacist can either arrange to have a medication specially compounded, or do so himself if the situation allows.

One goal in hospice is to avoid the use of parenteral medication administration if possible. Consider the following example:
Mrs. Smith is an 82 year old female with history of breast cancer receiving Hospice care. Mrs. Smith has occasional "anxiety" attacks, and the only thing that has helped measurably is lorazepam .5 mg po prn. Several months later, however, Mrs. Smith was unable to swallow her lorazepam tablets. The pharmacist suggested one of two alternatives: first, lorazepam is available as an intensol, which is a highly concentrated liquid (2 mg/ml). The patient may be able to swallow 1/4 ml. The second alternative is to administer the oral lorazepam tablet sublingually, which has been done with good results.[6] Both of these alternatives are preferred over IM diazepam injections, which is what the physician ordered.

Other types of recommendations that the pharmacist may make as part of the team include to identify monitoring parameters to assess the therapeutic or toxic effect of medications, to advise the team about medication costs, and to facilitate the provision of medications needed by the patient.

Home Visits

In some instances the nurse may request that the pharmacist make a patient home visit. The purpose of this visit may be to assess the patient's pain or other symptoms, or to educate the patient and/or caregivers. Patient and family/caregiver fears are often a barrier to pain control, which may be alleviated in part through education.

Quality Assurance/Drug Use Evaluation

Pharmacists may play a role in the development of criteria to assess documentation of pain and symptom control,[7] as well as criteria to assess patient outcomes (pain or symptom control achieved). Similarly, the pharmacist may draft criteria for a drug use evaluation, and share the results with the team. For example, when transdermal fentanyl first became available, there were times when it was inappropriately prescribed. Because fentanyl can be expensive, its proper use is important to patients and hospice programs.

Education

Opportunities for the pharmacist to educate in a hospice program, include answering drug information questions and providing formal inservice presentations. Possible audiences include the nursing staff, home health aides, volunteers, and other health care providers on the team. Pharmacists may also educate prescribers, through consultation in selecting appropriate medications for pain and symptom control.

Educational objectives may also be achieved by producing a newsletter that reviews new medications, adverse effects, and other medication-related issues relevant to hospice care.

Protocol Development

The pharmacist may serve as a member of the pharmacy and therapeutics committee, if one exists in the hospice. Even if the program does not have such a committee, the pharmacist may help write protocols related to medication use, such as the use of an emergency drug box, drug storage and disposal, and protocols on pain and symptom control (e.g., a bowel protocol).

DISTRIBUTIVE FUNCTIONS

Hospices that do not have a staff pharmacist may establish a relationship with a community pharmacist. This may be an informal relationship, or a contractual arrangement, such as is seen with Medicare-certified hospices. Services that the hospice program will look for in a pharmacy include 24-hour emergency medication access, hospice formulary, patient profiling, delivery services, competitive pricing, and specialty drug compounding.

The hospice nurse may anticipate when a patient is going to require a dosage increase or different medication for pain or symptom control, or if the patient will soon be unable to swallow. However, sometimes these events cannot be predicted, and they occur in the middle of the night, or on a weekend. If the pharmacy is closed, the nurse needs to have access to either an emergency drug box, or be able to contact a pharmacist on call.

While most hospices do not actually have a formulary, there are certain medications that the pharmacy should routinely stock in order to meet the needs of the patients. Additionally, the pharmacist should carry these medications in a variety of dosage formulations to meet the patients need. A partial listing of hospice medications is shown in Table 8-1.

Along with a medication formulary, the pharmacy may offer a variety of parapharmaceuticals, including pressure sore supplies, incontinence supplies, ostomy supplies, enteral feeding supplies, and home medical equipment. It would be useful to have the pharmacy provide home infusion pain therapy as well.

Occasionally the patient requires a medication that is not available in an acceptable dosage formulation. In this instance, it is very helpful to have a pharmacist who can extemporaneously compound prescriptions. Some examples of requested compounded formulations include phenytoin suppositories, multiple ingredient suppositories, and morphine suppositories containing more morphine than what is commercially available. Medications compounded as intensols (highly concentrated liquids), and troches are also desirable.

ADMINISTRATIVE SERVICES

The pharmacist may be asked to serve as a volunteer member of the administrative team of the hospice program. For example, it is not uncommon for the pharmacist to be asked to serve on the Professional Advisory Board of the hospice program. The Board establishes policies and procedures for the hospice, and sets the philosophy for the team.

RESEARCH OPPORTUNITIES

There are several research opportunities for the pharmacist involved in hospice care. One example is research that addresses optimal drug therapy in pain and symptom control. Another possibility is the investigation of reasons why patients do not achieve good pain control.

Another new area for research opportunity involves the growth in extemporaneous compounding. Clinical evidence is needed of the efficacy of these extemporaneously compounded dosage forms. This evidence may include blood level data, as well as clinical outcome evaluation.

GETTING INVOLVED WITH A HOSPICE PROGRAM

The first step in providing hospice pharmacy practice services is to identity local hospice programs. Many hospitals have a home HHC and/or hospice department. If the hospital does not have a HHC or hospice program, the discharge planner or social worker at the hospital may be able to identify hospice programs in the area.

Table 8-1 Hospice Medication Formulary

Hospice Medication Formulary

Analgesics:
- acetaminophen
- aspirin
- ibuprofen
- naprosyn
- codeine
- oxycodone
- oxycodone/aspirin
- oxycodone/acetaminophen
- hydromorphone
- morphine
- transdermal fentanyl

Antiemetics:
- prochlorperazine
- metoclopramide

Laxatives, stool softeners, enemas:
- senna (Senokot line)
- docusate
- lactulose
- phosphate enema

Anxiolytics, antidepressants, antipsychotics, sedatives:
- lorazepam
- alprazolam
- amitriptyline
- fluoxetine
- haloperidol
- diphenhydramine
- hydroxyzine
- chloral hydrate

Miscellaneous:
- B & O suppositories
- nembutal suppositories
- dexamethasone
- loperamide
- scopolamine (injectable and transdermal patch)

Getting Paid For Hospice Consulting

If the patient is receiving care under the Medicare hospice benefit, the per diem that the agency receives from Medicare includes providing the patient's medications, but the hospice program is not specifically obliged to provide or pay for clinical pharmacy services. In some situations the hospice program operates under capitation and is able to pay for clinical pharmacy services out of the general operating fund. If patients are receiving hospice care through the Medicare home care benefit (vs. the hospice benefit), the agency may increase their administrative and general fee per patient visit to enable them to pay for a clinical pharmacist. Other pharmacists have sought and received grant support, which has enabled them to get paid for working with a hospice program.

REFERENCES

1. Lukashok H. Hospice care under medicare - an early look. Pre Med. 1990; 19:730-6.
2. Magno JB. Hospice care: an overview. Henry Ford Hosp Med J. 1991; 39(2);72-3.
3. Magno JB. Management of terminal illness: the hospice concept of care. Henry Ford Hosp Med J. 1991; 39(2):74-6.
4. Lipman AG. Pharmacy service in hospice care. Wellcome Trends in Hosp Pharm. 1990; 6:2-5.
5. World Health Organization Expert Committee. Cancer pain relief and palliative care. WHO, Geneva, Switzerland, 1990.
6. Greenblatt DJ, Divoli M, Harmatz JS, Shader RI. Pharmacokinetic comparison of sublingual lorazepam with intravenous, intramuscular, and oral lorazepam. J of Pharm Sci. 1982; 71(2):248-52.
7. Lee DS, McPherson ML, Zuckerman IH. Quality assurance: documentation of pain assessment in hospice patients. Am J of Hospice and Palliative Care. 1992; 9(1):38-43.

Appendix 8-A Hospice Rounds Notes

NAME: **MD:** **RN:**

SOC: **AGE:** **DIAGNOSIS:**

Date	History/Progress		Date	Medications
			Aller:	

Appendix 8-B Hospice Rounds Notes (Example)

NAME: Betty Jones **MD: Dr. Smith** **RN: Cindy**

SOC: 9-15-93 AGE: 74 **DIAGNOSIS: Breast CA**

Date	History/Progress		Date	Medications
9/15	Pt. diagnosed Feb 92 with R-breast CA after		9/15	Tylenol 1g q4h
	finding a lump while showering. Pt. s/p		9/15	Diabeta 5 mg qd
	R-mastectomy and chemotx. Despite tx, disease		9/16	D/C Tylenol
	has progressed, with new mass in L-breast. Pt.		9/16	Percocet 1-2 q4h
	elected hospice care, does not want active tx.		9/16	Colace bid
	Bowels, skin integrity ok. Pain - 2/5 on VAS,			
	L-breast, on Tylenol 6 grams qd.Rec: start		9/22	D/C/ Colace
	Percocet 1-2 q4h, Colace 1 bid			
9/22	Pt's pain relieved, 0-1/5 per VAS. Now c/o		9/22	Senokot S bid
	constipation (stool not hard, but difficult to pass).			
	Rec: Senokot S 1 tab bid			
10/18	RN says pt. c/o left rib pain, 3/5 per VAS. RN		10/19	Ibuprofen 400mg
	discussed with MD, agreed it sounds like bone			q4h
	pain per description. Rec: Ibuprofen 400 mg q4h			
10/25	RN says pt c/o weakness, dizziness, palpitations,		Aller:NK	
	sweating. AM FBG 50-60. Rec: hold Diabeta,		10/25	D/C Diabeta
	check BG3 x qwk.			
			DATE	**PROBLEMS**
11/8	RN reports good pain relief. Diabeta on hold,		'83	NIDDM
	FBG between 100-120 with no further c/o.		9/15	L-breast pain
			9-22	constipation
			10-18	bone pain
			10-25	hypoglycemia

Key to abbreviations used:

Pt. - patient
s/p - status post
tx - treatment
rec - recommendation
CA - cancer
chemotx - chemotherapy
VAS - visual analog scale
FBG - fasting blood glucose

Appendix 8-C Pharmaceutical Care Plan (Example)

Betty Jones - Pharmaceutical Care Plan

Medical/Drug Related Problem	Desired Therapeutic Outcome/Goals	Pharmacist Intervention	Monitoring	Resol. Date/Ini
1. Pt. presents with breast CA, per history and X-ray, referred for palliative care. Pt. c/o L-breast pain per 2/5 on VAS.	1. Pt. without c/o L-breast pain. VAS 0-1/5.	1. Rec. d/c tylenol. Begin Percocet 1-2 q4h around the clock. Begin Colace 100 mg po bid for prophylaxis vs. constipation.	1. Status of pain qd. Status of bowels qd.	
2. Pt. c/o constipation, per difficulty in passing stool.	2. To alleviate ptÆs c/o constipation.	2. Rec. d/c Colace, and begin Senokot S bid.	2. Status of bowels qd.	
3. Pt. developed bone mets, as seen by left rib pain, and d/w MD.	3. Pt. without c/o left rib pain, VAS 0-1/5.	3. Rec. begin Ibuprofen 400 mg po q4h.	3. Status of pain qd.	
4. Pt. c/o hypoglycemia, as per sx of weakness, dizziness, palpitations, FBG 50-60.	4. Normalize blood glucose, with FBG less than 150 mg.dl.	4. Rec. hold Diabeta, check FBG 3 x qweek until stable.	4. Three times weekly.	

Appendix 8-D Pharmacy Progress Notes (Example)

MEMORIAL HOSPICE PROGRAM
PHARMACY PROGRESS NOTE

September 15, 1993 Patient: Betty Jones

S: Patient is a 74 year old female with history of R-breast CA, s/p mastectomy and chemotherapy treatment. Two weeks ago, patient was diagnosed with additional tumor in L-breast. Patient has elected palliative care, and declines further active therapy. Current problems include patient complaint of pain (2/5) in L-breast, and history of NIDDM.

O: Medications on admission:
Acetaminophen 1 gram q4h
Diabeta 5 mg qd

A: Patient finds her current level of discomfort unacceptable, and she is currently on a maximum dose of acetaminophen. The next logical step is mild opioid therapy. Due to risk of constipation, patient should also be placed on prophylactic bowel protocol.

P: Contacted Dr. Smith with recommendations, that were accepted:

1. Discontinue acetaminophen use.
2. Begin Percocet 1-2 tablets every four hours.
3. Begin Colace 100 mg po bid.
4. Assess pain and bowel status daily.

September 22, 1993 Patient: Betty Jones

S: Per nursing notes, patient's complaint of pain is decreased to 0 or 1/5, and this is acceptable to the pain. The patient is currently using 6-8 Percocet tablets per day. Patient now complains of difficulty passing stool; RN documents that stool is not hard, but patient is still experiencing difficulty.

O: Current medications:
Percocet 1-2 tablets q4h
Colace 100 mg bid
Diabeta 5 mg qd

A: Stool softener probably insufficient to treat constipation, which is probably exacerbated by opioid therapy.

P:

1. Continue with bowel protocol, and either add Senokot 1 bid to Colace therapy, or discotinue Colace and begin Senokot S, 1 tablet bid.
2. Assess pain and bowel status daily.

October 18, 1993 Patient: Betty Jones

S: As discussed at rounds today, RN states that patient is complaining of a new type of pain. Patient states that the pain is in her left ribs, has an "achy" quality, is worse with movement, and is only partially relieved by Percocet. Patient currently evaluates the pain as 3/5 on VAS. RN feels patient's description is consistent with bone metastases, and MD agrees.

O: Current medications:
Percocet 2 tablets q4h
Senokot S 1 tablet tid
Diabeta 5 mg qd

A: Percocet will be of limited usefulness in treating bone metastases, and increasing the dose will increase the acetaminophen component (on which there is a ceiling), and the increase in opioid may make the patient sleepier. NSAID therapy would probably benefit the patient more to treat this new pain.

P: Contacted Dr. Smith with recommendation, which was accepted:

1. Begin ibuprofen 400 mg po q4h; continue Percocet 1-2 tablets q4h.
2. Assess pain status daily.

October 25, 1993 Patient: Betty Jones

S: Per nurses notes, patient does not complain of pain at either site, and has no problems with bowels. Patient has had continued complaints of dizziness, weakness, palpitations and sweating for the past 7-10 days. RN documents that patient has been eating less, and is probably taking in about 400 calories per day.

O: Current medications:
Percocet 1-2 tablets q4h
Senokot S 1 tablet bid
Ibuprofen 400 mg po q4h
Diabeta 5 mg qd

Fasting Blood Glucose over past two weeks: 50-70 mg/dl

A: Due to patient's decreased nutrient intake, patient probably does not require Diabeta therapy.

P: Contacted Dr. Smith with recommendation, which was accepted.

1. Hold Diabeta, and check AM fasting blood glucose three times weekly for one week. If FBG remains less than 140 mg/dl, discontinue Diabeta, and check BG once a week, or with patient complaints related to hyperglycemia.

9 Pharmaceutical Care for Home Health Care Patients

Charles C. Schraa, Pharm.D.
Ralph E. Small, Pharm.D.

Hepler and Strand[1] introduced the pharmaceutical care concept to the pharmacy profession as an opportunity for the profession to mature by accepting responsibility to reduce preventable drug-related morbidity and mortality. As the role of the pharmacist in home health care (HHC) continues to evolve the integration of the pharmaceutical care model into HHC practice will enhance patient care and pharmacy practice.

DEFINITION OF PHARMACEUTICAL CARE

Hepler and Strand[1] defined pharmaceutical care as the responsible provision of drug therapy for the purpose of achieving definite outcomes that improve a patient's quality of life. These outcomes are to cure a disease, eliminate or reduce a patient's symptomatology, arrest or slow a disease process, or prevent a disease or symptomatology.

Pharmaceutical care involves the process through which a pharmacist cooperates with a patient and other professionals in designing, implementing, and monitoring a therapeutic plan that will produce specific therapeutic outcomes for the patient. This process in turn involves three major functions: (1) identifying actual and potential drug-related problems; (2) resolving actual drug-related problems; and (3) preventing potential drug-related problems.

Pharmaceutical care is a necessary element of health care, and should be integrated with other elements. However, pharmaceutical care is provided for the direct benefit of the patient, with the pharmacist directly responsible for the quality of that care. The fundamental relationship in pharmaceutical care is a mutually beneficial exchange in which the patient grants authority to the provider, and the provider makes a commitment (accepts responsibility) to provide competent care to the patient.

The fundamental goals, processes, and relationships of pharmaceutical care exist regardless of practice setting, and therefore should be provided for HHC patients.

To assist the pharmacist in understanding pharmaceutical care, the American Society of Hospital Pharmacists has published a statement on pharmaceutical care. The statement defines the principal elements of pharmaceutical care as medication-related care that is directly provided to the patient, outcomes that are intended to improve a patient's quality of life, and services provided by the pharmacist who accepts personal responsibility for the outcomes.[2]

PHARMACEUTICAL CARE: THE PROCESS

The essence of pharmaceutical care is that component of pharmacy practice that can be performed by no one other than a competent pharmacist. In this capacity the pharmacist is committed to establishing a reciprocal relationship of truthfulness, confidentiality, and loyalty with patients whose pharmacotherapeutic needs are met through the application of knowledge and humanistic principles.[3] Pharmacists perform the pharmaceutical care process using the sequence of events listed in Table 9-1.

Four factors have been defined that influence the pharmaceutical care needs of a patient and the pharmacist-patient relationship: (1) the patient's medical condition (related to diagnosis, acuity of illness, physiological status, clinical response to previous pharmacotherapy, and number of physicians involved); (2) the patient's drug therapy (also related to diagnosis, acuity of illness, physiological status, and clinical response to previous pharmacotherapy); (3) the degree of action required by the pharmacist (as determined by the clinical situation); and (4) the interprofessional relationships (e.g., drug knowledge, judgement, communication skills, and cooperation) between the pharmacist and other health-care providers.[5]

Table 9-1 Pharmaceutical Care Process: Sequence of Events[4]

Pharmaceutical Care Event	Needs and Skills
Establish a pharmacist-patient relationship.	Requires intimacy, cooperation, and trust with the patient.
Collect, synthesize, and interpret the relevant patient-related information.	Establish a database on each patient. The pharmacist must have relevant, comprehensive, and timely data for appropriate pharmacotherapeutic decision analysis.
List and rank the patient's drug-related problems.	All actual and potential drug-related problems are stated as specifically and clearly as possible. Drug-related problems are ranked with regard to severity, risk to the patient, and patient-related factors.
Establish a desired pharmacotherapeutic outcome for each drug-related problem.	Each outcome should be as specific as possible and clearly identify the desires of both the patient and pharmacist.
Determine feasible pharmacotherapeutic alternatives.	Development of a specific list of all possible pharmacotherapeutic alternatives that will resolve the drug-related problems.
Select the ideal pharmacotherapeutic solution and individualize the therapeutic regimen.	Review the possible pharmacotherapeutic solutions with the patient and select the most desirable.
Design a pharmacotherapeutic monitoring plan.	Determination of whether the desired pharmacotherapeutic outcome has been achieved. Identification of additional patient-specific information (e.g., blood pressure, fever, pain assessment) or laboratory tests may be required to determine patient response.
Implement the individualized regimen and monitoring plan.	Communication with patient and patient care providers information regarding the pharmaceutical care plan. A mutual commitment from the patient and patient care providers is essential.
Follow up to measure success.	Determination of whether the pharmaceutical care plan was successful. Identification of new drug-related problems. The pharmacist must take responsibility for the patient's drug therapy.

A graded system of pharmaceutical care based on the medical model (e.g., primary, secondary, tertiary) has been described to provide a framework for the delivery of pharmaceutical care.[5] Primary pharmaceutical care begins when it is first determined that drug therapy is needed for a patient but that hospitalization is not. Many HHC patients are candidates to receive primary pharmaceutical care. Secondary pharmaceutical care is provided to patients in acute care hospitals, skilled nursing facilities, and to certain patients receiving specialized care in HHC settings, such as parenteral oncology and pain control. Tertiary pharmaceutical care is provided in institutional settings that render critical care services.

The three levels of pharmaceutical care also have a common set of pharmacist functions. Each level of pharmaceutical care differs with regard to the intensity of pharmaceutical care needs and requires pharmacists to demonstrate unique patient-oriented skills. The basic pharmacist functions common to all levels of pharmaceutical care are described in Table 9-2.

The pharmacist must determine the level of pharmaceutical care required in each patient's clinical situation. One belief is that the needs of the patient differentiates the level of pharmaceutical care required by and provided to a patient.[3] If patient need is expressed in terms of risk associated with the patient's pharmacotherapy, appreciation of the nature of patient need and pharmacist responsibility become clearer. To determine the type and potential magnitude of pharmacotherapeutic risk experienced by a patient, delineation of the factors that place a patient at risk is required. Three categories of factors affecting the type and level of pharmacotherapeutic risk have been defined: (1) risk factors associated with the patient's clinical characteristics (e.g., age,

Table 9-2 Basic Pharmacist Functions Common to All Levels of Pharmaceutical Care[5]

- Pharmacist Functions
- Develop and utilize patient medication profiles
- Interpret, question, clarify, verify, and validate all drug-related orders
- Provide a safe and efficient drug-dispensing system
- Monitor drug therapy for safety, efficacy, and desired clinical outcome
- Screen for drug allergies, drug-drug interactions, drug-food interactions, and concomitant drug use
- Detect and report drug allergies and adverse reactions
- Recommend initial or alternative drug therapies
- Respond to drug information requests from physicians, nurses, and patients
- Teach health-care providers and patients about drug use
- Obtain medication histories by interviewing patients
- Assist in the selection of drugs of choice and dosage forms
- Conduct drug use evaluations to assess the appropriateness of drug use and achievement of desired therapeutic outcomes
- Apply pharmaceutical principles for selected drug therapies

gender, ethnicity, race, pregnancy status, immune system status, renal function, hepatic function, cardiac function, nutritional status, and outcome expectations); (2) risk factors associated with the patient's disease (e.g., rate of disease progression, severity of disease, and patient perceptions of progression and severity); and (3) risk factors associated with the patient's pharmacotherapy (defined as toxicity profile, adverse drug reaction profile, route and technique of drug administration, and the patient's perception of the toxicity, adverse reaction profile, and appropriateness of the pharmacotherapeutic regimen). The interaction of the pharmacotherapeutic risk factors and the risk factors associated with a patient's specific pharmacotherapy determines the level of pharmaceutical care required by the pharmacist.[3]

PHARMACEUTICAL CARE PRACTICE MODEL

Once the philosophy, concepts, goals, processes, and relationships have been established, a pharmaceutical care practice model must be developed.[6] General characteristics of an ideal pharmaceutical care practice model have been identified.[7] An ideal pharmaceutical care practice model: (1) is highly integrated within the overall health care process; (2) is predicated on the pharmacist's drug-based knowledge and expertise; (3) is based on a close pharmacist-patient relationship, in which the pharmacist shares in a meaningful way, the responsibility for patient-care outcomes; (4) requires that the pharmacist develops the discipline of documenting everything done on a patient's behalf; and (5) provides for continuity of care as the patient moves from one health care delivery site to another or from the care of one pharmacist to another (presupposing an adequate communications system between pharmacists).

A pilot pharmaceutical care program is an excellent method to identify and resolve practical problems and test functional elements associated with the implementation of such a program. Some practical questions related to implementation have been identified.[6-8]

- What specific changes in the way pharmacists practice will be required to implement a pharmaceutical care model?
- How much time will be required for each patient?
- How many patients can each pharmacist adequately care for?
- How many pharmacists will be needed?
- What type of training will pharmacists require?
- How can continuity of care be ensured (between inpatient and ambulatory care/home health care practices)?
- What obstacles will be faced upon implementation of a pharmaceutical care practice model?
- What functions that pharmacists perform currently could be performed by others?
- What system problems require resolution?

HOW TO PRACTICE HOME HEALTH PHARMACEUTICAL CARE

To provide a HHC pharmacy service (i.e., primary pharmaceutical care) requires the availability of information provided by the patient (ideally), family members, or caregivers. Medication-specific information could also be obtained from an accurate patient profile. This vital demographic information, including patient age, gender, drug allergies, smoking and alcohol history, weight, non-prescription and prescription drug use, medical conditions, and history of adverse drug reactions is needed to provide pharmaceutical care for the patient in a HHC practice. The following questions should be answered for each patient:

- Is the medication (or drug product) necessary?
- Is the medication (or drug product) the correct one for this patient?
- Is the patient receiving the right dose and dosing regimen?
- Will the patient be able to take the medication properly?
- Is the drug being administered by the optimal route?
- Does the medication interact with other drugs or foods the patient is using?
- Can the medication cause significant adverse drug reactions in this patient?
- Does this patient have any potentially harmful drug-disease interactions?
- Does the patient require more or less pharmacotherapy?

If answers to the first five questions above are yes, and answers to the last four questions are no, then the magnitude of pharmacotherapeutic risk is minimal and pharmaceutical care is complete. If not, then the actual and potential drug-related problems must be listed, and ranked with regard to severity, risk, and patient-related factors.

Pharmaceutical Care Plans

Desired pharmacotherapeutic outcomes for each drug-related problem must be established and feasible pharmacotherapeutic alternatives should be selected. A pharmacotherapeutic monitoring plan must also be designed and implemented with appropriate follow up to measure successful outcomes. An example of a pharmaceutical care case study is described in Appendix 9-A. (An example of a pharmaceutical care plan for a hospice patient is included in Chapter 8.)

It is necessary to record actions that have been taken during the provision of pharmaceutical care for a HHC patient (see Figure 9-1). This documentation is necessary to provide high quality care, to minimize liability, to provide proof of service, to report the patient-specific interventions that were conducted, and to justify reimbursement.[6]

Because the use of care plans by pharmacists is based upon a relatively new concept, designing a care plan model based upon the experience of other professions with care plans would be useful. The nursing profession has used care plans for over thirty years to document the nurse's contribution to patient care. A model nursing care plan documents six elements of nursing care: initial assessments and reassessments, nursing diagnoses and patient care needs, interventions, nursing care provided, the patient's response to and the outcomes of care, and the ability of the patient to manage continuing care needs after discharge.[9,10] A problem with the nursing care plan model is that it is labor intensive, often neglected, and not worth the time spent writing the plans.[11]

Chase and Bainbridge[9] tested a pharmaceutical care plan that used traditional patient profile information (e.g., demographics, allergies, drug name, strength, dose) and nontraditional indicators (e.g., desired outcomes, interventions, time devoted to monitoring). Although this care plan was useful as a documentation tool, the process was time consuming. Further research is needed to define a care plan model that facilitates the provision of pharmaceutical care.

CONCLUSION

Providers of pharmaceutical care are concerned with the outcomes of their services and not merely with the act of providing those services.[8] Because of the pharmacist's responsibility for the outcome of pharmaceutical care, documentation is an important requirement. Major pharmacist functions related to the achievement of pharmaceutical care outcomes are to identify therapeutic objectives, design a therapeutic care plan to meet objectives, implement the plan, and monitor progress.

Pharmaceutical care is a cooperative activity that should not diminish the role of other health care providers in the drug use process. Pharmaceutical care augments the effectiveness of other health care providers and improves the quality of patient care. It is provided in cooperation with physicians, nurses, dentists, physical therapists, optometrists, podiatrists, and other health care providers who treat illnesses, and prescribe or administer drugs. The ultimate purpose of pharmaceutical care is improved patient outcomes, and this objective can only be achieved through interdisciplinary cooperation in the HHC setting.

Figure 9-1. Pharmaceutical Care Record

Name:__________________________Prescription/patient Number:______________________

Address: __________________________

____

____

Age:___ Sex:___ Wt:___ Smoking:___ Alcohol:___ Allergies___________ Temp._______ Pulse______ Blood Pressure________

Drug Problem/Medical Condition:____

____

____

Review of Systems:

Renal _____________	GI/GU_______________	Cardiovascular ________
Hepatic_____________	Musculoskeletal_______	Neurology____________
Pulmonary _________	Psychiatric___________	Endocrine ____________
Skin _______________	EENT_______________	Hematology___________

Medical/Drug Related Problem	Outcome/Goals	Pharmacist Intervention	Monitoring Parameters	Resolution Date/initials

Appendix 9-A Pharmaceutical Care Case Study

BAB, a 45-year-old male, was admitted to a local hospital because of confusion, disorientation, and headache. He had been well until one month earlier when he developed intermittent fever and a dull, constant headache that had progressively worsened during the two weeks prior to admission. Four days prior to admission the patient became anorexic, agitated, and confused. The patient's medical record was significant for a positive HIV test done eighteen months before this admission. Social history was notable for homosexuality.

Physical Examination

Thin, pale, Caucasian male who was alert but disoriented. Vital signs: blood pressure 130/80 mmHg, pulse 80 beats per minute, respirations 20 per minute, and temperature 39.9°C rectally. No cutaneous signs of rash or vasculitis were seen, and no lymphadenopathy was found. Examination of the head, ears, eyes, and nose was unremarkable. Scattered white plaques on the tongue and pharynx were visible. The neck was supple. Lungs were clear to auscultation and percussion. Cardiac examination revealed a regular rate and rhythm with no murmurs, rubs, or gallops. The abdomen was relaxed and nontender, with normal bowel sounds; the liver and spleen were not felt. There was no peripheral edema, clubbing, or cyanosis, and the articular examination was normal. Rectal examination was normal. The stool specimen was negative for occult blood. Neurologic examination revealed fluctuating mental status. Cranial nerves II-XII, motor function, and sensation were intact. Tendon reflexes were 2+ and equal, plantar responses were flexor. Pulses were 2+ throughout.

X-Rays/Labs

Chest roentgenogram revealed no apparent disease, and a computed axial tomography scan of the head demonstrated no lesions or masses. Lumbar puncture showed an opening pressure of 20 cm of water with clear, colorless cerebrospinal fluid (CSF); 7 ml of CSF was obtained. CSF evaluation revealed a glucose of 63 mg/dL (serum glucose 90 mg/dL), protein of 134 mg/dL, and a leukocyte count of 48/cu mm (40 lymphocytes, 8 polymorphonuclear leukocytes, and 2 monocytes). An India-ink test demonstrated many encapsulated budding yeast cells. A latex agglutination test for CSF cryptococcal antigen was positive (1:128). Culture of the CSF was positive for Cryptococcus neoformans.

Hospital Course

A Hickman catheter was inserted, and the patient was started on intravenous (IV) amphotericin B (0.3 mg/kg/day) and flucytosine 2 gm (150 mg/kg/day) every six hours. Despite pretreatment with diphenhydramine 50 mg orally and acetaminophen 650 mg orally, BAB experienced rigors with amphotericin B administration. The rigors subsequently resolved with administration of IV hydrocortisone 25 mg and IV meperidine 50 mg. Three weeks later his mental status had returned to baseline, and repeat lumbar puncture demonstrated a decrease in cryptococcal antigen titer (1:16). The patient was discharged on oral flucytosine 2 gm every six hours and 50 mg IV amphotericin B every other day.

Pharmaceutical Care Events

The level of pharmaceutical care required by BAB can be characterized as a slow progression from secondary to primary. BAB retains many secondary pharmaceutical care properties such as the need for IV antifungal therapy and aggressive follow up by the health care team to achieve beneficial outcomes. The potential magnitude of pharmacotherapeutic risk associated with BAB's clinical characteristics, disease processes, and drug therapy regimen must also be appreciated.

The pharmaceutical care process begins with the establishment of a pharmacist-patient relationship. Since pharmaceutical care requires a meaningful level of intimacy, cooperation, and trust with a patient, a commitment by the pharmacist to develop this pharmacist-patient relationship is essential.

A database of patient-related information must be established, including objective, patient-specific information obtained from the patient and patient's medical record. A complete medication history is obtained. The patient's past medical and hospital records can be utilized to gather pertinent drug-related information. Nephrotoxicity is a predictable consequence related to amphotericin B administration. Collection of additional information regarding renal function (serum creatinine, BUN, creatinine clearance, and concomitant administration of other nephrotoxic drugs such as aminoglycosides and pentamidine) is recommended for initial evaluation and continued monitoring. Since flucytosine dosages must be reduced in the presence of impaired renal function, renal function monitoring will decrease the potential for flucytosine toxicity. Baseline complete blood count, serum potassium, serum bicarbonate, serum magnesium, and liver function tests should be obtained and monitored during combination amphotericin B/flucytosine therapy. The patient should be interviewed for perceptions related to adverse drug reactions from previous amphotericin B administration, and perceptions of the overall drug regimen. A patient educational needs inventory should be established. Information regarding the patient's disease processes (AIDS, Cryptococcal meningitis) should be collected. The severity, prognosis, functional impairments or disabilities, and patient's perception of the disease process should be collected. All information collected must be evaluated and a patient summary recorded.

All actual and potential drug-related problems must be stated as specifically and clearly as possible. All drug-related problems must be ranked according to severity, risk, and patient-related factors. Since BAB has experienced rigors with amphotericin B administration, this should be included. The potential for amphotericin B-induced nephrotoxicity, thrombophlebitis, electrolyte disturbances (e.g., hypokalemia, hypomagnesemia), and anemia should be documented. Flucytosine may cause bone marrow suppression and gastrointestinal adverse effects. Hickman catheter complications must also be considered.

Desired pharmacotherapeutic outcomes for each drug-related problem must be defined. Did the patient receive the appropriate medication and appropriate dose? Is the patient free from amphotericin B-related adverse effects? Is appropriate prophylaxis for opportunistic infections, as determined by the patient's T-helper/inducer (CD_4) lymphocyte count or previous infection history, being administered (e.g., Pneumocystis carinii pneumonia prophylaxis with cotrimoxazole if CD_4 count is below 200 mm^3)? Outcomes should reflect desires of both the patient and the pharmacist (e.g., eradication of signs and symptoms of the cryptococcal infection in a HIV positive male while avoiding medication-related morbidity). Relapse rates for cryptococcal meningitis in AIDS patients may be as high as 50-90% and lifetime anticryptococcal maintenance therapy may be required for optimal outcomes.

Feasible pharmacotherapeutic alternatives that will resolve drug-related problems should be developed. Alternatives to combination amphotericin B/flucytosine therapy for the treatment of cryptococcal meningitis in HIV positive patients are currently being evaluated.

A review of the possible pharmacotherapeutic solutions and selection of the most desirable option(s) should follow. The patient should be an integral part of the decision process and the pharmacotherapeutic treatment plan must be individualized. The medication administration guidelines should be considered, especially in light of the needs of the HHC patient. (See Table 9-3.)

Design of a pharmacotherapeutic monitoring plan will ensure that desired outcomes have been achieved. Identification of patient-specific information to determine outcomes will augment the plan. The weekly determination of renal function, hepatic function, hematology tests, and serum electrolytes could be established and followed by the HHC pharmacist. Patient education related to HIV disease and prevention of opportunistic infections should be included.

Implementation and follow up of the above actions in concert with the patient and patient's other health care providers is essential for successful outcomes. The pharmacist must take responsibility for the patient's drug therapy.

Table 9-3 General Guidelines for Administration of Amphotericin B

- Administer a test dose of 1-10 mg in 25-50 ml of dextrose 5% and infuse over 20-30 minutes.
- Observe for untoward effects and monitor vital signs.
- If a reaction to the test dose or cardiopulmonary impairment develops, cautiously try a second test dose (smaller dose with longer infusion interval).
- If test dose was tolerated, prepare a 0.1 mg/ml solution in dextrose 5% (for peripheral administration).
- Central line administration of amphotericin B in concentrations up to 0.25 mg/ml is well tolerated.
- Initiate therapy with 0.25 mg/kg administered over 2-6 hours.
- Adjust dose to patient's tolerance.
- Gradually increase daily dose on subsequent days to desired level (i.e., usually 0.5-0.6 mg/kg).
- Adjust infusion rate to patient's tolerance.
- Duration of treatment for most deep seated infections is 6-12 weeks.
- Severe infections may require daily doses of 1mg/kg for many months.
- If the patient is critically ill or immunocompromised, the first dose of 0.25 mg/kg may be given 2-4 hours after the test dose.
- The next two or three doses can be given at 8-hour intervals, not to exceed 0.6 mg/kg over the first 24 hours.
- Amphotericin B can be given on alternate days by doubling the daily dose up to a maximum of 1.5 mg/kg.
- Total daily doses of amphotericin should not exceed 1.5 mg/kg.

REFERENCES

1. Hepler CD, Strand LM. Opportunities and responsibilities in pharmaceutical care. Am J Hosp Pharm. 1990; 47:533-43.
2. American Society of Hospital Pharmacists. ASHP statement on pharmaceutical care. Am J Hosp Pharm. 1993; 50:1720-3.
3. Strand LM, Cipolle RJ, Morley PC, et al. Levels of pharmaceutical care: A needs-based approach. Am J Hosp Pharm. 1991; 48:547-50.
4. Strand LM, Cipolle RJ, Morley PC, et al. Drug related problems: their structure and function. DICP 1990; 24:1093-7.
5. Smith WE, Benderev K. Levels of pharmaceutical care: A theoretical model. Am J Hosp Pharm. 1991; 48:540-6.
6. Strand LM, Cipolle RJ, Morley PC. Documenting the clinical pharmacist's activities: back to basics. Drug Intell Clin Pharm. 1988; 22:63-7.
7. Lee MP, Ray MD. Planning for pharmaceutical care. Am J Hosp Pharm. 1993; 50:1153-8.
8. Penna RP. Pharmaceutical care: Pharmacy's mission for the 1990s. Am J Hosp Pharm. 1990; 47:543-9.
9. Chase PA, Bainbridge J. Care plan for documenting pharmacist activities. Am J Hosp Pharm. 1993; 50:1885-1888.
10. Nizioleck C, Shaw S. Professional practice, whose plan - whose care? J Prof Nurs. 1991; 7:145.
11. Brider P. Who killed the nursing care plan? Am J Nurs. 1991; 35:9.

10 Establishing a Home Medical Equipment Pharmacy

Martin M. Rosner, Ph.D.

Home medical equipment (HME) covers all products that are used by patients to treat or recover from an illness at home as opposed to professional settings, such as the hospital, nursing home or physician's office. HME has replaced durable medical equipment (DME) as the term of choice, although confusion arises because the word equipment does not usually imply consumable supplies. It should be understood that supplies are an integral part of the HME product mix. The classification may include but is not limited to the following:

- Aids to daily living
- Hospital equipment for the home
  - Bathroom equipment and supplies
  - Bedroom equipment and supplies
  - Physical therapy and exercise equipment and supplies
- Ambulatory Aids
  - Mobility equipment and walking aids
  - Wheelchairs and accessories
- Ostomy supplies
- Incontinent supplies
- Self monitoring equipment and supplies
  - Diabetes supplies and urine and blood monitoring equipment
  - Blood pressure devices
  - Thermometers
  - Pregnancy tests
  - Ovulation tests
  - Apnea monitors
- Dressings
- Prostheses and supplies
- TENS and back support products
- Parenteral, enteral and nutrition supplies

The discussion that follows will exclude infusion devices, which are covered in Chapter 19.

UNDERSTANDING THE HME MARKET

Composition of Home Health Care Spending

Total spending on home health care (HHC) has risen dramatically during the past ten years.[1,2] Spending on HHC services grew at an annual rate of 18% between 1980 and 1990. Growth has been even more dramatic since then. From 1990 to 1991 HHC services expenditures grew by 23.8% annually; between 1991 and 1992 it declined slightly to 21.5% annually but is expected to grow by 19.8% annually between 1992 and 1995. HME market growth has been slightly less, 17.6% annually between 1980 and 1990, 18.3% annually between 1990 and 1992 and 19.8% annually between 1992 and 1995. Table 10-1 shows the pattern of growth between 1980 and 1992 with estimates for 1995.

Table 10-1 Total Market for HHC Services and Products[3,4]

	1980	1990	1992	1995
Home Health Services (billions)	$1.3	$6.9	$10.3	$16.4
Home Medical Equipment (billions)	$1.0	$5.0	$7.0	$12.0
Total	$2.3	$11.9	$17.3	$28.4

Nurses in home health agencies (HHA) provide medical services while home makers and other non-medical personnel provide housekeeping and other services to the homebound. Of the total market for HHC services, over 50% is spent on services.

Specific product market estimates for 1993, given in current dollars, are shown in Table 10-2. The 1995 estimates in current dollars are based on adding average annual growth rates between 1985 and 1992 to annual medical equipment inflation, estimated at 3% annually. The product market estimates can also be used to evaluate potential opportunities in individual markets.

Areas of faster than normal growth include all facets of nutritional therapy, rehabilitation products, and diabetic and incontinent supplies. Technological advances are likely to increase the usage of patient monitoring equipment, self testing devices and communication equipment.

Home Medical Equipment Distribution Patterns Full Service vs Specialization

Full service HME facilities differ from location to location. They include both single and multi-location (chain) operations which may be national, or more likely, regional in scope. The full service or more comprehensively stocked operations may have 24 hour service, usually employ between 5 and 25 people, many of whom are health care professionals such as nurses, enterostomal and/or physical therapists. All stores rent and sell equipment. HME dealers must accept third party billings in order to be competitive.

Although larger HME distributors lay claim to being full-line, one-stop shopping outlets for HME, this is largely a myth. More typical is specialization in only one or a few business segments supplemented by the use of catalogs, or referrals to other specialist HME distributors. Specialty HME dealers usually cater to a specific type of HHC patient such as ostomates, or those needing rehabilitation, suffering from pain, or with respiratory or nutritional problems. Although it would seem that specialization limits income potential, specialists actually do better financially and professionally than full line dealers because they do a better job of serving their clientele, can promote more intensively to a limited number of referral sources and master reimbursement regulations for their product lines. In Table 10-3, "full line " dealers may be those who specialize in multiple areas rather than dealers who stock a complete line of HME and supplies, enteral and parenteral nutrition, and intravenous therapy.

Table 10-2 Estimated Markets for Home Care Products[4]

Product	1993 (millions)	1985-1992 Nominal Growth (a)
Wheelchairs	$490	13%
Electric Scooters/Carts	130	18
Exercise equipment	770	13
TENS	185	13
Respiratory	1,000	12
Ostomy	300	7
Self testing	500	22
Diabetic testing	595	12
Incontinence	612	15

(a) Estimated constant annual growth plus inflation

Medical Supply Dealers

HME dealers are in the retail business. Medical supply dealers run a similar operation but their primary client is the physician, and strictly speaking, act as wholesalers. However they sell the same items as HME dealers and many patients shop for their HME needs at the medical supply house.

TABLE 10-3 Home Care Equipment Dealers by Degree of Specialization[1]

Type	Percent
Full line	40%
HME or specialty products only	25
Respiratory only	6
Pharmacies with significant HME	24
Others	5
Total	**100%**

The Role of the Pharmacist in HME Distribution

Pharmacist participation in the HME market starts with setting up a HME department in the pharmacy and if business warrants expanding into free-standing businesses. The free-standing units compete directly with non-pharmacy HME outlets and with hospital HME operations. The role of the pharmacist in the distribution of HME has varied over time. At one time, pharmacists were respon sible for founding about half of the outlets for HME equipment and supplies.[1] Some of these pioneers have moved on to establish large HME outlets, have joined the ranks of manufacturers of HME or have moved on to specialty areas such as consultant pharmacies, enteral and parenteral nutrition and renal dialysis. Those who have succeeded have been rewarded financially and professionally. Others have abandoned the market because profits did not justify the investment required, because of reimbursement hassles, or because of perceived unfair competition from HME organizations with captive referral clients.

Characteristics of the HME Market

Third Party Reimbursement

Third party payers of HHC services are an important determinant of the HME services and product market. Medicare pays much of the cost of HHC services and products for their clientele while Medicaid may pay for non-medical services and products for both the elderly and non-elderly needy HHC patients. Table 10-4 shows the trend in the percent of coverage by third party payers between 1980 and 1992 and estimates for 1995.

Rental vs Sale of HME Equipment

The HME business involves both rental and a sale. Analyses of pharmacy HME operations indicate that rentals account for 39% of total revenue. The Health Industries Distributors Association indicates that the higher the proportion of rentals the more profitable is the HME operation, regardless of size. Table 10-5 shows charges for commonly rented items.

Table 10-4 Insurance Coverage for HHC Expenses[2,4],1980 - 1995 (Percent of Total Expenses)

		% Out of Pocket	% Private Insurance	% Medicare	% Medicaid
1980	Home Health Care Services	10.2	7.6	55.3	17.0
	Home Med. Equip./supplies	77.1	9.7	10.2	3.0
1990	Home Health Care Services	12.1	7.3	41.8	31.4
	Home Med. Equip./supplies	67.4	10.4	17.8	4.2
1992	Home Health Care Services	11.6	7.0	41.9	32.4
	Home Med. Equip./supplies	65.1	9.4	21.2	4.0
1995 (est)	Home Health Care Services	10.1	6.2	29.5	41.9
	Home Med. Equip./supplies	64.1	8.6	23.9	2.6

Trends In The HME Market

Growth in Hospital HME Operations

An ongoing trend in the industry is expansion of hospitals into HHA, parenteral therapy, enteral and parenteral nutrition and HME distribution. The justification for this expansion is the need for alternate sources of income to compensate for decreased bed utilization, the need for maintaining continuity of care for their patients and the ease of obtaining captive referrals as patients are discharged.

Table 10-5 Commmonly Rented Home Medical Equipment (* indicates Medicare-reimbursable items)

	Average Rent/mo.	Average Sale
Bathroom Aids		
Bath seat w/o back	Sale only	$34
Bath seat w/ back	Sale only	52
Bath seat w/back pad	Sale only	73
*Commodes	Sale only	<150
Bedroom Equipment		
*Semi-Electric Bed w/rails	$127	1,200
*Hosp. bed, manual w/mattress	82	725
*Pressure pad and pump	50	180
*Trapeze for bed	41	135
*Patient Lift w/sling	76	823
Wheelchairs and Accessories		
*Standard wheelchair w/footrest	29	252
*Standard wheelchair w/legrests	55	369
*Standard wheelchair w/footrests and removable arms	68	602
*Lightweight, fixed arms, swing-away leg rest	55	560
*Electric w/charger	220	2,500+
Respiratory Equipment		
Pulmo-Aide	31	180
Oxygen Concentrator	189	790
Miscellaneous HME		
*Transcutaneous Electric Nerve Stimulator	90	600
*Food Pump w/strand	75	550
*Electric Breast Pump	56	320
Apnea Monitor	150	n/a
Stair lift	250	2,200

Patients have the right to select any dealer for their HHC needs but may find it more convenient and have more confidence in hospital sponsored organizations.

Joint Ventures and Contractual Arrangements in HME Distribution

Instead of actually owning and operating HME distribution outlets, many institutional and cooperative providers of health care prefer to enter into contractual arrangements or joint ventures with independent HME distributors. Examples are hospital discharge planners and HHC coordinators, HHA, health maintenance organizations, skilled nursing facilities and even third party insurers. They do so in the interest of containing costs and maintaining product quality for their patients or of profiting financially. Contractual relationships for nursing homes and long term care facilities would probably call for suppliers of HME to take on the function of purchasing departments for the clients. Other agencies would provide price discounts for patients.

Joint ventures offer hospitals, HHA and other institutions a financial stake in HME without the risks and burdens of start-ups and acquisitions. Contractual arrangements without an ownership stake may be made in order to establish quality control for the patients, reduce costs, or provide specialized HME products. The health care provider or insurer might prefer to do business with a full line HME dealer. This m... or may not be possible. Specialized HME p companies have the advantage of a great... entory and selection within the product class.

In return the HME product provider gets controlled patient referrals. However, this may not work out to the HME provider's satisfaction. Despite the best efforts of the referring source, patients do have the right to select their own HME product provider. The stream of referrals should be monitored and the marginal profits from the cooperation evaluated. Table 10-6 is an overview of contractual or joint venture by type of health care provider and the form of the arrangement.

OPENING AN HME PHARMACY

The process of opening an HME pharmacy involves identifying the areas of HME that the proprietor would like to sell, estimating the market, developing a time and action plan, and providing the capital, personnel and facility to house the operation.

Selecting HME Niches

Before entering into any aspect of HME, it is wise to discuss areas of patient need with referral sources, physicians, nurses and potential customers. It is also of value to survey the product lines of competitors in the area. A good surrogate for the

Table 10-6 Contractual Arrangements and Joint Ventures

	Hospitals	HMO, PHP, PPO (a)	Home Health Agencies	Managed Care Plans	Nursing Homes	Long Term Care Facilities
Patient referrals	✔	✔	✔	✔	✔	✔
Contract bids		✔		✔		✔
Special HME programs, e.g., oncology home care	✔	✔				
Joint ventures/ partnerships/ on-site facilities	✔	✔				
For profit ventures within non profit organizations	✔	✔	✔			
Purchasing agency					✔	✔

(a) HMO = Health Maintenance Organization: PHP = Prepaid Health Plan; PPO = Preferred Provider Organization.

customer group is the local self help disease association. These are also good sources of information on usage patterns for the patient group especially the types of products and brands that are favored locally. It also could be used to identify product needs that are not being met in the area.

Estimating the Market

Methods for determining HME market potential vary. They all should be considered means of arriving at a rough estimate since extraneous factors can come into play which affect the actual result. One approach is to use a geographical hospital discharge model. Total hospital discharges in a given area are multiplied by the average amount spent per patient on HHC and products ($92.50). Add to this figure 10% for the amount spent by non-hospitalized products and 28% for rental equipment and reordered items. Finally divide this figure by the number of dealers in the area.

Another method is to use per capita spending on health care. The population of the store's market area should be multiplied by $3,150 and then by 0.015. In 1993, it is estimated that $3,150 is the per capital personal health care expenditures and 1.5% is the proportion spent on HME. This basic approximation should be weighted by the average age of the community, the availability of quality medical care, regional health care problems and characteristics of local competition and referral sources.

The core of the HHC patient base is the population with two or more impairments to daily living. In 1993, this would be 2.5 million, 7.6% of the population aged 65 or over. The latter can be determined by examining census tract data for the store's primary market area for HME. These are the primary recipients of HHC services. One rough way to establish this area is to determine where the dealer is situated in relation to its closest HME competitors. Another method of determining this core population is to visit a local HHA and make inquiries of the visiting nurse and social workers. Discharge planners at local hospitals could be contacted to determine how many patients are discharged annually with prescriptions for HHC services and supplies. Even then, the homebound patient comprises only 4 of the 10 patients that are consumers of HME and supplies.

Inventory for Establishing an HME Pharmacy

Table 10-7 gives the maximum and minimum inventory by class of product. The details of the inventory in each class are not shown. It is based on model inventory planograms offered by major pharmaceutical wholesalers.

The total merchandise investment to establish an HME pharmacy depends first on which HME lines are selected, and secondly on the degree of specialization for that product class. Even then, these are merely opening inventory estimates. In time, customer requirements will dictate which lines should be expanded and which ones should be cut back or even eliminated. Limitations on both space and capitalization may prevent the ownership or display of a full line of merchandise. The use of catalogs from suppliers who offer prompt delivery will allow a small store to be able to meet the needs of its clientele.

The question of sourcing involves the decision as to how much should be bought directly from manufacturers versus buying from full line HME wholesalers. A start-up operation will use a full line wholesaler extensively. However, as volume expands opportunities to buy from manufacturers will become economically feasible and they should be explored. Some pharmacists prefer to concentrate their purchases with a single wholesaler in order to reduce administrative costs. Offers will be made to lock into contracts in return for extra discounts. These should be entered into with care, especially if they contain provisions which may preclude the pharmacist from getting products at the lowest possible cost.

Other Capital Requirements

All start-up businesses have initial capital expenses. Major initial expenses for entry into the HME business include equipment, delivery vehicles, personnel, marketing and facility expenses. Total dollar allocation of the initial investment is dependent upon the pharmacist's business strategy. Most pharmacies start their HME operations as in-store departments and expand into free standing premises. For these stores, the initial start-up requires an analysis of existing departments to identify those that are not carrying their own weight and for which space might be freed for the new department.

Other capital expenses relate to administration. These include office equipment and supplies, telephone installation, stationery and forms and the inclusion of computers and the appropriate software for HME billing, inventory and reimbursement. Others involve the cost of acquiring or remodeling an

Table 10-7 Initial Inventory Levels by Product Class

	Maximum	Minimum
Aids to Daily Living	$500	$125
Hospital Equipment for the Home		
Bathroom equipment and supplies	4,400	843
Bedroom equipment	14,200	440
Physical therapy and exercise equipment and supplies	8,850	500
Ambulatory Aids		
Mobility equipment and walking aids	1,200	600
Wheelchairs and accessories	19,200	535
Ostomy Supplies	4,700	1,500
Incontinent Supplies	2,300	1,100
Respiratory Equipment and Supplies	8,820	300
Self-monitoring Equipment and Supplies	4,200	1,600
Dressings	1,600	500
TENS and Back Support Products	2,400	800
Prostheses and Supplies	35,000	200

existing business. Telephone expenses may initially be quite high. Many HME distributors install toll-free numbers as both a convenience for customers and as a marketing resource. This would seem most appropriate for large specialized or full-line dealers but not for in-store departments.

Personnel

No business can succeed without qualified people. The HME industry is a specialty, multi-faceted business requiring personnel of various professional backgrounds and training. At its inception, a simple HME business servicing a limited patient base and having no significant respiratory care services, can function with a minimum staff of three people, namely the pharmacist, the billing/customer relations person and a delivery/sales person. When respiratory equipment is added to the HME operation, at least one additional person may be required. In those HME operations expanding beyond this base, specialty personnel such as fitters for patients with mastectomies, and respiratory and enterostomal therapists are required. Salaries vary by geographic area. A salary survey of hospitals, trade associations, and newspaper employment advertisements should be made.

Professional boards in many states also dictate the qualifications of personnel delivering certain medical products and services, such as respiratory and nutritional services. Contact individual state licensing boards prior to making the decision to enter these markets.

Personnel should be imbued with a sense of personal commitment to the store. They should be made experts in the equipment that they sell by attending manufacturers' seminars, training sessions and continuing education programs. The staff must be able to discuss every aspect of product use with patients and health care professionals. Their primary goal should be to serve the customer to the best of their ability.

Facilities

A moderately stocked, fairly full line HME business can be operated out of as little as 1,200 square feet. A well stocked, finely displayed business with fitting rooms, office, repair and storage facilities may require 3,000 to 4,000 square feet. Full service, full line HME businesses grossing over $1 million dollars per year will require 5,000 to 7,000 square feet. In addition to the product display area, space must be allocated for office and billing functions, patient fitting rooms, merchandise storage, equipment cleaning and sterilization, oxygen tank filling and outside tank storage.

Delivery Vehicle

A vehicle is mandatory for delivery and servicing of respiratory patients but it is also a must for delivery and installation of hospital beds and other bulky items. It should be designed to be a workshop on wheels. Presently, many major oxygen therapy equipment manufacturers offer fully equipped HME vans with product usage contracts. A fully equipped delivery vehicle suitable for the delivery and storage of liquid oxygen can cost up to $30,000.

Time and Action Plan for Opening an HME Pharmacy

Table 10-8 is a timeline and action plan associated with the opening of a free standing HME pharmacy. The time line for an in-store department can be appropriately shortened by eliminating those steps that are associated with planning and implementing an entire new store and having all functions within the store itself. Identifying and contracting for appropriate support personnel may be substituted for hiring them. A priori, the development of an in-store department may require between 75 to 90 days less than this timeline.

OPERATING AN HME PHARMACY

Operating Expenses

The largest expense of any HME suppliers is the cost of goods sold. This will range from 44 to 46% for very large or specialty suppliers to 45 to 50% for the smaller suppliers. Salaries and wages are the second largest item. A small, under $1 million business, can be run by 4 or 5 people: a manager, a sales person, a billing/customer service clerk, a delivery person and an ancillary medical professional. The total costs associated with all

Table 10-8 Timeline and Action Plan for an HME Pharmacy (Free Standing Premises)

Function	Pre-opening schedule (Days Prior)
Business plan	180
Site location	150
Banking arrangements	150
Building identification	150
Lease negotiation & signing	120
Facility planning and layout	120
License and permits	90
Truck(s) ordered	90
Site construction bids	90
Manager on premises	90
Contact vendors	90
Telephones ordered	90
Yellow Pages advertising	90
Marketing/advertising plans	90
Medicare Provider number	90
Utilities	90
Remodeling	90
Insurance	75
Signs ordered	75
Drivers hired	75
Sales people hired	75
Office and showroom equipment	75
Office furniture ordered	60
Office machines ordered	60
Warehouse and cleaning equipment ordered	60
Oxygen supplier contacted	60
Inventory ordered	60
Warehouse racks ordered	60
Office stationery & forms ordered	60
Shop tools ordered	30
Begin promotion and marketing	30
Miscellaneous supplies	15
Grand opening preparation/publicity	5

personnel will be between 37 to 45% of gross sales.

Assuming a moderate facility cost, the costs associated with delivery and service vehicles is the next highest expense. General and administrative expenses such as interest, depreciation, rent, insurance, utilities and office expenses are not unusual for an HME business. Costs associated with inventory are freight, repair and maintenance. Especially important are costs for travel and education. These can be considered part of the capital cost of a business, human capital. Well trained employees are assets that are a necessity for an HME business. Other costs to anticipate, especially when starting a free standing facility are professional fees, taxes, licenses, and possibly the cost of leasing equipment. A final major expense to anticipate is the cost of bad debts. Because of third party reimbursement, bad debt expense may be as high as 5 to 8% of gross revenues.

The Health Industries Distributors Association annual survey[5] of free-standing HME distributors, not necessarily pharmacy oriented, show that pre-tax profits of 5.6% of sales and 9.5% of total assets. The analysis by size shows that the most profitable groups were those whose volume was between $1 million and $3 million; those with less than $1 million dollar volumes were slightly less profitable; those with volume between $3 million and $10 million had profit margins 1/2 of the industry average; and, super stores, whose volumes exceeded $100 million had negative average profits.

Comparisons of distributors by profit margins show that the most profitable group concentrated on better management of expenses. They had low debt and interest expense, better gross margins, and a greater percentage of their volume from rentals rather than sales. The most profitable distributors concentrated on high tech rather than traditional HME products and services and were more likely to cater to Medicare rather than Medicaid clients.

Promotion And Marketing

Model of HME Purchasing Behavior

All marketing plans require the identification of the customer, the product or service to be sold and the vehicle to unite the two. The audience for HME communication is three tiered: referral sources, families and caregivers, and patients. The model of HME purchasing behavior assumes that patients and/or caregivers at first operate out of a state of ignorance of the characteristics of products, services and sources of supply. The role of promotion for the HME pharmacy is to acquaint customers with its product lines, and its specialized personnel and services. This can be done via messages beamed directly to the customer group or indirectly via the customers' sources of information. Referral sources are persons who interact with them therapeutically or administratively. The motivational factors influencing the purchasing decision are shown in Table10-9.

Product refers to the variety of product lines, store product specialization, inventory levels of specific product lines, as well as the quality and technical characteristics of individual products. Also included in the definition of "product" are the reputation, the services and warranties of the manufacturer.

Services are essentially those offered by the pharmacy itself. They range from technical support services, response time, billing procedures, rentals, and educational support. This is regarded by some experts as the most important ingredient of all. For some items it is necessary to have private fitting rooms, and areas for holding discussions between patients and store personnel and for showing videotaped patient information from manufacturers. It is extremely important that the patient be given the time and attention to communicate with the store's technical and professional personnel.

As a motivational factor, convenience encompasses both accessibility and promptness of delivery. Price refers to the absolute prices of particular items, and the overall discount posture of the store. It also refers to the balance between prices, product quality and services. The HME pharmacist should communicate the concept of price in relation to the value or benefit to the patient. Specialized personnel include health personnel such as respiratory therapists, enterostomal therapists, physical therapists or HHC nurses available to the store, either as employees or contractors.

Referral Source Marketing

Referral sources are used by the patient and caregivers to overcome their initial ignorance of HME products and HME distributors. They include physicians, hospital social workers, discharge planners and HHC coordinators, social service agencies, community service organizations, and medical ancillary personnel. The importance of health care oriented referral sources to the consumer varies directly with the sophistication of the HME

Table 10-9 Motivational Factors Influencing the Purchase of HME

Referral Source (Initiator/Influencer)	Caregiver (Influencer/Buyer)	Patient (Buyer/User)
Product	Urgent Need	Urgent Need
Service	Product	Product
Personnel	Convenience	Convenience
Price	Personnel	Price
Convenience	Services	Personnel
Promotion	Price	Services
	Promotion	Promotion

Table 10-10 Potential Referral Sources for HME

Adult Day Care Centers	American Cancer Society
Rehabilitation Hospitals	Nursing Homes
Churches	Cerebral Palsy Association
Rehabilitation Nurses	Occupational Nurses/Therapists
Hospital Discharge Planners	Easter Seal Society
Senior Citizen Centers	Physical Therapists
Enterostomal Therapists	Disease Oriented Association
Social Service Directors	Physicians
Health Maintenance Organizations	Muscular Dystrophy Association
Community Social Workers	Preferred Provider Organizations
Home Health Agencies	National Spinal Cord
Spinal Cord Trauma Centers	Public Health Departments
Hospitals	Injury Foundation
Veterans Hospitals	Registered Nurses/Physicians Assistants
Industrial Nurses	Ostomy Clubs
Visiting Nurses Association	Rehab. Centers/Clinics/Schools
Insurance Companies	Self-Help Organizations
Vocational Rehabilitation Programs	Rehabilitation Therapists
Local Health Officials	Spina Bifida Foundation
Volunteer/Service Associations	Non-HME Pharmacies
Medical Agencies Clinics	March of Dimes

product group. This is especially relevant for the first purchase. As the patient and caregivers become familiar with the HME they use, their reliance on prescribers and medical personnel decline. With time, a reversal will occur - the medically oriented referral source may rely on patients, caregivers and patient self-help associations for product evaluations.

A survey of customers of HME pharmacies show the following sources of information: professionals, 35%; their own family, 17%; advertising, 15%; and friend, word of mouth 5%. Table 10-10 shows the variety of referral sources. Table 10-11 shows the range of influence of major referral sources in relation to specific product lines.

Another group of referral sources are institutional health care providers. Examples are hospital discharge planners and HHC coordinators, HHA health maintenance organizations and skilled nursing facilities. Insurance company case managers often have to approve coverage of HHC products and services and they can refer patients to distributors whom they trust and whose prices are acceptable.

Marketing to Families, Caregivers and Patients

Families, caregivers and patients are promotional targets for both the existence of the HME establishment as well as its individual product lines. They may be reached through ads in such general circulation media as the Yellow Pages or through local chapters of patient self-help groups. Local chapters of volunteer and self-help organizations are listed in Table 10-10 as referral sources. They are important sources of market information, often knowing more about local purchasing preferences than physicians, nurses and other referral sources. They are interested in information on new product developments that are relevant to their needs. Displays at their meetings is an effective way of reaching patients and opinion leaders who would refer the pharmacy to their fellow users.

Promotional Media

Promotion of the HME pharmacy is a never ending task. The HME business is narrowly specialized in that the population that uses and needs HME is limited and the products are diverse. In addition, the promotional message must be directed at primary referral sources, caregivers and patients. For simplicity, patients and caregivers will be grouped together because a majority of caregivers are members of the family. Paid caregivers can range from aides to registered nurses. The latter group requires a different promotional approach than those that are, at most, extensions of the patient. The media that are used are personal detailing, public relations, brochures, direct mail and paid advertising. Each has its place. Table 10-12 shows the relevance of each of these to major promotional targets. The two stage approach to the development of the purchasing decision envisions a consumer who will consult a referral source for information on what products to use and where should they be obtained. In addition, patients will undertake their own search for sources.

Detailing

The use of detailing and personal sales calls requires the HME pharmacist to make a special effort to get out from behind the prescription counter and tell the audience, whether they be physicians, nurses and allied health professionals, or discharge planners at hospitals how the HME pharmacist can help referral sources fulfill their responsibilities to their patients. Whatever common connection the pharmacist shares with the physician or the professional should be exploited to set up the appointment and to gain their confidence. It is important to approach the front office personnel with as much respect and courtesy as will be shown the physician. Come prepared with business cards, product samples and brochures that describe the HME product lines and the qualifications of the specialized personnel in the store.

Have a well prepared presentation. Be goal oriented and be informative without being overly aggressive in seeking business. The important thing is that what is being sold is the organization rather than any particular product. The amount of time that will be available to you may be as little as five minutes so it is necessary to get your message across in this time. It will require limiting the message to only a few basic concepts preferably those that will provide new information to the audience such as a new product with definite advantages to the physician. One recommendation is that the call should be limited to two new products or services. End up with a description of staff qualifications and an invitation to drop in anytime to meet them. A follow up call or letter is necessary and plan a reason to return.

Detailing should not be confined to physicians. Physical therapists, respiratory therapists and occupational therapists are valuable referral sources and are often more accessible to the patient than physicians are. Indeed some may be hired on a contractual basis to help in the education of patients and to fit particular devices for patients. HHC agencies can be sources of referrals. Some pharmacies leave HME equipment on consignment at the agencies so that they will have something to give the patient immediately, pending a final choice.

Hospital discharge planners should be detailed regularly to keep them informed of new lines and new developments in the store. The constant turnover in personnel requires that discharge planners be called on a regular schedule. Point out services that are consonant with a hospital's patient population.

A survey[1,4] of a successful group of HME pharmacists who practice in independent and free standing premises, indicated the popularity of detailing various referral sources: physicians 89%; nurses 75%; hospital discharge departments 67%; physical/occupational therapists 43%; home health agencies 86%; and self-help groups 57%. Those with in-store departments primarily detailed physicians and nurses. Only a minority of them detailed the four other referral sources.

Public Relations

Planned public relations activities that stress activities for the disabled and senior citizens are an inexpensive and very effective means of promoting the HME pharmacy. Such events as free blood pressure checks, demonstrations of self monitoring equipment and supplies, and diabetes detection drives can center around the HME pharmacy. The purpose is to provide needed volunteer service and keep the name of the store in the public's mind and relate it to HME products. The same kind of efforts can be expended to professional referral sources. Contacts with self help organizations for arthritis, lupus, diabetes, cancer and participation in their activities will reach patients who need HME products. Press releases should focus on specific activities or interesting patients, and should be of interest to the general public, especially to the potential clientele of the store. At the same time, it might be worthwhile for the HME pharmacy to distribute an in-house publication that stresses new health news

Table 10-11 Promotional Target—Home Medical Equipment Pharmacies Referral Source Influence by Product Group

	Physicians	HHC Agency Nurses	O.T. P.T. R.T. (a)	Hospital Discharge Staff (b)	Pharma-cies	3rd Party Insurers Case Mgr.
Business Existence	✔	✔	✔	✔	✔	✔
Specific Lines:						
Aids to Daily Living		✔	✔	✔	✔	✔
Hosp. equip. for home:						
Bathroom equip. and supplies		✔	✔	✔	✔	✔
Bedroom equip. and supplies		✔	✔	✔	✔	✔
Physical Therapy/exercise equip. and supplies	✔	✔	✔	✔	✔	✔
Ambulatory Aids:						
Mobility equip. and walking aids			✔	✔	✔	✔
Wheelchairs and accessories			✔	✔	✔	✔
TENS/back support products	✔	✔	✔	✔	✔	✔
Ostomy supplies	✔	✔	✔	✔	✔	✔
Incontinent supplies	✔	✔	✔	✔	✔	✔
Respiratory equip. and supplies	✔	✔	✔	✔	✔	✔
Self-monitoring equip. and supplies	✔	✔	✔	✔	✔	✔
Dressings	✔	✔	✔	✔	✔	✔
Prostheses and supplies	✔	✔	✔	✔	✔	✔

(a) O.T. = Occupational Therapists, P.T. = Physical Therapist, R.T. = Respiratory Therapist

(b) Discharge planners, HHC coordinators, social workers

for the store's clientele on a regular basis. The lead story can be supplemented with information on new products or features of older products and information on new personnel in the store. The important thing is to stress the new and the interesting.

Brochures

Brochures issued by manufacturers are important sources of information to referral sources and to patients. Ideally they should be an educational tool. These should be distributed to referral sources, be made available in physicians' offices and to hospital discharge planners and HHC coordinators. Professional caregivers can use them to gain information about the products that they use. The important thing is that they have an educational content. A commonly used HME sales medium is the catalog. Catalogs have traditionally consisted of manufacturers' product sales sheets inside of a dealer's binder. These are distributed to referral sources to be used as a reference prior to the time of purchase.

Advertising

Advertising to the public is best achieved through the local Yellow Pages with ads in the hospital equipment, oxygen, ostomy or any other category of products that the store carries. Patients in need of HME are in fact likely to "let their fingers do the walking," as the advertising jingle suggests.

Advertising in local and regional professional publications of nurses, allied health personnel and physicians who are both customers and referral sources keep the store's name before opinion leaders and at the same time support their organizations. The same kind of ads can be inserted in newsletters of self help organizations.

REFERENCES

1. Rosenberg J L. Establishing a Durable Medical Equipment Pharmacy. in Catania P N and Rosner MM, eds: Home Health Care Practice, Palo Alto; Health Markets Research. 1986.
2. Anon. Home Health Care Sales. Drug Topics. 1992; 11:50.
3. Anon. Health Care Financing. Health Care Financing Administration. Fall 1992.
4. Unpublished Data. Health Markets Research, Palo Alto. 1993.
5. Anon. Health Industries Distributors Association. 1993.

Table 10-12 Promotional Media

	Physicians	Nurses and Therapists	Hospital Discharge Staff	Home Health Agency	Self Help Groups	Patient Care-Givers
Detailing/sales calls	✔	✔	✔	✔		
Public relations	✔	✔		✔	✔	
Brochures		✔	✔	✔	✔	✔
Direct Mail Campaigns	✔	✔	✔	✔	✔	
Advertising						
Yellow Pages						✔
Professional publications	✔	✔	✔	✔	✔	

11 Home Medical Equipment

William E. Fassett, Ph.D., RPh
Barbara Fotheringill, B.A.

Home medical equipment (HME) includes a variety of devices that the home health care (HHC) pharmacy practitioner may provide to help maintain patient independence and self-determination. HME includes ambulatory aids, hospital equipment, and related convalescent aids. (See also Chapter 10.)

Ambulatory aids are mechanical helpers that provide their users with mobility and independence. Some, like canes, offer minimal physical support but encourage patient confidence. Others, like wheelchairs, become their owners' waking-hour living environments, as important to them as the automobile is to the daily commuter. All must be selected to meet patient needs and adjusted or fitted to individual dimensions and circumstances.

Hospital equipment for the home is frequently the essential accoutrement that enables the patient to be transferred from institutional to home care. It helps family members create an environment that lets them efficiently care for their loved one. The proper bed, mattress, and aids for decubitus prevention are important for patient comfort and well-being. Patient safety is enhanced by bed rails and bathroom safety equipment. Patient comfort and convenience are aided by commodes and elevated toilet seats. Caregivers are helped by patient lifters, plastic and enamel ware, rubber goods, and means of administering heat, cold, and other physical treatments. The many benefits of HHC—financial, physical, social, and spiritual—are more difficult to obtain in the absence of proper facilities.[1]

The selection of hospital equipment for the home is largely determined by the nature of the patient's condition. However, the HHC pharmacist must also carefully evaluate the needs of the caregiver when recommending equipment. The caregiver is part of a team (which may include the pharmacist, physician, nurse, occupational and physical therapists, respiratory therapist, social worker, and psychologist, among others) that must plan and implement care that will meet the patient's needs and choices, and his or her ability to carry out the care plan is crucial to its success. Further, the caregiver is often the principal point of contact between the HHC pharmacist and the patient care team. Two major sections of this chapter will discuss these devices, their proper selection and adjustment for patient use, steps necessary to maintain the equipment in good condition, and information consumers should know to use the devices safely and effectively.

AMBULATORY AIDS

Ambulatory (or mobility) aids are often classified into five major groups. In order of the amount of physical support they provide, they are: canes, crutches, walkers, wheelchairs, and motorized chairs and scooters. They range in the same order from relatively simple devices selling for under $10 to complex, even computerized, equipment costing tens of thousands of dollars. The HHC pharmacist may not be the provider of the entire array of these devices, but, as an adviser on HME, he or she should be conversant with their variety and availability.

Disability and Barriers to Access

An injury can be measured in absolute terms. Joint dysfunction, for example, is expressible as diminished range of motion, and measurable in degrees of movement before and after the illness episode. Disability is a relative term, however, and the degree of disability can be different in two individuals with same absolute injury. Disability measures the extent to which an individual is restricted or at a disadvantage because of injury (or other impairment). The disadvantage is a function of bodily limitations, but also of perceptions. Therefore, a disability is lessened by removing the physical restriction, by improving the patient's ability to cope with the disability, and may also be diminished when others view it in a new light.

Under the Americans with Disabilities Act (ADA)[2] an "individual with a disability" is defined as a person who "has a physical or mental impairment which substantially limits a major life activity." Major life activities include walking, seeing, hearing, speaking, breathing, learning, working, caring for one's self, and performing manual tasks. Institutions, businesses, programs, or other activities receiving federal financial assistance may not exclude an otherwise qualified individual with handicaps from employment or participation solely because of his or her disability, and must provide reasonable accommodation to allow that individual to participate. This is a legislative enactment of the ethical principle that we should act when reasonable to remove barriers preventing our fellow citizens with disabilities from having fair access to society's benefits and burdens.

Many reasonably removable barriers to access exist in our environments. Curbs at crosswalks, for example, are easily replaced by ramps. Doors and hallways can be made a little larger in public places. Controls on elevators can be placed at chair level. These are just examples; other barriers have been described elsewhere.[3,4] Even health practitioners who wish to serve the needs of patients with disabilities may work in environments that present barriers to access.[5] The HHC pharmacist should make certain that his or her practice environment is barrier-free. Equally important, the HHC pharmacist should begin to think differently about access, removing barriers, and just how relative a disability can be. Changes in the pharmacist's awareness of access issues can also eliminate barriers to communication with patients.[6] When barriers to access and communication are eliminated in the HHC pharmacy practice site, the HHC pharmacist will be better positioned to recommend devices to improve the patient's mobility.

Canes

Canes provide, as do other ambulatory aids, the ability to transfer weight from a weakened limb or body hemisphere to the device. Their most important function, however, may be to provide balance, and an increased sense of security, rather than significant physical support. They are generally made of wood or metal, but other materials, includ-

Figure 11-1 Canes

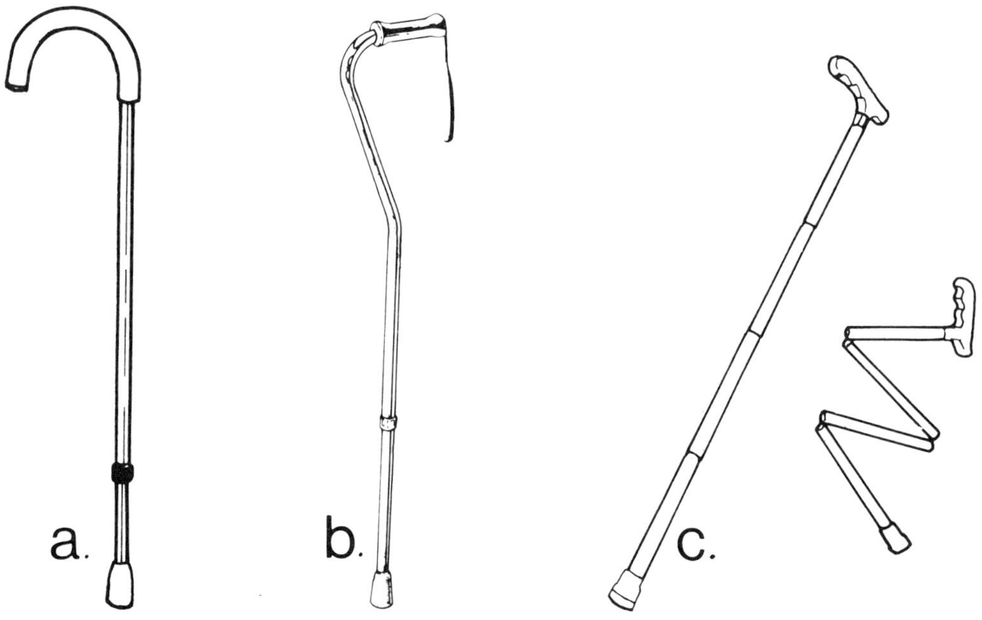

a. standard adjustable aluminum monopod cane;
b. adjustable aluminum monopod cane with offset handle and handgrip;
c. T-handled folding monopod cane.

Figure 11-2 Aluminum Quad Canes

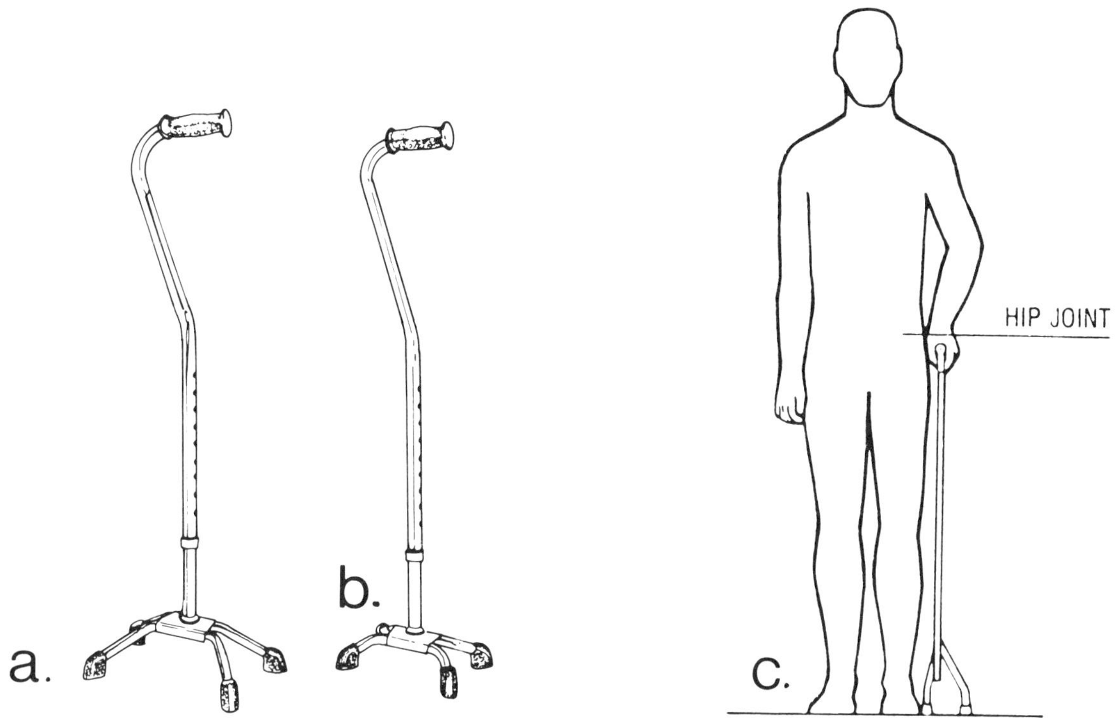

a. large base cane;
b. small base cane;
c. proper placement of quad cane.

ing fiberglass and Lucite, are also used. The most common designs are either single point canes or quad canes (see Figures 11-1 and 11-2).

Important considerations in cane selection are choice of single point or quad style, proper adjustment of cane height, selection of a comfortable and utilitarian handle, and maintenance of the tip(s). Other factors include weight, portability, cost, and appearance. Patients should understand on which side the cane is best carried, the importance of tip inspection, and safety precautions for certain environments or when in the presence of others. Cane users must have good arm, wrist, and grip strength on at least one body side. The HHC pharmacist should ensure that a cane will provide support appropriate to a given patient's circumstances.

Single Point Canes. The standard, wooden, "crook-handled" cane is well known. Its chief advantage is its low cost: standard wood canes can be purchased for under $15. However, its handle may be uncomfortable for some users and may be undesirable for patients with arthritis. Although the tight curve of the handle may not actually promote hand deformities, it is unlikely to mitigate them. More serious, perhaps, is that the weight of the user's body cannot be placed directly above the shaft of the cane, thus reducing the device's stability. Finally, adjusting the cane requires removal of part of the base end; it can only be shortened, never lengthened.

Some wooden canes are fitted with a "T" handle, which is regarded as more comfortable, albeit more expensive. The handle also allows more of the patient's weight to be distributed directly over the shaft. Wooden canes also have a variety of lengths and shaft diameters. Canes designed for smaller persons are generally lighter and have thinner shafts, which may taper toward the base.

Freed from some limitations imposed by wood, aluminum canes offer several advantages. Some feature the traditional crook-handle, but many have an offset handle that places the weight in a line with the shaft. Aluminum canes are generally lighter than wood canes of the same size and strength. Handle designs include foam or padded grips, and may be flattened to spread pressure more evenly across the palmar surface.

Telescoping canes consist of a two-part shaft, the lower portion sliding within the upper, and are easily shortened or lengthened. Their adjustment is made possible by spring loaded buttons on the inner tube that engage into holes drilled on the outer portion. A threaded bushing is usually located on the base end of the upper tube; it is loosened prior to adjustment and then tightened to add stability to the cane and prevent rattling.

Several manufacturers produce a folding aluminum cane composed of several sections that can be taken apart. The sections are linked by an elastic cord that keeps them tightly nested when the cane is assembled. The manufacturers claim strength and stability equivalent to tapered aluminum canes of the same shaft diameter.

Quad Canes. Quad canes, with four tips, provide increased stability due to their widened base, and users may transfer more weight to these canes than to single point models. However, quad canes are generally heavier and less easy to handle than single point canes. The laterally-extended tips of these canes are also more likely to catch on furniture, corners of walls, or other obstructions. Depending on the patient's needs, strength, and environment, the HHC pharmacist must help the patient choose among varying base sizes. Larger sizes provide greater stability, but are more unwieldy. Another choice regarding the base is between traditional metal base plates and newer bases made of composite materials that are less likely to deform under the weight of a heavy patient.

The shaft of the quad cane is not centered on the base plate, but is located closer to one pair of tips than the other. It is important that the cane is carried so that the tips nearest the shaft are also closest to the patient's body. Otherwise, stability is lessened and the user is more apt to trip on a cane tip. The hand grip must be rotated 180° about the shaft to adjust the cane for one side of the body or the other.

Adjustment. Except for the cutting required for wood or certain metal canes, adjustment is relatively easy. A general rule can be followed for canes, most crutches, and walkers: when the user stands with his or her arms hanging loosely at the side, the top of the hand grip should be at the same level as the crease on the inside of the wrist. Some authors recommend adjusting the cane so that the top of the handle is level with the patient's greater trochanter.[7] Either method will result in 20° to 30° of flexion (the interior angle between the upper arm and forearm will therefore be between 150° and 160°) in the patient's elbow during normal use.

If a cane must be cut to fit, the device should be turned upside down with the hand grip resting on the floor next to the patient's foot. Mark where the crease in the wrist crosses the cane shaft. Cut the cane approximately 1/4" shorter than this to allow for the thickness of the crutch tip. Wooden canes may be cut with a fine-toothed crosscut saw, assisted by a miter box. It is tempting to use a hacksaw for aluminum canes, but a tubing cutter is less likely to deform the shaft and readily produces a true right angle cut.

Most persons' arms are of unequal length. This is seldom significant for the user who wishes to switch the cane from one hand to another. However, some individuals with skeletal deformities (e.g., scoliosis) may need to be measured on both sides, particularly if two canes will be used.

Tip care. The tip is the part of the cane most subject to wear, and most likely to cause injury if not properly maintained. Tips on rented canes must be carefully inspected each time the cane is returned and before being rented again. Ideally, new tips should be provided each time a cane is rented. Users must be instructed to inspect their tips periodically, and replace them if the base is no longer flat or if the circular grooves in the base have disappeared. When replacing tips on metal canes, it is imperative that metal slugs are placed at the inside base of the tip to keep the raw edge of the shaft from cutting through.

Although the tips provided by the manufacturer are sometimes somewhat rounded at the base, a tip with a flat or concave base is preferred. The tip should be sufficiently flexible so that the base remains in contact with the ground as the shaft pivots through a step.

Tips are sized by inside diameter, which corresponds to the outside diameter of the cane shaft. If too small a tip is chosen, the base of the shaft will not firmly contact the inside base of the tip, and the tip will feel "spongy" in use. The American Standards Association (ASA) has established a scale for cane, crutch, and walker tips. Cane and walker tips typically range between ASA sizes 15 and 19, while crutch tips are more commonly sized between ASA 18 and 21. Table 11-1 lists typical ASA sizes and corresponding inside diameters (also called the plug size) for cane tips, along with standard overall widths for the base.

Patient instructions. A cane aids balance

Table 11 - 1 Cane Tip Dimensions

ASA SIZE	PLUG SIZE	BASE WIDTH
15	3/8"	1-1/8"
16	1/2"	1-1/8"
17	5/8"	1-1/8"
18	3/4"	1-1/4"
19	7/8"	1-1/2"

and lets the user transfer weight from the injured or weakened side to a stronger side or limb. Unless the physician or therapist has instructed otherwise, the pharmacist may counsel the patient to carry the cane on the side opposite the affected limb or joint. The goal is to provide the patient with a gait that is as close to natural as possible, thus minimizing subsequent hip and back problems. When a cane is used for balance only, the patient may carry it on either side. When walking with the cane held on the strong side, the patient will transfer weight to the cane and move the good foot forward, then transfer weight to the good leg and move the weak leg and cane forward.

Examples of worn tips are useful to demonstrate to the patient when tips should be replaced. In addition users should understand how to adjust cane height, how to adjust a quad cane for the alternate side of the body, and how to take advantage of canes with adjustable hand grips. Folding cane users must understand how to inspect the cane for complete fit of each section prior to placing weight on the device.

Cane users must have a strategy for using their canes on stairs. Quad canes may not fit on the step if used in the normal manner, but may fit if turned sideways. As with crutches, the cane should be kept below the user's center of gravity at all times. It is best to depend on the handrail rather than the cane whenever possible.

Crutches

The wrist and hand provide most of the stability and weight transfer when using a cane; crutches depend more fully on the forearms and upper arms. Crutches clearly provide more stability than canes, and may be used where there is more severe involvement of the lower body, such as patients who must avoid bearing weight on one limb. Principal varieties of crutches are forearm crutches, platform crutches, and axillary crutches. As with canes, crutches are usually made of wood or aluminum. Quad crutches are also available. See Figure 11-3.

Forearm crutches. Forearm crutches provide extra support to the forearm and elbow because they have a cuff that fits around the fleshy portion of the forearm (see Figure 11-3). They are usually made from aluminum. A handgrip is attached at right angle to the shaft, and points forward in use. The portion of the shaft above the handgrip is usually angled back to allow for an elbow bend of about 30°. Forearm crutches with open cuffs may also be called Canadian or Lofstrand crutches, and the cuffs open to the front or the side. Kenny sticks are forearm crutches with closed cuffs, and are named after Sister Elizabeth Kenny, an Australian nurse who first used them in the 1920's for patients with poliomyelitis. One advantage of forearm cuffs is that the user may let go of the hand grip and the cuff will prevent the crutch from falling. This frees the user's hand for other purposes. To be effective in this way, the cuff must fit snugly around the forearm and must swivel freely over 180° of arc. Side opening cuffs are less apt to fall off than are front opening cuffs.

Forearm crutches are more expensive than underarm crutches. They are selected most frequently for persons who will use crutches on a long-term basis, rather than for the patient with a temporary need (e.g., with a broken leg). However, their greater ease of use makes them more ideal for patients with good upper body strength; they would be the rental crutches of choice for young people with legs on the mend if it weren't for their higher cost.

Platform crutches. Platform crutches are used for persons with inadequate grip strength or other inability to use a handgrip. A forearm rest (the platform) is mounted at right angle to the shaft, and the forearm is firmly bound to the platform with wide nylon and Velcro straps. The platform may be fitted to the top of a shaft from a forearm crutch (in which case it may be called a forearm cane) or a platform attachment is available for use on aluminum axillary crutches. In use, the elbow is bent at 90° so that the forearm is parallel to the ground, and the user's weight is transferred to the upper arm.

Axillary crutches. Axillary crutches extend from the ground to the underarm (axilla) and have both a handgrip and an axillary support. The traditional axillary crutch is made of wood or aluminum, and the handgrip is mounted between two upright supports. The axillary support spans the upright supports at their upper ends, and the uprights remain

Figure 11-3 Crutches

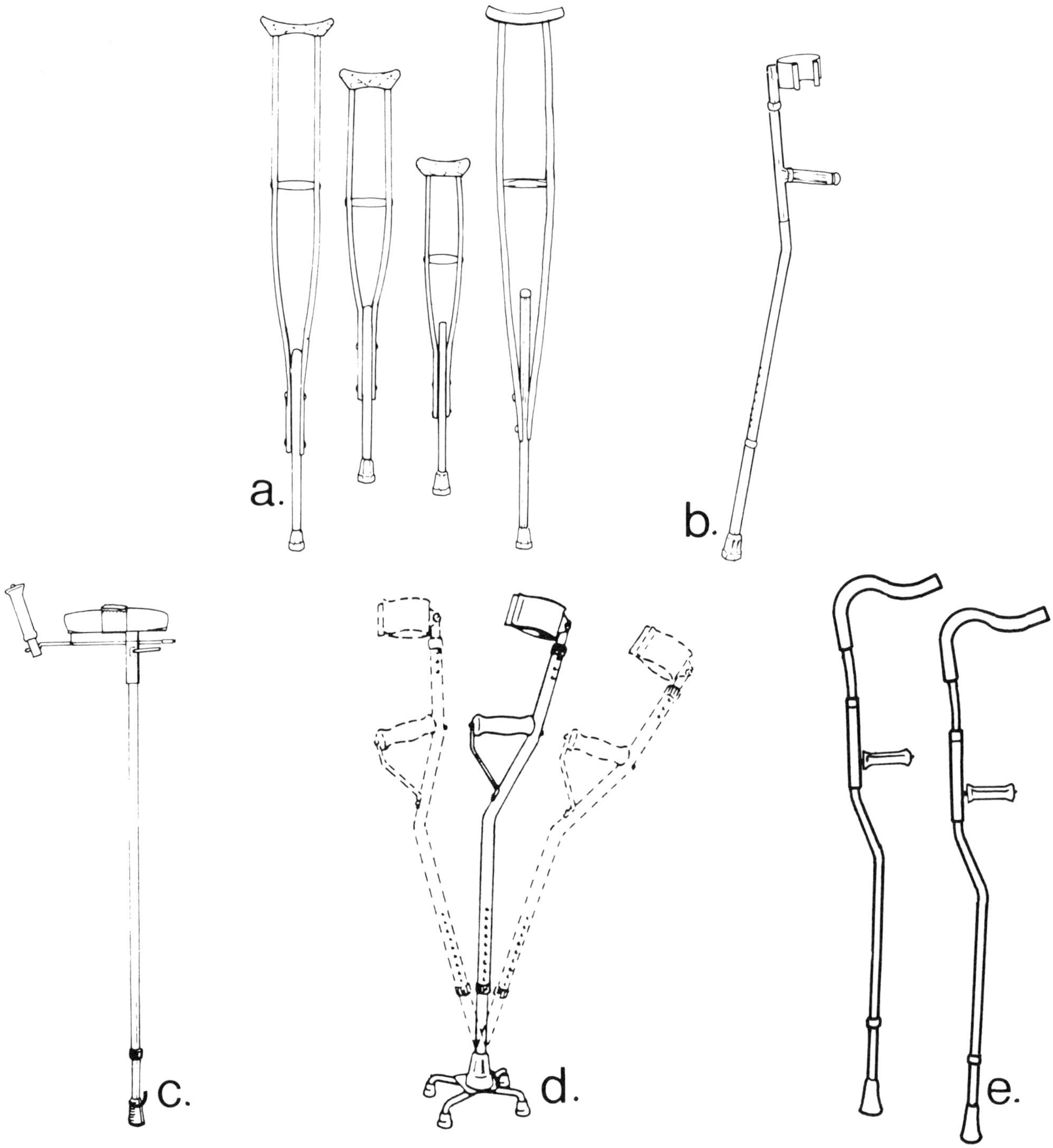

a. wood and aluminum crutches;
b. forearm crutch with side-opening cuff;
c. platform crutch;
d. forearm quad crutch;
e. shepherd's crook axillary crutch.

parallel until just below the handgrip, where they curve toward each other. At their lower ends, the pair of uprights join to a single lower support whose position between the uprights can be adjusted to shorten or lengthen the crutch.

Single shaft axillary crutches are also available. One type is made from laminated wood; the single upright curves forward above the handgrip to position a wooden axillary support directly over the handgrip. The length of this crutch is modified by trimming the lower end of the shaft. Aluminum single shaft axillary crutches are sometimes called "shepherd's crook" crutches. The lower portion of the shaft, from the handgrip down, is identical to that of a forearm crutch. An axillary support replaces the forearm cuff. Unlike the forearm crutch, single shaft axillary crutches are usually used with the handgrip pointing toward the rear.

Quad crutches. Forearm crutches with quad bases are useful for persons with upper body spasticity, or balance and stability problems, as in patients with multiple sclerosis (MS). These individuals may have difficulty predictably placing the crutch near their side. Quad crutches have a four-footed base attached to the crutch shaft by a flexible rubber mount. As the user walks, the flexible mount permits all four feet to remain in contact with the ground, even if the crutch is positioned at widely divergent points.

Precautions when purchasing crutches. Crutches are frequently rented items in the HME pharmacy. They must be sufficiently durable to withstand treatment by renters, and the crutch must survive for enough rental cycles to be able to return a profit to the renter. Crutches should be easily and quickly adjustable so as to minimize labor costs associated with fitting. Replacement parts should be readily available, because a crutch in poor repair when rented poses serious legal liability for the pharmacist. Finally, the crutch's finish must resist nicks, scratches, and discoloration; no customer wants to rent a beat-up looking pair of crutches.

There are several characteristics of an acceptable forearm crutch. The cuff should be adjustable so it may be worn without sleeves as well as with a jacket. It should pivot 180° to allow freedom of arm movement. A comfortable and appropriately padded handgrip should be welded (not riveted) securely to the crutch shaft. The upper portion of the shaft must adjust to allow the cuff to be placed over the fleshy part of the forearm while avoiding any pressure on the medial or lateral epicondyles of the elbow. The lower shaft adjustment should be enabled by a pair of spring-loaded buttons, not just one. The buttons should be bullet-shaped so they continue to fit snugly as the adjustment holes enlarge slightly over time. A bushing should be used to keep the inner shaft from rattling within the outer shaft as the user walks with the crutches. As with all crutches, the tips should be large, with a "suction" base, flexible, and in good repair.

Adjustment. Crutches are available to fit most people, from toddler to large adult. Depending on the manufacturer, they may be labeled by size category (e.g., CHILD, YOUTH, ADULT), or may be marked with a range that corresponds to the user's overall height (e.g., 4'6" to 5'0"). The first step in fitting a crutch is to select one from the proper category. Some pharmacists find it useful to wrap colored plastic tape (e.g., blue for child, green for youth, etc.) around a portion of the shaft for quick recognition of the approximate size of the crutch. Table 11-2 provides a quick reference guide to initial selection of a basic axillary crutch, according to the user's height. The length range shown for a given type is the typical range over which adjustments can

Table 11-2 Guide to Initial Crutch Size

Patient Height Range	Type	Crutch Length Range
48-55 in (122-140 cm)	Child	30-38 in (76- 97 cm)
56-63 in (143-160 cm)	Youth	36-48 in (91-122 cm)
64-69 in (163-175 cm)	Med. Adult	42-55 in (107-140 cm)
70-75 in (178-191 cm)	Adult	48-60 in (122-152 cm)
76-79 in (193-201 cm)	Tall Adult	54-66 in (137-168 cm)

(Adapted from "Crutch Scale" in Canes, Crutches, and Sick Room Supplies, p. 42, Harvy Surgical Supply Corp., Flushing, NY, 1979.)

be made to that type. As a rule, the required axillary crutch length is approximately 16 inches (40 cm) shorter than the patient's overall height.

The patient's weight should primarily rest on the forearms, hands, and wrists during use. Axillary and forearm crutches, therefore, should be adjusted to place the patient's elbow in approximately 30° of flexion. As with canes, the handgrip will be at about the level of the crease in the user's wrist when the arms hang loosely at the side. The axillary bar is intended as a stabilizer parallel to the rib cage. It is not designed for primary weight bearing. Clearance must exist between the axilla and the top of the axillary support, so that when the user walks with the crutch there is no pressure on the nerves, glands, and blood vessels in the arm pit.

With forearm and single shaft axillary crutches, the pharmacist should first adjust the handgrip height by lengthening or shortening the lower shaft. The cuff or axillary support may then be adjusted. The cuff on a forearm crutch should be positioned at the fleshy part of the forearm, with the upper edge of the cuff approximately one inch (2.5 cm) below the medial and lateral epicondyles of the elbow. If the cuff is too high, pressure on these bony prominences will eventually result in painful irritation that resembles tennis elbow. If the cuff is positioned too low (i.e., greater than 1 1/2" or 4 cm below the elbow), the stability of the crutch will be compromised. Likewise, when adjusting the upper portion of an axillary crutch, two or three finger breadths of clearance should remain between the axillary support and the underarm area. If one or both of the user's shoulders are forced to rise up when walking with the crutch, it is a clear sign that the crutch is too long.

The order of adjustment should be reversed for a standard axillary crutch. The overall length of the crutch is modified first, then the handgrip height is adjusted. Many aluminum axillary crutches have lower supports that adjust with spring loaded buttons. For these, the overall length is first adjusted by placing the crutch under the standing individual's arm and moving the lower shaft in or out. The handgrip bolt may be removed and the handgrip adjusted to the level of the wrist.

In wooden and some aluminum models, the lower support is held in place by two machine bolts that must be removed to adjust the length. Since this is more time consuming than for crutches with button adjustments, it is better to measure the person with a cloth tape, then adjust the crutch to fit these measurements. The procedure is:[6]

Overall length—Have the user stand at ease with his or her arms at the side. Mark a spot on the floor that is six inches in front of the toe of the user's shoe and two inches laterally from the side of the shoe. Now measure the straight-line distance from this spot to the user's axilla. Deduct two inches from this measurement to obtain the desired overall length of the crutch.

Handgrip height—Measure from the crease in the individual's wrist to the floor to obtain the desired distance between the handgrip and the base of the crutch tip.

Adjusting the length—Lay the crutch on a flat surface and remove the two machine bolts holding the lower upright support in place. The two parallel uprights will spring apart. Place the lower upright next to one of the paired uprights and slide it up or down until the distance between the crutch tip and the top of the axillary support matches the desired overall length of the crutch. Insert the machine screws through the holes in one side support and the lower upright support to temporarily hold the lower upright in position. Now remove the machine bolt holding the handgrip in place, and move the handgrip to a new position so that the desired distance between the handgrip and the crutch tip is realized. Reinsert the handgrip bolt and replace the wing nut. The two side supports may now be brought together and the position of the lower support permanently fixed.

Repeat the steps for the other crutch and, by having the user place the crutch under the arm, verify that the elbow bend is approximately 30° and that there is sufficient clearance under the arm. In general, the topmost hole in the lower support of a wooden crutch should not be used; select the next larger crutch instead.

As with other ambulatory aids, crutches should be adjusted with all intended attachments and accessories (e.g., tips, pads, cushions) in place. When adjusting aids used in walking, the user should be wearing normal footwear. Figure 11-4 illustrates fitting guidelines for axillary and forearm crutches.

Crutch tips are generally larger than cane tips, but should otherwise meet the same criteria. For a given diameter of tip, "standard" and "oversize" varieties are available, referring to the surface area in contact with the ground. Like cane tips, the inside diameter can be stated by ASA size number or by plug size. Table 11-3 lists typical measurements for crutch tips. Tips for aluminum crutches with cut shafts require metal slugs in their bases. Oversize tips are preferred. Crutch tips must be inspected regularly prior to rental or sale. Both handgrip and axillary support pads are available. For hygienic reasons, axillary cushions and handgrip pads should not be rented or resold; they are inexpensive enough that each consumer should purchase his or her own.

Instructions to patients. Patients should know how to inspect the crutch tips, and how to adjust the devices. There are several ways of walking with crutches, called gaits, and the patient may be helped to select the most suitable one. Finally, the patient must know how to negotiate stairs and other special locations.

A gait used with a single crutch is called the hemiplegic gait. The cane or crutch is carried on the user's strong side, and weight is transferred to the crutch while the good leg is moved forward. The weight is then transferred to the good leg, and the crutch and the weak leg are brought forward. The user alternates these two steps in a manner identical to the use of a walking cane.

Figure 11- 4 Fitting Guide for Crutches

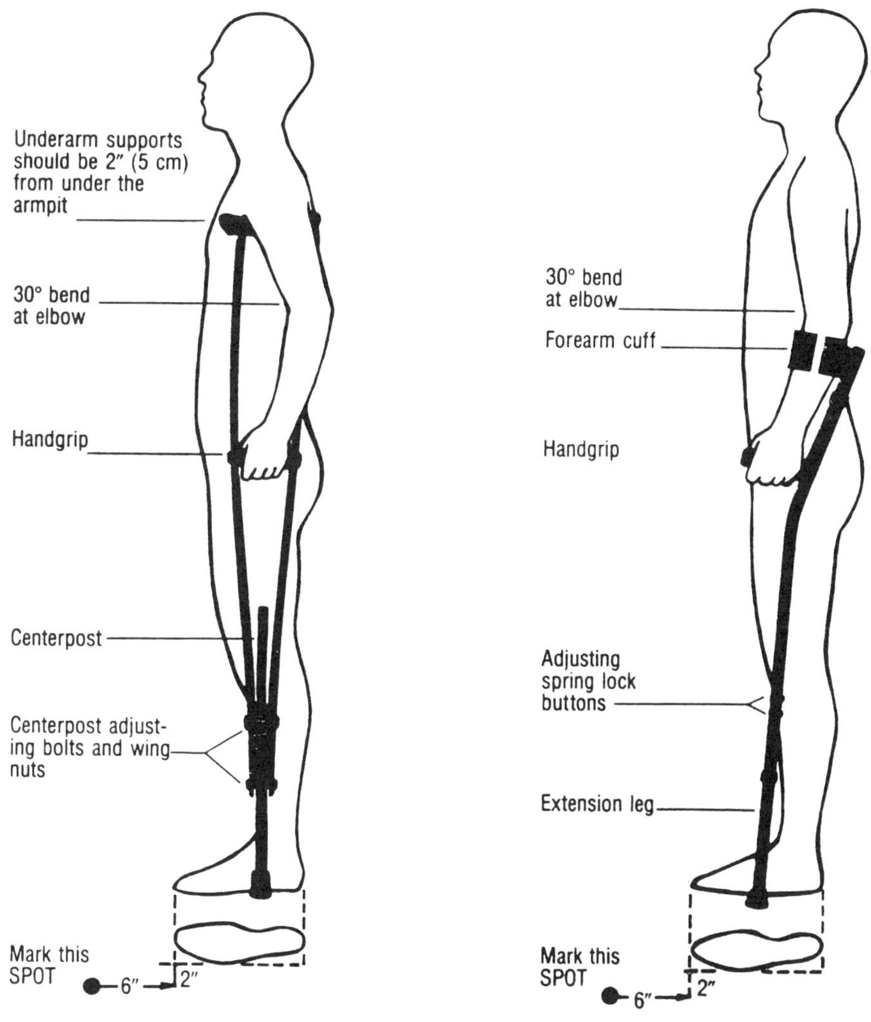

(Modified with permission of Futuro.)

Table 11-3 Crutch Tip Dimensions

ASA Size	Plug Size	Width for Normal Base	Width for Extra-Large
18	3/4	1-1/2	1-3/4
19	7/8	1-1/2	1-3/4
20	1	1-1/2	1-3/4
21	1-1/8	1-1/2	1-3/4

Adapted from "Cane and Crutch Tip Information and Technical Conversion Scale," in Canes, Crutches, and Sick Room Supplies, p. 47, Harvy Surgical Supply Corp., Flushing, NY, 1979.

The two-point gait (which keeps two points—one crutch and one foot on the ground at all times) is used with two crutches, and is also used with double canes. As the user moves one leg forward, he or she simultaneously moves the crutch on the opposite side: right crutch-left leg, then left crutch-right leg, and so on.

There are two versions of the three-point gait: swing-to and swing-through. These are often used when the patient has one leg in a non-weight-bearing cast. In the swing-to version, the crutches are moved forward together, then the legs are brought forward to a point even with the crutches. In the swing-through version, the legs are brought forward to a point ahead of the crutches. The swing-through gait is probably the fastest crutch gait, but it requires good strength and balance. A youth with a broken leg will almost naturally adopt the swing-through gait.

The most stable gait is the four-point gait. The user moves one crutch forward, then brings the opposite foot forward. The other crutch is brought even with that foot, then the remaining foot is brought even with the first crutch. A typical repeating pattern would be: right crutch - left leg - left crutch - right leg.

Stairs can be negotiated by holding the crutches in one hand and holding to the handrail with the other. When using crutches instead of the handrail, the patient should keep the crutches below the center of gravity. Thus, when ascending, the legs go up one step first, then the crutches are brought up to that step. When descending, the crutches are first placed on the next lower step, then the legs brought even with the crutches. The swing-through gait should be avoided on stairs.

First-time crutch users may be oblivious to the danger that crutches may pose to others. A tactful reminder should be given that when seated on a bus, in a restaurant, or similar public place, the crutches should be held vertically at the side, or laid on the floor at the base of the wall where others cannot stumble over them.

Walkers

Walkers provide a more stable platform of support than canes for the patient with reasonable strength in hands, wrists and arms. To provide this stability, however, the walker must be adjusted so that all four feet will be in contact with the floor whenever weight is placed on the device. In use, the patient picks up the walker and moves it forward, then walks toward the device. The pharmacist should reinforce the safe use of a walker by teaching the patient to walk "into" a walker, but never to walk "in" it.

Walkers may be standard (i.e., non-folding), folding, reciprocating, and/or wheeled. All types are available with adjustable legs, but non-adjustable standard walkers are also available. Walkers are available in adult (31-37" or 80-95 cm high), youth (28-32" or 70-80 cm), and child (20-26" or 50-65 cm) sizes. See Figure 11-5.

Folding and non-folding walkers. Walkers typically consist of two side frames connected by upper and lower bridging tubing in the front. The side frames are often molded from a single piece of aluminum tubing, and are strengthened by a cross brace near the lower end of the tubing. Extensible legs are formed from smaller diameter tubing that inserts into the bottom ends of the side frames. In non-folding walkers, the lower portion of the front bridge is often continuous with the side braces, and the top bridging tubing is of one-piece construction. Folding walkers differ in that the bridging tubing is not continuous with the side bracing, is attached to the side frames using a collar that allows the side frames to fold, and the top bridge can lengthen or

Figure 11-5 Walkers

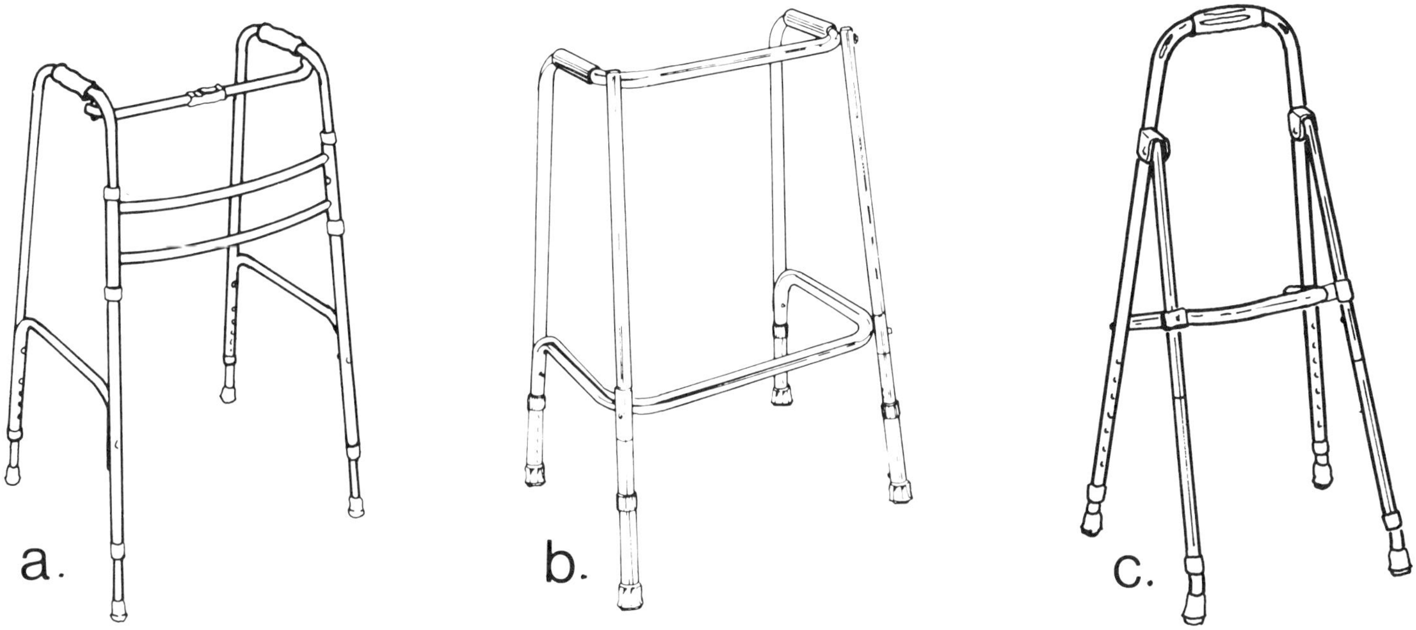

a. adjustable, folding walker with bridge style frame;
b. adjustable walker with modified physical therapy style frame;
c. side walker.

shorten as the side frames are folded together. The height of the lower bridging tube and side-frame bracing varies; most popular walkers have the bridging tubing high enough to allow them to be used in front of a toilet.

Folding walkers are easily portable, but are more expensive, and may be slightly heavier. They have the additional advantage that one side only may be folded in, forming an L-shaped device that may fit in narrow spaces. Most users wanting to rent walkers need to transport them in a car, and will prefer a folding walker for that reason. Modern folding walkers are virtually as durable as non-folding types, so the primary basis for choosing between the types is cost.

Wheeled walkers. Both folding and non-folding walkers may be equipped with wheels, which are indicated for patients who need a walker but cannot or should not lift the walker to use it. Two-wheeled models have wheels at the base of the front legs only, and the rear legs must be picked up to roll the walker forward. Four-wheeled models are also available. Early designs for wheeled walkers were criticized as being inherently unstable and unsafe.[7] Modern wheeled walkers have safety features such as adjustable wheel drag, caliper brakes, and large wheels that allow outdoor use; these seem to satisfy the requirements of more recent writers.[8]

Reciprocating walkers. Reciprocating (or reciprocal) walkers are similar to folding walkers, except that the sides never fold completely flat. Rather, one side may be moved forward at a time, leaving at least two legs constantly on the ground. Their use is similar to two canes, and the two-point gait is utilized. Reciprocating walkers require the ability to tilt the walker slightly from side to side, and do not provide the stability of standard walkers. Infrequently purchased, they are used primarily during rehabilitation to retrain the patient in the mechanics of walking.

Side walkers. Side walkers are also called hemiplegic or hemi walkers, or walkanes. They are carried, one-handed, on the user's side. The two legs nearest the user are formed from one piece of tubing, and the handgrip is located on the transverse portion of the tube. A second set of legs are attached to this frame and extend further to the side. Side walkers provide greater stability than quad canes, but are less cumbersome than full walkers. Most can be folded for transport. The patient should be instructed by the physician or therapist on which side to carry the device. Normally, it will be used, like a cane, on the strong side.

Adjustment and maintenance. The height adjustment for walkers is made in the same fashion as for canes. When the user is standing up to the front of the walker with his arms at the side, the handgrips should reach to the crease on the inside of the wrist. In use, therefore, the elbow will be in about 30° of flexion.

A few users may tend to lean into the front of the walker, and can tip it forward. As a result, some authors show walkers with the front legs (those away from the user) adjusted one or two inches (2.5 to 5 cm) longer than the rear. In this case, the adjustment for handgrip height should be made at the rear legs. Most individuals, however, will have their walker adjusted with all four legs set at the same length.

As with other walking aids, tip care is of paramount importance. Walker tips are generally rounded at their base, in contrast to the flat base of cane and crutch tips. This minimizes the tendency for the tips to catch on the floor as the walker is moved. A steel insert in the base of the tip is essential. Tips range from ASA sizes 15 through 21. The wheels and braking systems on wheeled walkers should be regularly inspected, lubricated as appropriate, and kept free of debris which might affect their operation.

Wheelchairs and Scooters

As noted in the title of a publication of the American Rehabilitation Association, wheelchair selection is "More than Choosing a Chair with Wheels." Available models range from an inexpensive "standard" chair, useful for temporary transportation and costing a few hundred dollars, to complex high technology wheelchair systems at $75,000 or more. The HHC pharmacist must exercise the same care in selecting a wheelchair as in filling a prescription for a legend drug; Veterans Administration studies show an equivalent potential for patient harm from a misprescribed wheelchair as from an inappropriately ordered medication.[9]

Engineering and technological advances have greatly increased the complexity and variety of wheelchairs and scooters,[10] and new wheelchair testing standards are resulting in better information for selection and prescription of wheelchairs.[11] Increasingly, provision of wheelchairs for chronic use is becoming highly specialized, and the HHC pharmacist is more likely to be a referral agent than a primary provider. To be effective in the referral role, however, he or she must possess a basic understanding of wheelchair technology and options.

Patient factors. The most obvious patient factor in wheelchair selection is size, but several other considerations are also important. Among these are:

1. General physical condition. In spite of the particular disability that mandates the use of a wheelchair, users vary in their strength and endurance. Thus, one patient with paraplegia may actively participate in various sporting activities, while another may not. In addition to the patient's current condition, it is helpful to consider the likely progression of the patient's underlying disorder, particularly in degenerative diseases, so as to predict future needs during the normal life of the wheelchair.
2. Focal paralyses. Individuals with hemiplegia may require a chair with a one-handed drive mechanism, a special axle that links both main wheels, and/or seat height adjusted to allow the patient to place a foot on the floor for propulsion and steering. Most patients with paraplegia retain their upper body functions, but require special attention to seat design and fitting to minimize decubitus ulcer formation. Users with quadriplegia will often require motorized chairs; they may have sufficient use of an arm to allow hand controls, but some need fairly exotic steering and control mechanisms.
3. Spasticity. Patients with cerebral palsy or multiple sclerosis will need chairs equipped with belts or supports to aid their positioning. When motorized chairs and electronic controls are used, an adjustable level of tolerance must be available in the control to minimize erratic chair movement.
4. Systemic disease. Rheumatoid arthritis may be eased by greater seat height, elevated leg rests to minimize contractures, and projections on the wheel rim to compensate for lack of grip, among other chair adaptations. Diabetes mellitus may predispose patients to pressure sores, particularly on their heels, and they may have reduced rate of wound healing. Users with respiratory difficulty may require special positioning features; formerly they were fitted

with reclining chair backs, but newer "tilt-in-space" designs allow positioning for postural drainage while retaining the optimum relationship between head, trunk, and legs to allow patient comfort.

5. Amputation. A change in frame design is needed to compensate for the loss of the weight of the lower extremities in patients with above-the-knee amputations. For these reasons, an outdoor style chair will be modified so that the large rear wheels are set further back, thus reducing the chance of backward tipover. Amputation of one arm will necessitate a one-wheel drive chair.

Chair Types. Most modern wheelchairs feature large drive wheels at the rear of the chair and smaller pilot wheels in the front. These are derived from a general design that has been called an "outdoor chair" to distinguish it from an older and rarely used design (the "indoor chair") that had drive wheels in the front. Modern chairs can be roughly placed in three categories: Standard Weight, Lightweight and High Strength Lightweight, and Custom Ultralight. All chairs may be adapted, either in design or with accessories, to accommodate a variety of operating environments and user preferences and needs.

Standard Weight Chairs. Featuring chrome-plated steel frames, these chairs have push handles and frame extensions ("tipping levers") that allow an attendant to provide propulsion, steering, and manipulation of the chair over a variety of terrains, both indoors and out. Figure 11-6 depicts a standard weight chair.

These chairs are generally available with seat widths ranging from 16 to 22 inches (40 to 55 cm) in roughly 2-inch (5 cm) increments. Some manufacturers produce 14-inch (35 cm) wide chairs, and some produce "hemi-height" chairs with lower seat heights. Other major options are fixed or detachable arm rests, amputee adapters, and specification of overall chair, seat, and back rest height as well as seat depth and leg length.

Lightweight Chairs. Lightweight chairs are similar in design to standard weight chairs, but of lighter construction from chrome plated steel. They are an appropriate option for users who are not physically active and have limited strength. High strength lightweight chairs are made from aluminum, and offer greater durability at a higher price. Similar options in features are found in these chairs, except seat widths are typically limited and range between 16 and 20 inches (40 to 50 cm).

Properly included among lightweight chairs

Figure 11-6 Standard Outdoor Wheelchair Showing Major Parts and Terminology

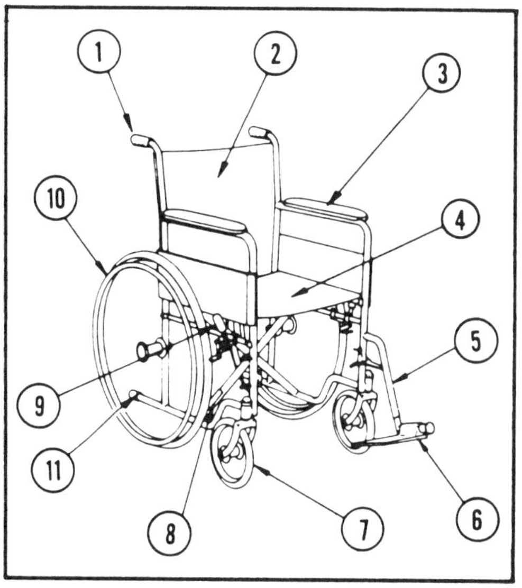

1. Handgrips/Push Handles
2. Back Upholstery
3. Armrests
4. Seat Upholstery
5. Front Rigging
6. Footplate
7. Casters
8. Crossbraces
9. Wheel Locks
10. Wheel and Handrim
11. Tipping Lever

(Courtesy: Everest & Jennings)

is the compact travel chair, which is designed for temporary use, such as taking a patient shopping. It is a folding chair with four small wheels, and requires an attendant. The absence of the large drive wheels is especially helpful when the chair is transported in a compact car.

Custom "Ultralight" Chairs. Featuring both rigid and folding frames, these chairs are constructed from high strength but lightweight materials such as aluminum, titanium, and carbon fiber. These chairs are intended for active users who seldom depend on others for propulsion, and often lack hand grips or tilting aids. These designs feature a low profile and minimal arm and back support, and require good upper body strength. A common feature is quick release axles on the drive wheels, so the wheels may be removed for transportation. See Figure 11-7.

Ultralight chairs are frequently custom-designed for a particular user, and may cost as much as a compact car. A special variety of custom chairs includes high performance chairs for athletic use. Sports chairs are even more streamlined than their counterparts used for daily transportation, and are often modified for particular sports. The variety of wheelchair sports is exemplified by the many sports organizations listed in Sport 'N Spokes magazine.[12] A list of the affiliated governing bodies for major wheelchair sports is available from the National Wheelchair Athletic Association (3595 E. Fountain Blvd., Suite L-1, Colorado Springs, CO; 719-574-1150).

Special Considerations for Young Users. Children are not "miniature adults," especially because the body proportions in adults and children are not the same. For example, the ratio of arm height (the height of the arm rest above the seat) to back height is 0.6 for adult chairs, 0.5 for a child's chair, and 0.33 for a toddler's chair. Thus, wheelchairs and similar mobility aids for young people cannot simply be downsized from the adult version. Except for strictly limited short-term use, an adult chair should not be sold or rented for a child's use.

Interaction with the environment may be more critical to growth and development in child-

Figure 11-7 Ultra Light Chair

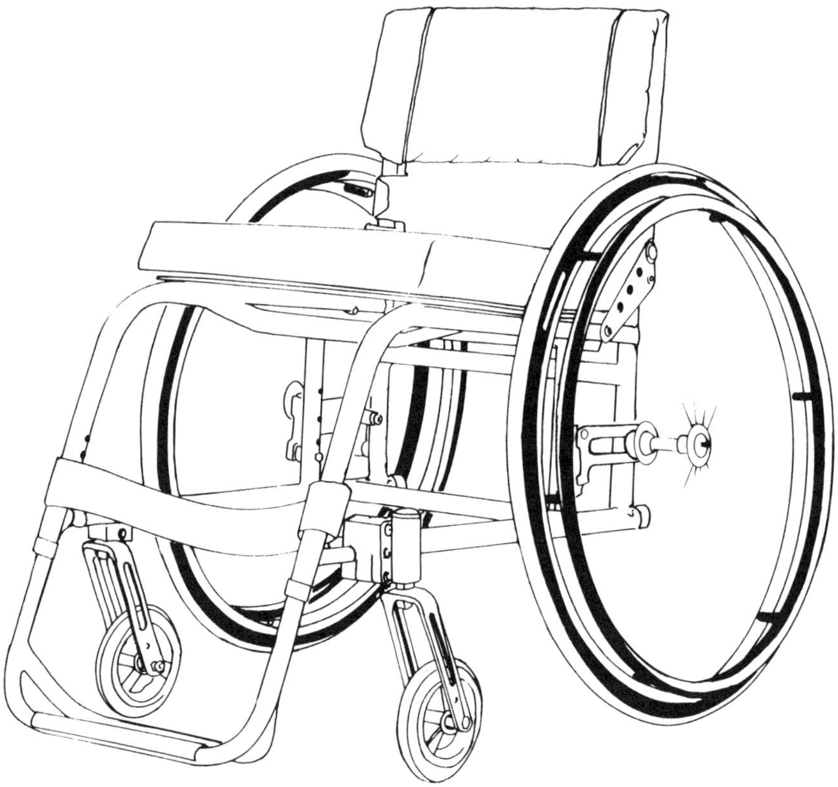

(Courtesy: Sunrise Medical, Quickie Designs, Inc.)

hood than later in life. Thus, manufacturers of devices for pediatric rehabilitation have introduced products that allow the child to stand as much as possible. Included in this category are four-wheeled "walkabouts" whose frame surrounds the child. The child is supported by wide straps around the trunk. Another device is a motorized "MotoStand." The child leans against a vertical front, and is held upright by straps around the buttocks. The front stand and supports can be raised as the child grows. The common element in these devices is to provide the child with greater independence of movement than is possible with wheelchairs. There may be an added psychological benefit that comes with being able to "stand up and look around." There are also mobility devices modeled after scooters, tricycles, and bicycles. These may provide better physical activity than a wheelchair, and also mimic the forms of locomotion used by other children in the user's environment.

Motorized Chairs. Motorized devices comprise two major categories: scooters and chairs. Scooters are three- or four-wheeled powered mobility aids that are most suitable for indoor transportation for a person who would otherwise need a cane or walker, or who lacks sufficient endurance for extended walking (e.g., the patient on portable oxygen). They are poorly suited to outdoors use, and the user must be ambulatory or sufficiently stable to transfer in and out of the scooter. They are not suitable as a day-long user environment. They are lighter, somewhat speedier, and less expensive than motorized chairs. Like motorized chairs, they are normally powered by electric motors and use rechargeable batteries with either liquid or gel electrolyte.

Motorized chairs can be relatively simple; one manufacturer makes a conversion unit that provides motive power to any standard wheelchair. Alternatively, the motorized chair can form the basis of a complex wheelchair system costing tens of thousands of dollars. Some motorized chairs use large rear drive wheels; these are especially useful in outdoor travel. Others, particularly for indoor use on mostly level surfaces, have four wheels essentially the same size. Motorized chairs usually feature an electronic control system with a "joystick" type controller. Chair motion is selected by moving the joystick in the desired direction, and speed will be proportional to the amount of pressure placed on the stick. Computerized control mechanisms can be very sophisticated, however, allowing for chair movement control via a mouthpiece or eye movements.

The HHC pharmacist who wishes to feature motorized chairs and scooters will need additional training (or must hire a trained technician) to adjust and maintain the electrical and electronic parts of the chairs. Additional accessories, including batteries, special tires, battery covers, cables, and belts, are needed to backup the sale of a powered chair. Because motorized chair systems are complex and quite expensive, the user may well expect more support from the supplier than for standard chairs.

Training and Certification. Opportunities for training, certification, and continuing education regarding wheelchairs and related devices are also provided through professional associations interested in assistive technologies, including the following:

NARD
205 Daingerfield Road
Alexandria, VA 22314
(703) 683-8200

National Registry of Rehabilitation Technology Suppliers
625 Slaters Lane, Suite 200
Alexandria, VA 22314-1171
(703) 836-6263

RESNA
1101 Connecticut Ave. N.W., Suite 700
Washington, DC 20036-4303
(202) 857-1199

A variety of publications regarding assistive technologies, including ANSI standards documents, is available from RESNA Press (Dept. 3113, Washington, DC 20042-3113). Included in their listing are such titles as: Assistive Technology Sourcebook, Childhood Powered Mobility, Interactive Robotic Aids, and Managing a Rehabilitation Technology Practice.

Measurement and Fitting. Wheelchairs must be selected from available designs according to patient age, size, and general needs. Each manufacturer's literature will show a range of dimensions for each style of chair it makes. If the user's needs are met within these dimensions, one of the standard types will be preferred, and the HME supplier will often have the chair in stock. If the standard types are not appropriate, however, an individual prescription should be developed and the manufacturer can create a chair unique to the individual.

The following include the important chair dimensions that must be provided to the manufacturer, or that must be adjusted on chairs already in stock. These measurements are best taken with the patient sitting in a straight-backed chair. A principal consideration in fitting a wheelchair is to avoid pressure on several areas of the body that are prone to irritation and decubitus formation, such as shoulder blades (scapulae), the area behind the knees (popliteal space), bony buttock protuberances (ischial tuberosities), and outside femur bone points (greater trochanter).

1. Seat Width. The purpose in setting the seat width is to allow adequate clearance to avoid pressure on the greater trochanter, while keeping the chair width overall as narrow as possible. An overly-wide seat provides less side-to-side support for the patient. See Table 11-4.
2. Seat Depth. The objective in determining seat depth is to distribute the weight evenly over the thighs and buttocks. This minimizes pressure on the ischial tuberosities. Too shallow a seat depth places more weight on the ischia and may lead to decubiti. If the seat is too deep, pressure on the popliteal areas will cause irritation and may interfere with circulation to the lower legs.
3. Leg Length and Seat Height. The leg length must be adjusted to distribute the leg weight over the thighs, without placing undue pressure on the popliteal areas. If the foot rests are set too low, popliteal pressure will increase. If the foot rests are set too high, the knees rise up and weight is transferred from the thighs to the buttocks and ischia. The seat height must be adjusted to allow at least two inches (5 cm) of clearance between the foot rests and the ground, otherwise the foot rests will hit on rocks or curbs. The seat height includes the width of a cushion, but compression of the cushion must be considered. If the seat height is too high, the chair will not fit easily under tables or desks.
4. Arm Rest Height. The goal in setting the arm rest height is to provide support for the user's

Table 11-4 Measurements for Fitting the Wheelchair Patient

Seat Width	
Patient Measurement	Width of hips or thighs, whichever is wider.
Chair Measurement	Add 2" to patient measurement to provide at least 1" clearance on each side.
Seat Depth	
Patient Measurement	From behind calf to back of buttocks.
Chair Measurement	Subtract between 2" and 3" from the patient measurement.
Leg Length and Seat Height	
Patient Measurement	From the heel of the shoe or foot to just under the thigh.
Chair Measurement	The same as the patient's. The leg length is the distance from the seat to the foot rest. The minimum seat height is obtained by adding 2" to the leg length, and is the distance from the floor to the top of the seat cushion.
Arm Rest Height	
Patient Measurement	With elbows flexed at 90°, measure distance between elbow and chair seat. The patient should be seated on the cushion that will be used in the chair.
Chair Measurement	Add 1" to patient measurement.
Back Support Height	
Patient Measurement	With patient seated on the cushion that will be used in the chair, measure from the chair seat height to just under the arm as it is extended forward.
Chair Measurement	Subtract 4" from the patient measurement.

forearms without unduly elevating his or her shoulders. Too low an arm rest will cause the user to hunch forward, while too high a setting will place undue pressure on the elbows and also elevate the shoulders uncomfortably. Chairs may be ordered with adjustable, rather than custom arm rests.

5. Back Support Height. The back height measurement determines how high the chair's fabric back will ride on the user's back. If the chair back is too low, insufficient postural support will be provided to the user's trunk. If the chair back is too high, the ability of the patient to reach around behind the chair, or to look around to the rear, will be impeded. This setting must be adjusted for the patient's level of activity and upper body strength. In any case, the chair back should be at least one inch (2.5 cm) above or below the inferior angle of the scapulae, to avoid pressure over these bony prominences. Some individuals will require a head rest or support accessory.

Important Options. Among the common options when ordering a wheelchair are: elevated leg rests; detachable, flip-back, and/or height-adjustable arm rests; solid seats or backs for positioning; solid, poly, or pneumatic tires; 5 inch (12 cm) poly pilot wheels with cast rims or 6 and 8 inch (15 and 20 cm) poly, solid rubber, or pneumatic casters; spoked or cast plastic rear rims; and plastic-coated hand rims. Accessories that are available from after-market sources include desk attachments for arm rests, various types of pouches for attachment to the back rest or under the seat, and cane, crutch, and IV holders.

Perhaps the most important accessory is a seat cushion, and most authorities recommend that every wheelchair user have one. In addition to the comfort it provides, the cushion is a critical aid in preventing pressure sores by spreading pressure evenly over thighs and buttocks. Depending on the user's physical condition and level of activity, a range of cushions from foam rubber to those filled with liquid silicone are available to accomplish this goal. New assessment techniques include a computer-linked matrix of pressure transducers to produce topographic maps of seat area contact pressure; these help clinicians select the best form of cushion. Recently developed is a new form of seat called the Total Contact Seat, which replaces the standard wheelchair seat altogether.[13]

HOSPITAL EQUIPMENT FOR THE HOME

There are two major functional differences between a bedroom in the home and a private hospital room. First, the hospital patient spends nearly 24 hours a day in the room, and second, the room and its equipment are designed to facilitate caregiving by hospital personnel. Thus, although short term illness is readily cared for in a regular bedroom, both the room and its equipment must be modified for long term care.

Resources for the Caregiver

The HHC pharmacist has little control over the home environment. The pharmacist may indirectly influence that environment, however, by giving advice to the caregiver, and also by directing the caregiver to other information sources. The American Red Cross formerly offered a course in Home Nursing, which included an excellent text, Family Health and Home Nursing;[14] the book is still available in many public libraries. Another text, Home Care: An Alternative to the Nursing Home,[15] is also useful for the caregiver. Its author recounts her experience in caring for her husband, a stroke victim, in the home, and provides step-by-step instructions for others. Step-by-step instructions, accompanied by clear illustrations, are also featured in the Manual of Home Health Care Nursing.[16] This latter text will be quite useful to the HHC pharmacist, as well.

Assessing Patients' Environmental Needs

Recommendations for equipment to be used in HHC must be relevant to the patient's condition and home environment. Thistle, et al.,[1] recommend that a **PULSES** profile[17] be developed. The PULSES acronym stands for six areas of evaluation:

- **P**— physical condition (basic health/illness status)
- **U**— upper limb functions (self care activities including drinking, eating, dressing, washing, etc.)
- **L**— lower limb functions (mobility and transferring, use of chair/toilet/tub/shower, walking, climbing stairs, propelling wheelchair)
- **S**— sensory components (sight, speaking, hearing)
- **E**— excretory functions (control of bladder or bowel)
- **S**— support factors (family, social, financial, psychological, and social support)

Although the actual PULSES numerical result (the patient is rated from 1 to 4 in each area) may be of little value to the HHC pharmacist, the six areas provide a useful inventory of factors to consider in making recommendations for homecare equipment and services.

The second portion of the evaluation is the home environment. At the very least, specific assessment of access, safety, and other limitations should be made for each of the following areas of the home: bedroom, bathroom, doors, hallways, furniture, entrances, stairways (if applicable), and kitchen.[1]

Beds and Accessories

If the patient will be spending most of the day in bed, an adjustable hospital bed is essential. It will allow the patient to sit up for feeding, reading, conversation, and other daytime activities. Changes in position are also important to minimize pressure sores, and to help relieve boredom and fatigue. The hospital bed may also be raised or lowered to aid the caregiver: raised for easy access to the patient, and lowered for ease in transfer. See Figure 11-8.

Manually-adjustable beds. Adjustments to a manual bed are made by cranks at the foot of the bed. Several styles are available, but the minimum adjustments should include head, feet, and total bed height. Beds are usually rented, and the pharmacy will need to deliver the bed and install it in the home. The pharmacy should therefore purchase beds with detachable head and foot boards, and a bedspring that can be split in half so that one person can transport it.

Electrically-adjustable beds. The principal advantage of the electric bed is that the patient can adjust positions easily. Electrically operated beds are available with head and foot adjustments, and may be either semi-electric or full-electric depending on whether overall height is manually or electrically adjustable. Third party payers, such as Medicare, may restrict payment for full-electric beds to situations where the patient must change the bed height independently (e.g., one height is needed to transfer into the bed and another height is needed to transfer out), and may pay for a semi-electric bed (instead of a manual bed) only if the physician certifies it is essential for the patient to be able to operate the bed.

Pharmacists should assure that any electrical equipment rented for use in the home meets local electrical codes. Certainly, the equipment should bear

Figure 11-8 Manually Adjustable Hospital Bed With Rails

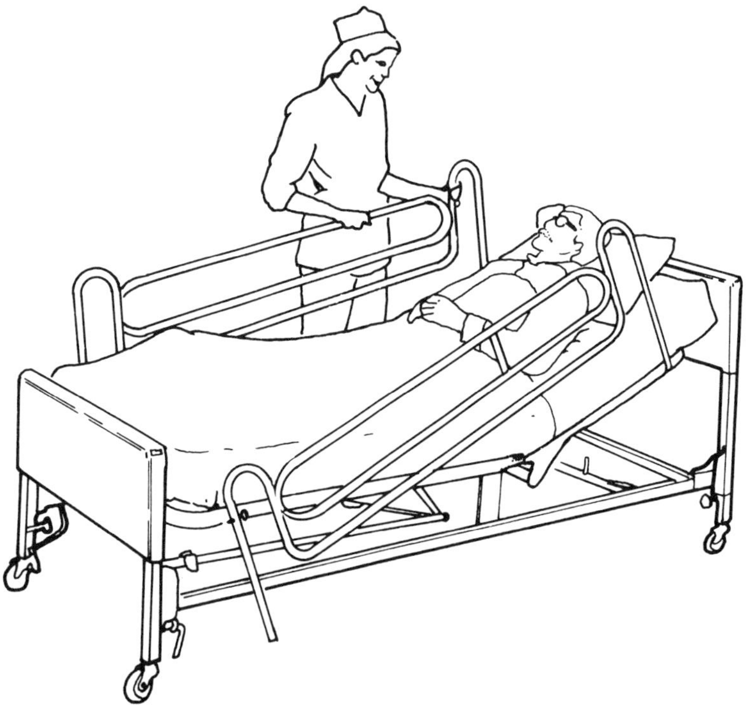

the Underwriters' Laboratories (UL) approval for use in patient care environments. Special precautions are necessary to prevent sparks whenever oxygen is used. The caregiver may also be advised to have the wiring of the patient's room and bathroom modified to include a ground fault detector. This type of circuit breaker is able to detect and interrupt abnormal current flow more rapidly than standard circuit breakers, and will provide additional security against accidental electric shock.

Mattresses. Many HHC pharmacists will prefer to rent foam mattresses because they are easy to transport. Inner spring mattresses are more durable under heavy use, but care should be taken to use types designed for adjustable beds; the springs must be hinged to allow the mattress to flex in conjunction with the bedspring. No rental mattress should ever be delivered without a suitable mattress cover made from material that is resistant to bacterial contamination.

Bed rails. Bed rails are an essential safety aid that may prevent the patient from accidentally falling. They also provide a handhold for the patient to aid in positioning. Rails that attach directly to the bed are available from the bed manufacturer, are preferred in most situations, and are essential with electric beds. "Universal" bed rails have their own frame, which may fit under a mattress or be a floor stand; they may be rented for short term use with a standard, non-adjustable twin bed. Because the upper portion of the universal rails do not move up or down as the head is raised, they are unsuitable for use with adjustable beds.

Blanket supports. No matter how light the bedding, its constant pressure over the feet and ankles becomes uncomfortable for the bedridden person. It may also contribute to foot drop and pressure sores. One type of bedding support is a wire frame that fits under the mattress on each side and forms a loop over the feet, thus "tenting" the sheet and blanket. Another device attaches to the foot of the bed and forms a shelf on which extra bedding may be folded when not needed. The shelf may extend either to the rear of the footboard or over the patient's feet.

Trapeze bar. Trapeze bars may either attach directly to the headboard or may have their own floor stand, enabling their use with any bed. The trapeze bar provides a horizontal support extending over the patient's head, from which is hung the trapeze. The trapeze is used as a positioning aid. Occasionally, the trapeze is placed at the foot of the bed, and used to elevate a leg. See Figure 11-9.

Overbed table. An adjustable-height

Figure 11-9 Trapeze Bar With Floor Stand

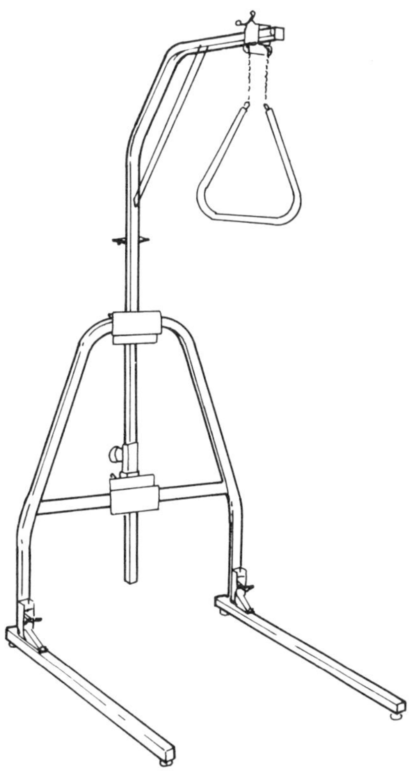

overbed table is much preferred to lap trays for feeding, and provides an easy-to-reach location for water carafes, tissue, and similar items. The table top may be tilted to form an easel on which a book may be propped. The tables are wheeled for easy removal when the patient must be transferred.

Commodes

Commode means "convenient." This device provides the user with a convenient portable toilet, and is used when a regular toilet is not readily accessible, or for the individual who is not confined to a bed but cannot go or be taken to a bathroom. The commode consists of a chair-like structure with a toilet seat and a removable basin beneath. See Figure 11-10.

Commode types. Several types of commodes are generally available:

1. Stationary commodes. These are usually made from tubular steel or aluminum, with adjustable legs. The arm rests may slope from rear to front to facilitate entry and exit. The toilet seat is similar in construction to a standard toilet.
2. Drop-arm commodes. These are commodes on which either armrest may be lowered to allow transfer to and from the side of the commode.
3. Chair commodes. These feature upholstered back rests and an upholstered seat that is placed over the toilet seat when the commode is not being used as a toilet. They thus can double as a chair in the patient's room.
4. Folding commodes. These are similar to stationary commodes, except that the frame folds flat for storage when not in use.
5. Transport commodes. These devices are wheeled versions of the above styles, and can be upholstered, with or without a drop arm, and may be folding. Varieties of transport commodes in which all surfaces and wheels are waterproof can be used to transport persons into walk-in showers, and are sometimes called shower chairs.
6. Over-toilet commodes. These commodes have a splash shield below their toilet seat, and can be used with a removable bucket or can be placed over a standard toilet. Their advantage when used in conjunction with a regular toilet is that they provide the user with arm rests as well as an elevated seat.
7. Elevated toilet seats. These are toilet seats that fit over the regular toilet to raise the seating height for the user. Some styles are in the form of regular seats with elevating supports; others are molded and several inches thick. Like the over-toilet commodes, they have splash guards that fit into the toilet bowl.

Commode use. The commode should be adjusted to a comfortable height, usually higher than the standard toilet. The rear legs may be set higher than the front to slightly tip the commode forward; this is especially helpful for patients with arthritis, hip problems, or certain patients with stroke, by reducing the patient's need to bend.

After the patient has used the commode, the bucket is removed from beneath the seat, and emptied in a toilet. Most commode buckets are equipped with lids for transportation. The commode is used as one would use a normal toilet; however, DuFresne offers the following specific comment regarding the use of the commode by males who cannot cooperate by raising up from the commode: With the male patient it will be necessary to remove the catch basin from the runners under the chair seat and place it on the floor on a towel under the patient. It is impossible to move the basin after the patient is seated, in order to check results, or to do the clean-up, without hurting the genital organs which drop below the basin rim.[13]

Commode care. The commode buckets should be rinsed thoroughly before returning to the commode. They are usually constructed of polypropylene and can be autoclaved. The commode itself must be routinely cleaned. One manufacturer[18] recommends the following procedures for pharmacies to use when cleaning commodes between rentals:

- Using detergent, water and sponge, wash the chrome plated frame, bucket holder, and toilet seat. Rinse with clean water. Wipe down with damp chamois.
- Add one half (1/2) ounce disinfectant to a gallon of clean water.
- With a sponge and the above disinfectant solution, thoroughly wipe the entire toilet seat.
- Always sell the pail and lid when renting commodes.

Note that some states or local health departments may have specific regulations for disinfecting reusable personal devices.

Figure 11-10 Commodes

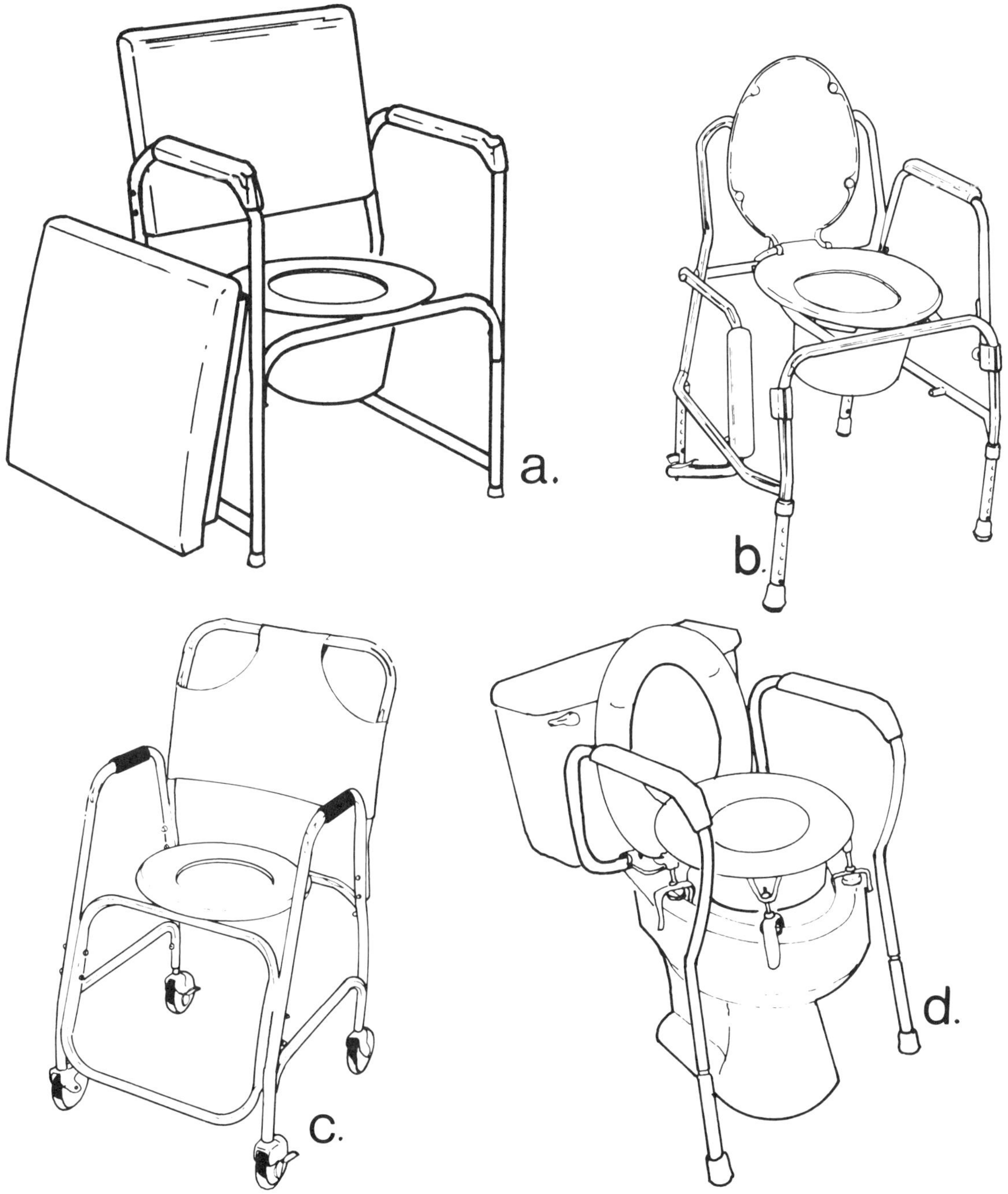

a. stationary aluminum commode;
b. drop arm commode;
c. shower chair transport commode;
d. adjustable toilet hand rails used with a raised toilet seat.

Bathroom Safety Equipment

The bathroom, particularly the tub or shower, is a common location for injury in the home. The individual being cared for in the home may need special protection against falls in the tub, shower, or while using the toilet. In addition, patients with diminished sensation in the extremities may be more prone to burns and scalds, so the water heater temperature setting should not exceed 120° F (50° C).

Safety rails and grab bars. Bathroom safety rails and grab bars attach to the walls of tubs and showers, or around toilets. Safety rails are typically 1 1/2" (4 cm) in diameter and are mounted with 1 1/2" (4 cm) of clearance. The user may grab them or rest a limb on them. Grab bars are generally 1" (2.5 cm) in diameter and are mounted with 3" (8 cm) clearance between the bar and the wall. A person thus may hook a limb behind the bar. The choice of one device over another depends on patient factors and the opinions of the patient's physician or physical therapist. See Figure 11-11.

The HHC pharmacist who sells or recommends safety rails or grab bars should generally refer the purchaser to a competent, licensed and bonded installer. Although the rails and bars are able to withstand a 500 pound (225 kg) lateral pull, the strength of the device when installed in the home depends on the quality of the installation. Selection of appropriate mounting hardware (rather than adhesive) and effective waterproofing require familiarity with various construction materials and with local building codes.

Tub rails are available that clamp over the side of the tub (see Figure 11-11C). For long-term care, they should be supplemented by permanently-installed rails and grab bars.

Aluminum hand rails are available to attach to the back of the toilet, using the same bolts that hold the toilet seat in place. Adjustable-height models may be used with or without elevated toilet seats, and are preferred.

Shower and tub accessories. Adhesive traction strips or spots should be applied to the bottom of the tub or shower. Types with roughened rubberized surfaces may be preferred to more abrasive surfaces. Also useful are various types of shower seats. Some fit across the tub sides, while others fit in the tub and have suction cups at the bases of their legs. Most are vinyl coated. A hand-held shower extension will allow the seated person the benefits of a shower, without the need to stand.

Patient lifters. Useful for transfer between wheelchair and shower, tub, or commode, patient lifters are valuable outside of the bathroom as well, for transfer between wheelchair and bed, or between wheelchair and automobile. The first of two common types is comprised of a sling type seat suspended from an overhead boom. The boom is raised or lowered pneumatically, and may be swiveled to move the person from chair to alternate location. This type of lifter is usually wheeled. The second type is mounted in the tub, and looks like a chair. The chair is raised or lowered either pneumatically or hydraulically, and when raised can pivot 90°. The chair is swung out over the edge of the tub, the patient is placed in the chair, then swung back into the tub and lowered into the water.

Plastic and Enamel Ware

Once commonly made of enamel or stainless steel, but now more often of plastic, this group of assistive devices consists of various containers useful in the patient care environment. Although considered disposable, most are made of dishwasher-proof plastic. In long-term use, however, they may retain odors. In some settings, therefore, stainless steel or enamel versions continue to be used. Included in this category are beverage carafes, emesis basins, bedpans, and urinals.

Carafe or water pitcher. Most carafes come with a lid, and commonly hold about one quart or liter. Larger sizes may be too heavy for the user. Companion items to the carafe include plastic tumblers and flexible drinking straws. In contrast to household pitchers, carafes have a translucent band on one side with graduations that can be used to help measure the patient's total fluid intake.

Emesis basin. This familiar kidney-shaped basin (sometimes called a "pus-basin") was designed originally to receive vomit from a bedridden patient. Its inner curve fits around the side of the patient's face when reclining. These containers are also useful in tooth brushing, or to catch the drainage from otic lavage. Thus, it is helpful to have several emesis basins on hand for different uses.

Bedpans. Two major types of bedpans are the standard, contour type bedpan, which is available in adult and child sizes, and the fracture pan. The latter is wedge-shaped and is designed to be more easily slipped under the patient who is immobilized by a body cast, is obese, in pelvic traction, or experiences other difficulty in being elevated onto the

Figure 11-11 Bathroom Safety Equipment

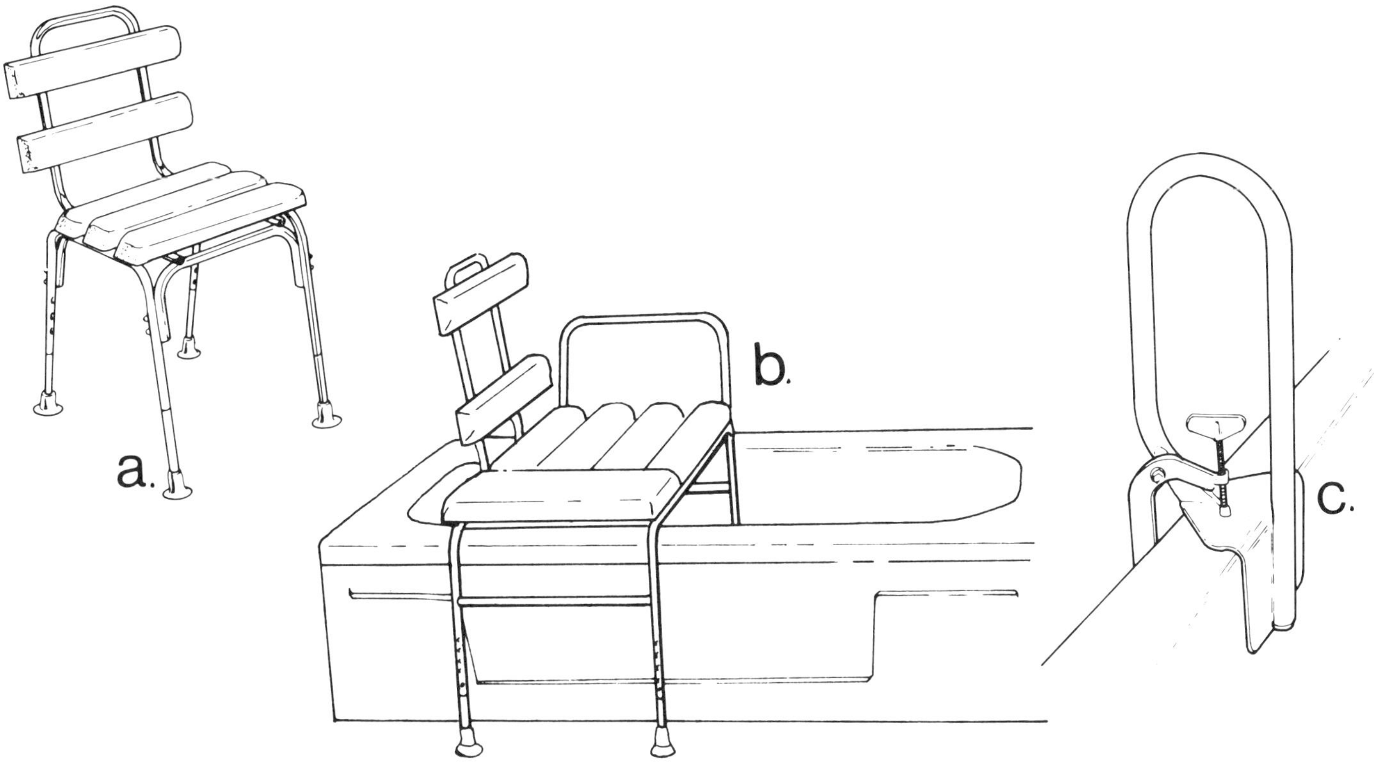

a. padded shower seat;
b. padded shower seat with transfer bench;
c. bathtub safety rail.

standard bedpan. The fracture pan also can serve as a female urinal. The following steps may be followed in bedpan use:

1. Bring enamel or stainless steel bedpans to body temperature with warm water prior to use.
2. Place a disposable underpad beneath the patient; the upper edge of the underpad should be at waist level. Place the pan between the underpad and the patient's buttocks, then draw the underpad up between the patient's legs to shield the bedding from any splatter. The underpad may be used as a cover when removing and transporting the pan to the bathroom.
3. It may help to place some water in the pan to wet the bottom and sides prior to giving it to the patient. This will aid in emptying the pan later.
4. After the pan is emptied in the toilet, rinse it first with cold water, and use a toilet brush to dislodge any feces that remain. Disinfectant solutions may be placed in the pan between uses to remove odors.

If the patient is in an adjustable bed, raise the head to elevate the patient into a sitting position, and raise the knees slightly. With a regular bed, pillows or a wedge may be placed behind the patient.

Urinals. Urinals are containers for receiving the patient's urine. They are used more commonly for males than for females; female urinals are available, but the fracture bedpan may be more suitable. Plastic urinals are imprinted with graduations to help measure urinary output.

Urinals should be used in conjunction with a disposable underpad to catch inadvertent spills. Their use is otherwise straightforward, except that caution should be used to avoid confusing them with carafes.

Urinals are cleaned and sanitized in the same manner as bedpans. Urinals and bedpans are personal care items that are never rented.

Rubber Goods

A miscellaneous group of useful products were traditionally made of rubber, but are now constructed of neoprene or other synthetic polymers. Chief among these products are various syringes, hot water bottles, and ice packs. The latter two types of devices are discussed below along with other devices for heat and cold therapy.

All rubber goods share common guidelines for care. Most will become brittle and crack over time if exposed to high heat or intense sunlight. Most are used to contain aqueous fluids, and are reservoirs for growth of mold and fungi if not dried thoroughly between uses. All bulb syringes are personal care items that should neither be rented nor shared between individuals (the possible exception is the ear syringe used only for irrigation).

Bulb syringes. Bulb syringes are so named because of a large rubber bulb that is compressed to eject the syringe's contents, and released to aspirate fluid from a body cavity. The type of syringe commonly used for injections is called, by contrast, a piston syringe. Whenever a bulb syringe is used to irrigate a body orifice, care should be taken to avoid excessive force when compressing the bulb. Thus, fountain syringes may be preferred for administering enemas or douches.

1. Asepto syringes. Asepto syringes are composed of a bulb whose opening is inserted into a barrel similar in appearance to a standard piston syringe. They are used primarily for aspiration, sometimes through a catheter. Typical volumes for the syringe barrel are from 50 ml to 150 ml, and the bulb is sized so that the fluid will not flow into the bulb as long as the syringe remains upright during aspiration. Graduations on the barrel are provided to measure the volume of aspirate.
2. Ear syringes. Ear syringes are one-piece bulb syringes with a long flexible tip. They are available in 30 to 60 ml capacities, and are intended for irrigation of the external auditory canal.
3. Nasal aspirators. Nasal aspirators are bulb syringes with a clear plastic tip shaped somewhat like a football. The opening thus can be inserted only slightly into the nostril to aspirate its contents, avoiding possible injury if the baby wiggles. Unfortunately, some infants' nostrils are too small to seal around the tip, thus thick mucus may not be aspirated effectively. In these cases a small ear syringe may be used, if done carefully.
4. Rectal syringes. Bulb syringes with rectal pipes are used to administer enemas. They are available in adult and infant sizes, and consumers should be cautioned that adult pipes should never be used for infants. Flexible rectal pipes are preferred over hard pipes, especially for infants. Most enemas are administered by fountain syringes if a commercially-prefilled enema syringe is not used.
5. Vaginal syringes. Vaginal bulb syringes use a vaginal pipe to administer a vaginal douche, which is a water rinse (with or without added ingredients) of the vagina. A movable shield slides along the pipe, and should be fitted against the vaginal opening to prevent leakage of the douche. The bulb is compressed and pressure is applied continuously for a short period, then the douche liquid is aspirated back into the bulb for disposal in a toilet. Douches also are commonly administered by fountain syringe.
6. Fountain syringes. A fountain syringe is a flexible bag that is filled with irrigation fluid and from which the fluid then flows through tubing to the desired body cavity. A tubing clamp is used to regulate the flow rate, and either a rectal or vaginal pipe is connected to the distal end of the tubing.

For an enema, the user hangs the syringe at shoulder level, while sitting on the toilet or commode. The rectal tip may be moistened or lubricated with a personal lubricant (note that petrolatum will dissolve rubber) and is inserted into the rectum. The flow rate should be controlled to prevent cramping. When the enema has finished flowing, the rectal pipe is removed. Similar procedures are used for irrigating a colostomy, but a special ostomy irrigation tip is used.

An individual may administer a vaginal douche via a fountain syringe in one of three ways. The first is while seated on a toilet or commode, with one leg raised on a small stool. The second method is to recline in a bathtub with both knees drawn up and parted. A third choice is to administer the douche while standing in the shower. In each case, the irrigation fluid is allowed to flow freely into and out of the vagina. The syringe should be no more than about 30" (75 cm) higher than the vaginal pipe; excessive fluid pressure could force liquid into or through the Fallopian tubes. In any irrigation, prior to insertion of the pipe into the body cavity, the tubing clamp should be opened and fluid allowed to run until all the air is expelled from the tubing.

Thc HHC pharmacist should discourage routine vaginal douching. Not only may douching adversely effect the vaginal environment, its use has been associated with increased incidence of pelvic inflammatory disease[19] and risk of tubal pregnancy.[20]

Although enema bags and douche bags are sold separately, a hot water bottle can also double as a fountain syringe, using a combination attachment kit. This kit contains a spigot replacement for the bottle stopper, approximately five feet (1.5 m) of flexible tubing, a tubing clamp, and rectal and vaginal nozzles. Some water bottles are sold with the combination attachment included.

Equipment for Heat and Cold Therapy

Applications of heat and cold are recognized treatment modalities for both chronic and acute painful conditions. (See also Chapter 22.) The choice between heat and cold for treatment of a given condition may be based on whether one wants to increase or decrease circulation in the area. Heat generally increases local hemoperfusion, whereas cold does the reverse. Other generally opposite reactions to heat and cold are seen with edema and metabolism, which heat increases and cold decreases. Thus, initial treatment for acute injuries generally features the application of cold. In the rehabilitation phase, either heat or cold may be used, and the choice is often made empirically according to patient response.[21]

Heat therapy. Heat is applied in one of two forms: dry or moist. Physicians or therapists may order moist heat in the belief that it provides "deeper" heating. The cheapest form of delivering heat, towels dipped in hot water and wrung out, is but one way to deliver moist heat. Dry heat can be provided by direct application, and also by radiation (e.g., sun lamps), electrical energy such as diathermy, ultrasound, or by friction (e.g., a back rub). Some medicinal agents (e.g., methyl salicylate) produce local heat through counterirritation that increases local blood flow.

1. Hot water bottles. The ubiquitous hot water bottle is the safest and least expensive source of dry heat in the home. Only two precautions are necessary to avoid burns: (1) after filling the bottle, check its temperature against the back of the hand, and (2) wrap the bottle in a towel to protect against direct contact between the skin and the rubber. Because the hot water bottle is "self timing" it may be used on a sleeping person or placed under a limb, unlike a heating pad. Excess air should be expressed from the bottle before use so that it will remain flexible.
2. Moist heat packs. Moist heat can also be delivered via commercially-available moist heat packs. These packs are compartmentalized cloth bags containing colloid beads. When the packs are placed in hot water, the beads swell, absorbing both water and heat. The heated pack retains high heat levels for 30 minutes or more. The best known bags are meant to be heated in "Hydrocollator" heating units, but they may also be heated in a pan on the stove. Once hydrated, packs may also be heated in a microwave oven. After several microwave reheatings, however, the pack must be boiled to rehydrate it. Maintaining hydration during storage is important; packs should be wrapped in plastic and stored in the refrigerator.

   The packs are available in several shapes and sizes, including special shapes for the neck, knee, shoulder, and face. Because of their high heat capacity, they must be wrapped in several layers of towel to prevent burns. Packs sold exclusively for home use may include a foam-lined terry cloth cover.

   Some moist heat packs are now marketed for dual use as either cold or heat packs, depending on whether they are stored in a freezer or are boiled or microwaved.
3. Electric heating pads. Electric heating pads are marketed for providing either dry or, if specially constructed, moist heat. They are a popular form of heat, but require cautious use to avoid electric shock or fires,[22] and prolonged application can result in severe burns. Consumers should be counseled to AVOID electric heating pad use:
   - on a sleeping or unconscious person;
   - on patients with impaired sense of touch or pain or with poor circulation;
   - under any body part (where heat can be

trapped between the body part and the bed and allowed to build up);
- on any skin that has been previously treated with a counterirritant;
- over a recent wound;
- in patients with diabetes, the elderly, or in patients taking corticosteroids, except with caution or under physician's orders.[22]

Pads should not be affixed with pins (which may penetrate wiring), and should never be used without their cover intact and in place. Consumers further should be instructed to inspect the pad frequently. If it becomes lumpy, or develops "hot spots," or the cord or control is damaged in any way, it should be replaced. Most pads have removable covers that are machine washable; the pad itself, of course, is not. To clean the interior plastic pad jacket, the user should unplug the device and sponge off the cover with a mild detergent and water, using a damp cloth, then dry thoroughly.

To minimize the danger of electric shock and household fire, all heating pads should meet Underwriters' Laboratories (UL) standards. Pads are considered safer as the number of thermostats per pad increases. Pharmacists can palpate pads to determine the number of thermostats. The Consumers Union encourages the sale of pads with at least four thermostats.[22]

Varieties of heating pads include "wrap around" pads for use on joints, "sinus masks" for application to the forehead and sinus area, and "moist heat" pads with sponge inserts that can be immersed in water and wrung out. As with moist heat packs, treatment with a moist heat pad should be limited to approximately 30 minutes.

4. Paraffin baths. Paraffin baths are used primarily to relieve arthritis pain in the hands, both for comfort and to allow passive range of motion exercises that otherwise would be painful. Safe use of paraffin requires a temperature-controlled heating unit that maintains the wax between 126° and 130° F (52° and 54° C). This also necessitates a paraffin mixture with a fairly low melting point, designed for medical use. Users should verify the temperature with a paraffin thermometer prior to immersing their hands.
5. Chemical packs. Several varieties of chemical "instant heat" packs are available. All are plastic pouches with two compartments. One contains water and the other a dry chemical that produces an exothermic reaction when mixed with the water. In use, the pouch is compressed to break the inner bag, and the reaction proceeds rapidly. Temperatures approaching 170° F (77° C) can be maintained for 15 minutes or more; if the bag does not include foam insulation it must be wrapped in a towel. Some packs are labeled as harmful or fatal if the contents are swallowed, a notice that should be brought to the consumer's attention.

   A different form of chemical heat pack consists of a saturated solution in a plastic bag that crystallizes when a catalyst button is "tweaked" in its corner. The heat liberated during crystallization produces instant warmth. The pack is returned to its liquid state by boiling or microwaving, then cooling, and is stored until it is again needed.
6. Gel packs. Packs containing flexible polymer gels can be used for either heat or cold therapy. They are immersed in hot water or stored in the freezer. As heat sources, they retain their heat longer than water bottles, and can be handled and stored more easily than colloid packs. When cold, they remain flexible; this is their major advantage. Pharmacists who sell the flexible cold packs find it useful to keep some in the freezer for immediate use.

Cold. Forms of cold therapy include the gel packs and colloid packs mentioned above, chemical cold packs that depend on an endothermic reaction to produce cold when their components are mixed, and ice bags. As with heat sources, insulation between the pack and the skin is essential to avoid damage to tissue, in this case from local freezing (chemical cold packs typically decline to 20° F or -7° C).

Ice bags are available in two styles: the round English ice bag (or "ice cap," due to its shape) and a long, narrow throat bag. These are made of latex rubber that is thinner than a normal water bottle, and usually have a cloth outer cover. To avoid puncturing the inner lining, ice cubes should be rinsed in tap water to melt any sharp edges before placing them in the bag.

The use of cold in sports injuries has resulted in special pouches designed to hold flexible ice packs in place. Some of these are combined with elastic bandages to create and ice/compression wrap. Typical styles are available for hand, shoulders, knees, neck, and one for a pitcher's arm and shoulder. Also available are cervical and lumbosacral supports with pouches for cold packs. These are normally sold to athletic departments and facilities, but can be obtained by the HHC pharmacist.

CONCLUSION

This chapter is an introduction to two classes of HME, ambulatory aids and hospital equipment for the home. Any caring pharmacist needs merely to observe crutch users at a local shopping mall, or talk with patients about their parents' and grandparents' experiences in hospitals or nursing homes, or attend a meeting of a wheelchair athletes' group, to understand both the need for quality services and the hope that those services can provide.

Perhaps the pharmacist will become excited enough about HME pharmacy services to investigate further. Even if the pharmacist chooses not to be a provider of HME products and services, the material in this chapter should provide the basis for intelligent referral to a HHC pharmacist.

Line art figures were adapted from the Lumex product line, courtesy of Lumex, Inc., unless specified otherwise.

REFERENCES

1. Thristle HG, et al. Preparing the physical environment. In: Bernstein LH et al. Eds. Primary care in the home. Philadelphia PA, Lippincott. 1987.
2. 29 USC Sec. 794, 1990.
3. Allan B and Small R. The environmental situation. In: Martin N, et al. Eds. Comprehensive rehabilitation nursing. New York: McGraw-Hill. 1981.
4. Allan B, Moffett FC and Small R. Accessibility design for all: an illustrated handbook. Olympia WA: Washington Council, AIA. 1992.
5. Kramer RA. Access to care for children and adolescents with disabilities. Conn Med. 1990; 54(8):428-430.
6. Eigen BN. Improving communication with the physically disabled. Amer Pharm. 1982; NS22(10):549.
7. Scharold FJ. Principles of home health care for the convalescent: patient aids. Cincinnati, OH: The FUTURO Company. 1977.
8. Knueppel RW. Health accessories. In: Genarro A, et al. Eds. Remington's pharmaceutical sciences, 18th ed. Easton PA: Mack Publishing Company. 1990; 1867-8.
9. McKibben C. Homecare/rehab resource guide. Homecare rental/sales. 1983; 5(9):27.
10. Geiger R, et al. Redefining wheelchairs -- not just redesigning them. Proc 16th Ann Conf. Washington, DC: RESNA. 1993.
11. Axelson P, et al. Clinical interpretation of wheelchair standards test results. Ibid.
12. Anonymous. Sports organizations. Sport 'N Spokes. 1993; 7-8:87.
13. Felton RM, et al. Force management system utilization in wheelchair seating. Proc 16th Ann Conf. Washington, DC: RESNA. 1993.
14. American Red Cross. Family health and home nursing. Garden City, NY: Doubleday. 1982.
15. DuFresne F. Home care: an alternative to the nursing home. Elgin, IL: The Brethren Press. 1983.
16. Walsh J, Persons CB and Wieck L. Manual of home health care nursing. Philadelphia, PA: Lippincott. 1987.
17. Granger CV, et al. Outcomes of comprehensive medical rehabilitation; measurement by PULSES profile and the Bartel index. Arch Phys Med Rehabil. 1979; 60:145.
18. Anonymous. Futuro patient-aids care & management. Cincinnati, OH: The FUTURO Company. 1977.
19. Wolner-Hanssen P, et al. Vaginal douching as an independent risk factor for acute pelvic inflammatory disease. JAMA. 1990; 263:1936.
20. Daling JR, et al. Vaginal douching and the risk of tubal pregnancy. Epidemiol. 1991; 2:41.
21. Sherman M. A primer on use of hot or cold therapy. US Pharm. 1987; 1:72.
22. Anonymous. Heating pads. Consumer Rep. 1981; 3:173.

12 Home Medical Diagnostic Products

Diane Nykamp, Pharm.D. and
Randell K. Miyahara, Pharm.D.

The willingness of consumers to participate in their own health care and to prevent disease coincides with the new era of biotechnology to produce in-home testing products.[1] Biotechnology has produced significant improvements in the specificity and reproducibility of diagnostic tests. Monoclonal antibody test kits are the most common type of biotechnology device. Monoclonal antibody test kits are used most commonly for the prediction of ovulation and the detection of pregnancy. Additional tests that will be described in this chapter include blood pressure monitors, thermometers, pregnancy kits, ovulation kits, occult blood tests, finger sticks for cholesterol monitoring, and dipsticks for urinary bacteria detection. Blood glucose monitoring will be covered in Chapter 14.

The cost savings of self-care is high. It is estimated that Americans would have spent 10.5 billion dollars more in 1987 for health care if nonprescription products which include the home medical diagnostic products were not available. The figure is estimated to rise to 34.1 billion in the year 2000.[2] Sales of home diagnostic products in supermarkets and drug stores totaled $462.9 million during the period between October 1, 1991 and September 30, 1992.[3] The kits that were responsible for the greatest amount of sales during this time period include blood glucose strips, pregnancy kits, blood glucose monitors, blood pressure meters, ovulation kits, and urinary test strips.[3]

BLOOD PRESSURE MONITORING

Blood Pressure Monitors

Blood pressure monitoring is important in the diagnosis and control of hypertension. Monitoring can detect high blood pressure or borderline hypertension, provide visual evidence that encourages patients to comply with a specific medical regimen, foster family support, and help the physician evaluate the efficacy of drug therapy.

Blood pressure is the amount of force required for the heart to circulate blood throughout the body. The systolic blood pressure is the maximum pressure the heart encounters while contracting the ventricles. The diastolic blood pressure is the least amount of pressure the heart experiences while the ventricles are relaxed and filling. Blood pressure monitoring may detect blood pressure greater than the Joint National Committee (JNC) criteria for diagnosis of high blood pressure. Current estimates are that approximately 50 million Americans have hypertension as defined as a diastolic blood pressure above 90 mm of mercury or systolic blood pressure above 140 mm Hg.[4] Refer to Table 12-1 for staging system for blood pressure.[4]

In the past, blood pressure monitoring has generally been performed in the physician's office by mercury sphygmomanometer. However, home monitoring can be especially useful for people with white-coat hypertension, those whose blood pressure is driven by the stress of having a doctor measure it. Additionally, one study indicated that when patients monitor their own blood pressure at home they can reduce costs by fewer physician visits without compromising blood pressure control.[5] Methods of monitoring blood pressure that can be used by patients themselves include mechanical aneroid home devices, electronic devices, finger oscillometric monitors, 24-hour ambulatory monitoring, and stationary automated blood monitoring devices.

Mercury Sphygmomanometer

The mercury sphygmomanometer (Greek for pulse-pressure measurer) consists of a vertical glass tube adjacent to a reservoir containing mercury. The reservoir is linked by rubber tubing to a compression cuff. The mercury sphygmomanometer detects blood pressure by auscultation (detection of sound).

Table 12-1 Classification of Blood Pressure for Adults[4]

Category[a]	Systolic, mm Hg	Diastolic, mm Hg
Normal	< 130	< 85
High Normal	130-139	85-89
Hypertension[b] (average blood pressure readings)		
Stage 1 (mild)	140-159	90-99
Stage 2 (moderate)	160-179	100-109
Stage 3 (severe)	180-209	110-119
Stage 4 (very severe)	≥ 210	≥ 120

[a] When systolic and diastolic blood pressures fall into different categories the highest category should be selected to classify the blood pressure.

[b] Not only is the stage of hypertension necessary, documentation should include any target organ damage (i.e., left ventricular hypertrophy, stroke, elevated serum creatinine, proteinuria, etc.) or risk factors (i.e., diabetes, dyslipidemia, stroke, etc.)

As the cuff is inflated the pressure from the cuff exerts a force on the mercury, causing it to rise in the tube. Korotkoff's sounds are detected when the cuff deflates allowing pressure to decrease.

Korotkoff sounds are a series of sounds heard through a stethoscope placed over an artery that has been occluded by a compression cuff. The sounds are divided into five phases. Phase 1 is the point when clear, tapping sounds are first heard and Phase 5 is the point when sounds disappear.

The mercury sphygmomanometer is the most accurate blood pressure meter and is the standard to which others are compared. In order for the monitor to give accurate readings, however, the monitor must be placed on a hard, level surface.[1] A disadvantage of the mercury sphygmomanometer is that it is a bulky device to use, and is fragile since it has breakable glass parts. This method of blood pressure monitoring also requires good vision, hearing acuity and good dexterity.

Mechanical Aneroid Sphygmomanometer

The mechanical aneroid monitor like the mercury manometer also measures blood pressure by auscultation. The aneroid has a needle that rotates clockwise as blood pressure increases and counter clockwise as blood pressure decreases. Mechanical aneroids are models without liquid to distinguish them from mercury manometers. A mechanical aneroid can also be described as a dial type meter and is connected by rubber tubing to an inflatable arm cuff pumped by a squeeze bulb. If the upper arm circumference is greater than 13 inches, an oversize cuff must be used. A needle on the gauge registers changing pressure as pulse sounds are listened to with a stethoscope.

The accuracy of an aneroid sphygmomanometer may be checked by observing if the needle of the gauge returns to zero when the cuff has been deflated. When using an aneroid monitor, the point of inflation (PIF) should be determined. The point of inflation is the maximum level to which the cuff should be inflated when measuring blood pressure.

When measuring blood pressure the left arm is bound with the cuff, while the same hand is holding the gauge. The right hand pumps the bulb and controls a thumb screw valve on the bulb to let the air out. Most mechanical monitors have the stethoscope sensor sewn into the cuff, making the self-monitoring process easier. Mechanical instruments are inexpensive as well as accurate as long as the person measuring the blood pressure is skilled. If dexterity, eyesight, or hearing is impaired this type of devise should be ruled out.[6,7] Tables 12-2 and 12-3 summarize general guidelines when using home monitors.[6,7]

Electronic Monitors

Electronic monitors are devices where the cuff inflates automatically, and pressure is displayed on a digital window. Electronic units are convenient, but not as accurate as a mechanical aneroid monitor.

Table 12-2 Recommendations for Blood Pressure Measurement at Home and Guidelines for Monitoring Devices

Equipment	Guidelines
Cuff	Adult/Regular size cuff should be used for average adult. Large size cuff should be used for an obese individual or person with muscular arms, greater than 13 inches circumference.
Inflation/Deflation Bulb and Valve	The pumping activity required to inflate a blood pressure cuff may increase systolic blood pressure by 12-13 mm Hg, therefore, it is important to pump it high enough so blood pressure is not recorded too soon after pumping. Or, the bulb should be able to produce a bladder pressure 30 mm Hg above the estimated systolic pressure within five seconds of rapid inflation and deflation should occur at a rate of 3 mm/sec or pulse beat, and not too fast.
Monitor	
Mercury	Column should be at zero before inflation with a clearly visible meniscus which should move freely when pressure is applied.
Aneroid	The needle should be at zero before inflation. Accuracy of the gauge should be checked by connecting the aneroid to one limb of a Y-piece connector, the other limb to a mercury manometer, and the bottom to a bladder, or accuracy checked by simultaneous comparison against another cuff with a mercury manometer used on the other arm.
Electronic	These devices should be checked with a Y-piece connector against a mercury manometer. Or, the accuracy should be checked by simultaneous comparison against another cuff with a mercury manometer used on the other arm.

Electronic monitors are void of a stethoscope and measure blood pressure by calculating changes in pressure (oscillometric) in the cuff that are due to a blood surge rather than sound detection. Electronic monitors are usually more expensive than the aneroid devices.

Movement of the arm that is being measured may produce an inaccurate reading when using an electronic monitor. Additionally, this monitor may give false readings in individuals who have heart rates between 45-60 beats per minute or if there is a slow deflation rate of the cuff.[8] As with the aneroid monitor, the starting systolic pressure should be 30 mm Hg higher than the estimated systolic reading. The patient must also be instructed to sit quietly for the procedure. Repeated readings should be done if unusual blood pressures are noted.

An advantage of using an electronic monitor is its ease of use which usually is a consideration when selecting a specific product. A compromise to help reduce the cost of a monitor and increase the accuracy would be to select an electronic monitor that is manually inflated.

Finger Blood Pressure Monitoring Devices

Blood pressure measurement with a finger device is generally easier to operate when compared to other traditional monitors. Finger devices, however, are much less accurate and not as reliable as the standard brachial artery devices.

Blood pressure measurement with a finger monitor is calculated from the movement of blood, most commonly in the index finger. This type of measurement can result in inaccuracy since a finger

Table 12-3 Recommendations for Blood Pressure Measurement at Home and Guidelines for Individuals

Patient	Guidelines
Circumstances	Patients should be instructed to avoid: caffeine-containing beverages, cigarette smoking, strenuous exercise within one hour prior to measurement.
	Patients should be instructed to avoid sympathomimetic agents (including ophthalmic preparations).
	If the patient is currently taking antihypertensives, the time since the previous dose should be noted. Special note should be taken to attempt measurement at end of dosing interval.
Posture	Bare arm should be supported at heart level, patient may sit or lie quietly for five minutes before measurement.
Technique	At least two readings should be taken on each occasion, with at least one minute in between readings. If two readings vary by more than 5 mm Hg, additional readings should be taken until two are similar.
Arm	Blood pressure is commonly a little higher in the left arm than in the right arm. Whichever arm is initially used should be used again so comparisons of readings will be more accurate.
Other	A diary should be kept to explain blood pressure readings that may be higher or lower than expected. For long-term monitoring of therapy, readings should be taken routinely at the same time and circumstances in relation to meals and medications should be documented.

artery is smaller and more muscular than the brachial artery which is a large distributing artery. Systemic blood pressure is a reflection of brachial pressure, whereas, digital artery blood pressure may be affected substantially by local condition such as oxygen and carbon dioxide tension, temperature and pH changes. In addition, finger arteries are highly responsive or reactive to emotional changes.[9]

The finger monitor must also be held at heart level for readings to be accurate. However, for people who have visual, auditory, or coordination problems, the finger monitor remains an option in blood pressure monitoring as long as limitations are known.

Stationary Automated Blood Pressure Device

Stationary blood pressure monitors are often found in pharmacies. The arm is inserted into the machine, a cuff automatically inflates then deflates after a fixed period, and a reading is displayed on a liquid crystal display. Stationary automated monitors are a valuable service to the public, especially to those who are unable to afford a home monitor or a visit to a physician. When this type of monitor is used the blood pressure reading should occur at the same time of day so fewer variations result. Additionally, stationary monitors use a standard cuff so the size of the cuff may not be appropriate for those whose arms are significantly larger than average.

Evaluation of commonly used stationary blood pressure devices indicate blood pressure readings can vary considerably between machines. Machine recorded blood pressures may vary between 5-10 mm Hg. The majority of these monitors error on the high side. Ensuring the devices receive regular maintenance checks and posting the dates of calibration should provide confidence in these devices. Additionally, users may ask a health professional for help in interpreting readings and asking if they are accurate. One way to ascertain if the stationary monitor is accurate is to compare readings with a mercury sphygmomanometer.[10,11,12]

Ambulatory Blood Pressure Monitoring

Ambulatory Blood Pressure Monitoring (ABPM) makes it possible to automatically obtain multiple blood pressure readings over one or more days. The monitors are patient specific and use either oscillometric or auscultatory methods to obtain blood pressure readings. Data is collected and stored in a compact unit that is usually attached to the waist. Using computer software, data is then analyzed. Patient diaries are usually used in interpreting the results.

ABPM is expensive when compared to casual home or office measure and is most often used as a research tool. The National High Blood Pressure Education Program (NHBPEP) Working Group has judged the ABPM to be useful in certain clinical situations.[4,13] Table 12-4 summarizes the different blood pressure monitors used by the ambulatory population.[14,15,16]

TEMPERATURE MONITORING

Temperature monitoring has traditionally been accomplished with a mercury thermometer. Fever, an elevation of body temperature, is a symptom of various disease states. Causes of fever include infections, vaccines, tissue injuries, malignancies, medications, inflammatory diseases, and metabolic disorders. The normal range of temperature for older children and adults is from 97.7°F to 99.5°F. Normal temperatures in an adult include an oral temperature of 98.6°F, rectal temperature of 99.6°F, and axillary temperature of 97.6°F.

In children the range is wider, from 96.8°F to 100.2°F (oral). Temperatures over 104°F may precipitate a febrile seizure, although the literature states that instead of the actual height of the temperature, it is rate of rise that induces a seizure in a child. A child should be referred to a physician for evaluation if the child is less than 3 months of age and has a rectal temperature of greater than 100.4°F or temperature of less than 97.5°F. A child with a fever for more than 48 hours in duration without an explanation, or with a temperature greater than 102°F orally, should also be referred to a physician.

Table 12-4 Blood Pressure Monitors Used by Ambulatory Patients

	Accuracy	**Convenience**	**Cost**	**Comments**	**Special Considerations**
Mercury Manometer	++++	+	+++	Most accurate, standard to which other monitors are compared.	Very bulky, need flat surface to place the monitor on.
Aneroid Monitors	+++	+++	++	Accurate if used correctly; portable.	Requires frequent calibration or purchase of new unit.
Electronic Devices	++	+++	+++	Easy to use.	No stethoscope needed.
Finger Monitors	+	++++	+++	Should be used as a screening device rather than monitoring device.	
Stationary Monitors	++	++	+	Useful if average weighted individual.	Calibration date should be posted.
Continuous 24 Hour Ambulatory Monitoring	++++	+	++++	Used for research or special clinical considerations.	Dairy must be kept for interpretation of some readings.

++++ greatest
\+ least

The rectal temperature is the best method of taking a temperature for a child under three if the caretaker or parent is using a mercury thermometer. The rectal temperature is always one degree greater than the oral temperature. The axillary temperature is generally one degree less than the oral temperature. The main difference between oral and rectal thermometers is the oral thermometer has a long, thin end for an accurate temperature by mouth while the rectal thermometer has a short, stubby end for protection against breaking in the rectum.

Guidelines for Taking A Temperature

The lowest temperature in a child is usually found in the morning and highest in the late afternoon or evening. Ideally, a person should remain calm for approximately 30 minutes before a temperature is taken. Hot or cold drinks, and food should be avoided before taking an oral temperature. Each mark on a thermometer usually stands for two-tenths of a degree.

Taking an Oral Temperature

Manually shake the thermometer down so mercury is below 94°F, if using a mercury thermometer. Carefully place the end of the thermometer under the tongue, usually in a person over the age of three. Instruct the individual to keep the lips closed and to breath through the nose. Retain the thermometer in the mouth for a period of 3 minutes. Remove the thermometer and read the temperature.[14]

Guidelines for Taking an Axillary Temperature

After a child is two years of age, taking a rectal temperature may become awkward and at this stage an axillary temperature may be used for monitoring. Another reason an axillary temperature may be useful is when a child is vomiting or has diarrhea. Either an oral or rectal thermometer can be used to take the axillary temperature. When taking an axillary temperature the thermometer should be held high in the armpit. Additionally, the arms should cross one's chest so the thermometer is held tightly in place or have an adult "bear hug" a child for a period of 3-4 minutes for this type of temperature taking.[17]

Guidelines for Taking a Rectal Temperature

Rectal temperatures are often used for babies and children under the age of 3. Manually shake the thermometer down so mercury is below 94°F, if using mercury thermometer. The stubby bulb end of the thermometer should be lubricated with petroleum jelly. Bulb of the thermometer should be inserted approximately one inch into the rectum. The thermometer should remain in the rectum for a period of two minutes. A digital oral thermometer can be used rectally for a temperature reading.[14]

Basal Thermometry

Basal temperature monitoring is used to detect ovulation. This method is an economical way of keeping track of the ovulation phase of the menstrual cycle. The most satisfactory method of determining a temperature change is with a basal thermometer. A basal thermometer is designed to have an expanded scale in the normal range, i.e., 96-100°F. A basal thermometer should not be confused with a fever thermometer in that a fever thermometer is designed to detect abnormal temperatures. A basal thermometer will detect temperature changes of as little as 0.1°F. A temperature change alone will usually permit a female to predict ovulation; however, usually cervical mucous changes along with temperature monitoring are used when detecting ovulation. A woman's "basal" resting temperature is usually lower (less than 98.6°) during the first part of the menstrual cycle than it is during the last two weeks of the same cycle, and further, the shift from the lower level of temperature to the higher occurs about the time of ovulation. Therefore, in many cases, it is possible to determine the time of ovulation by keeping a graphic record of daily temperature. When using a basal thermometer the temperature should be taken upon rising while still in bed, after at least three hours sleep. Ovulation temperature readings are compared with each other so the same thermometer, route and time of day must be used every time. The temperature may be taken orally, rectally, or vaginally. Temperature should be taken for a period of five minutes if monitoring rectally or vaginally, or eight minutes if the temperature is being taken orally. The thermometer should be shaken down below 96.5°F before use. Temperature monitoring should occur the day after the last menstrual period which normally corresponds to day five or six of the menstrual cycle if day one is the first day of spotting or bleeding.[18]

Electronic Ear Thermometer

When using an ear thermometer, the ear

canal temperature is converted to the familiar frame of reference of oral or rectal temperature. With this device the probe is inserted in the ear canal, the button of the monitor is pressed, and a temperature is displayed in one second. The device senses infrared rays that are released from the ear drum and surrounding tissue.[19]

Electronic Digital Oral Thermometer

Electronic digital oral thermometers are very convenient, easy to use, and well accepted especially when taking a temperature in a child. The digital thermometer can be used orally as well as rectally. A recent advance in the electronic digital thermometers includes a flexible digital thermometer.

Forehead Thermometer

A "forehead strip" is a way of detecting temperature especially in a child who prefers not to have a rectal temperature taken. The forehead surface temperature is less than an internal temperature so a conversion scale is provided to aid in predicting actual temperature. The forehead strips utilize liquid crystals which are set to reflect different colors of light at specific temperatures.[20] Temperature strips are held against the forehead and give a reading within 15-60 seconds. They are mainly used as a device for temperature screening, i.e., a normal or elevated temperature. If the temperature is abnormal it is advised to verify the temperature using a mercury thermometer or an electric digital thermometer.

PREGNANCY DETECTION[21]

Pregnancy Tests

Most pregnancy test kits available today can detect a pregnancy as early as the first day after a missed period with ninety-five percent or better accuracy. An early confirmation of pregnancy gives a woman the chance to make early decisions concerning prenatal care and lifestyle changes to limit fetal exposure to drugs, alcohol, tobacco and radiation.

Since their introduction in the 1970's pregnancy tests have improved in several ways. The time to obtain results and the number of days after a missed period before the test could detect a pregnancy have decreased, and the results are easier to read. These improvements are largely due to a shift from the hemagglutination inhibition reaction test to monoclonal antibody technology. Today, the majority of home pregnancy tests are one-step and one-piece in design. Monoclonal antibodies bind to urine human chorionic gonadotropin (HCG), causing a distinct color change.

Hormonal Changes in Pregnancy

Human chorionic gonadotropin (HCG) is considered a diagnostic marker for pregnancy, since HCG is produced by trophoblast cells of the fertilized ovum and is secreted into maternal circulation at the time of implantation (i.e., 6-7 days post conception) and latter is detected in the urine. Chorionic gonadotropin preserves the corpus luteum in early pregnancy and maintains production of estradiol and progesterone, which are both important in maintaining pregnancy.[22] Levels of HCG reach a maximum level at 8-12 weeks of pregnancy.[23]

The concentration of HCG declines over the following 4-6 weeks and finally stabilizes for the remainder of the pregnancy. During the eighth to tenth week of pregnancy, the urinary HCG levels average 40,000-60,000 μ/ml and then decline to 10,000 mIU/ml, remaining low for the duration of the pregnancy.[24]

Human chorionic gonadotropin is a glycoprotein consisting of two different subunits, denoted alpha and beta. The alpha subunit of HCG is structurally similar to the alpha subunits of other glycoprotein hormones: luteinizing hormone (LH), follicle-stimulating hormone (FSH), and thyroid stimulating hormone (TSH). The beta subunits, however, are structurally unique to each of these hormones. Monoclonal antibody tests currently available are highly specific to the unique structure of the beta subunit of HCG. This specificity causes less false-positive test results than would otherwise occur due to cross reactions with other hormones such as LH that might be produced during menopause, or TSH, that is produced in thyrotoxicosis.[25,26]

Monoclonal Antibody Technology

The newest pregnancy and ovulation home test kits rely on monoclonal antibody technology that are antibody-specific. Initially, a mouse is injected with an antigen, such as LH or HCG, and is allowed to develop B-lymphocytes in response to the antigen challenge. Lymphocytes are harvested from the mouse spleen and fused with myeloma cells in vitro. This fusion of the plasma cells containing B-lymphocytes with an immortal cell line of myeloma cells is referred to as a hybridoma cell or combined cell.

Hybridoma cells are then screened for appropriate antibodies specific for target cells, LH or HCG. After identification, the hybridoma cells are isolated and grown in a culture to develop a clone of identical cells with specificity to the antigen that is used for home testing.[25]

Mechanism of Action of Home Pregnancy Test Kits

Monoclonal antibodies recognize and bind to various antigenic sites on the HCG molecule. Currently, the three most popular monoclonal antibody tests include: enzyme-linked immunoassay test (ELISA); colloidal sol particle immunoassay test; and a rapid assay delivery system (RADS). Older kits, the first being introduced in 1976, utilized hemagglutination inhibition reaction (ring or doughnut test).[25,26]

Pregnancy test kits are based on antigen/antibody reactions, with HCG being the antigen, and the antibody being a monoclonal antibody to HCG, referred to as anti-HCG. The widely used ELISA[26,27] test involves a "sandwich technique." Urinary HCG is first attached by a covalent bond to an anti-HCG to form an antigen/antibody complex. This anti-HCG is a specific monoclonal antibody (specific for the alpha subunit of HCG) that is fixed to a surface such as a test tube wall, plastic paddle, plastic bead or membrane. Next, a solution containing a second monoclonal antibody (specific for the beta subunit of HCG) is placed in contact with the membrane or plastic paddle and binds with any HCG that was attached in the previous step forming an antibody--HCG--antibody "sandwich." The second antibody is attached to an enzyme conjugate that produces a chemical reaction when a solution is added. This produces a color change if HCG is present.

The colloidal sol particle immunoassay test[6] consists of sol particles that are coated with monoclonal antibodies to HCG. Urinary HCG, if present, agglutinates the dispersed particles in a sandwich-type reaction. A washing or filtering step may remove any unbound compounds, and in the step an agent that produces a color change is added.

The Rapid Assay Delivery System (RADS)[28] produces a result for urinary HCG in approximately three minutes. Urine must saturate an absorbent test tip or test well. Urine then travels across three bands of monoclonal antibodies. When passing through the first zone, urine forms a complex with a monoclonal antibody labeled with a colored pigment. This complex then passes through a second zone where immobilized antibodies specific to HCG produce a colored line if HCG is present. The complex then moves by absorption to the third zone that confirms an accurate test by producing a colored line.[29]

The older "ring" or "doughnut" test kits utilize hemagglutination inhibition reaction. These tests are outdated, time-consuming, and cannot be used until 3-9 days after a missed period. Additionally, they produce false results with certain conditions and drug interactions. For example, with conditions that produce blood or protein in the urine, hypoglycemia, thyrotoxicosis, and with certain drugs such as oral contraceptives, phenothiazines, methadone, antidepressants, antiparkinsonian agents, and anticonvulsants, false-positive results may occur.

Generally, pregnancy test kits currently available are sensitive to 25 mIU/L[23] - 50 mIU/L[30] of HCG and will turn positive 24-27 days after the last menstrual period.[23,30] A negative result one week after a missed period almost always means a woman is not pregnant.[23]

Proper Testing Techniques

Although some tests do not require morning urine, first morning urine contains the highest concentrations of HCG and, therefore, should be used for testing. If a woman's schedule interferes with performing morning testing, her urine may be stored in the refrigerator for up to twelve hours and should be tightly covered. Sediment may settle to the bottom of the sample while in the refrigerator. The urine sample should not be shaken, and the urine to be tested should be removed from the sediment-free top layer of the sample after it has been brought to room temperature. This takes approximately 20-30 minutes.[31,32]

Although many of these kits have a toll-free number for patients to ask questions, it is important that the pharmacist be able to instruct the patient on basic steps involved in using a test kit and provide other helpful information. When counseling a patient, it is important to stress complete compliance with the test kit directions.

Additionally, the patient should be taught to use proper technique when urine testing for HCG and perform a practice run before the "real" test is attempted in order to become familiar with the basic steps. A practice run assures patient confidence and also assures the availability of proper testing equipment such as a clock or timer and water.

Some monoclonal antibody stick tests require a stream of urine to completely saturate the absorbent end of the stick and caution should be taken that urine not come in contact with or splash up on the test window. This problem can be avoided by turning the window away from the urine stream. Other tests provide the patient with a urine collection cup and urine dropper. The urine can then be dropped into a test well or test window.

The patient should also be taught to check the expiration date of the test kit before using it. Monoclonal antibody tests have shorter lives than the older ring tests, and expired test kits may produce unreliable results.

Drug and Medical Interferences

There are some conditions and drugs that produce an incorrect result with monoclonal antibody test kits for urinary HCG. For example, a HCG-secreting neoplasm may cause a false-positive reaction to occur due to an elevation of HCG.[31,32] Additionally, an intramuscular injection of HCG may cause a false-positive response with a home pregnancy test kit since exogenous HCG may still appear in the urine up to 14 days after the last dose. Fertility endocrinologists may administer HCG (Profasi, Pregnyl) to induce ovulation. Levels of HCG are higher following intramuscular than subcutaneous injection. In women receiving HCG injections a positive test may occur even if there is not a pregnancy.[33] Human chorionic gonadotropin may also be detected in the urine up to 60 days following a miscarriage in the first trimester.[23] Lastly, a false positive result may occur in post-menopausal women due to low circulating levels of HCG in non-pregnant women.

Complications of Pregnancy

Women with an ectopic pregnancy may have a positive pregnancy test when using a home test. An ectopic pregnancy may produce a false positive result since HCG is being produced, but not at concentrations that are as elevated as in an uterine pregnancy. Care should be taken to rule out signs and symptoms that may occur with ectopic pregnancy.[23]

Patient Information - Pregnancy Test Kits

- Women should familiarize themselves with the test kit components.
- Testing may usually be done on the first day of the missed period.
- Products commonly recommend first-morning urine for testing because it contains the highest concentration of HCG.
- If the test requires urine to be collected, the patient should use the container that is provided in the kit (some kits require a dipstick to be held under a stream of urine).
- If the test requires different timed stages, a watch with a second hand should be available (some kits do not involve times steps and simply are left to stand for a period of 3-5 minutes before the results can be read).
- A woman should be careful when opening the sealed package that contains the test strip or test cube/well. Many kits contain areas that are sensitive to skin oils and are not to be touched.
- A woman should read and then reread the test kit instructions. Proper technique is paramount for accurate results.
- If a woman does not have time to complete the test after her urine has been collected, she can refrigerate the urine sample. However, the urine must be brought back to room temperature (20-30 minutes) before proceeding with the test. The test urine should be removed from the top of the urine sample, avoiding any sediment that may have settled to the bottom of the sample container.
- The expiration date of the test kit should be checked before use. Outdated kits may produce inaccurate results.
- Test kits commonly contain two tests. If the first test result is negative, then the woman should repeat the test in 4-5 days using a second test. If the test results remain negative and menstruation has not occurred, a physician visit should be scheduled.
- If the test result is positive, a physician visit should be scheduled for proper prenatal care.
- A negative test result means that HCG was not present in the urine at a detectable concentration. If menstruation has not begun, then retest the urine in 5-10 days. If the test results still remain negative and menstruation has not begun, a physician visit should be scheduled.
- Abdominal pain or discomfort should be confirmed as a pregnancy and not an ectopic pregnancy.

Selecting a Pregnancy Test Kit

The FDA requires manufacturers to have at least a 95% accuracy rate. However, it has been estimated that up to 32% of patients who purchase home pregnancy test kits do not follow the instructions provided, thereby reducing the overall accuracy rate of 75.7%.[34] The accuracy of the home pregnancy test is also greatly affected by the user's technique and experience. One study reports an accuracy rate of 93.5%, which is still lower than the manufacturer's claim.[35] Additionally, reliability of a test depends on experience and competence of the user. Home tests have been shown to be more accurate when used by older patients or patients with higher incomes.[30] Therefore, when selecting a product, consideration should be based on the ease of use as well as precision and clarity of instructions. The best selection is the test kit that has specificity so there is no cross-reaction with other hormones such as LH; sensitivity that is 50 mIU/l or better; produces quick reliable results;[36] and is priced competitively. Refer to Table 12-5 for home pregnancy kit comparisons.

Table 12-5 Pregnancy Test Kits Using Monoclonal Antibody Technology

Product	Results	Total Assay Time	Manufacturer	Comments	Type of Test
Advance Pregnancy Test	Test stick; yes (if two lines) or no (if one line)	5 minutes	Advanced Care Products	One step test and control window to inform user the test is working properly.	Enzyme Immunoassay
Answer Quick & Simple	Test key; lower area changes to pink-purple if positive, remains white if negative.	3 minutes	Carter Products	Can be used one day after missed period*	Colloidal Gold Particle Immunoassay
Clearblue Easy Pregnancy Test	Wand with window; blue line in large window positive; absence of color negative. Control window	3 minutes	Whitehall Laboratories	For correct results test must be held with tip pointing down. Sample is collected by stick in urine stream.	ELISA
Daisy 2	Test cube displays (+) or (-) sign.	5 minutes	Advanced Care Products		ELISA
EPT Early Pregnancy Test	Wand with windows; pink or purple circle in large window positive; absence of color negative. Control window.	4 minutes	Parke-Davis Consumer Products	Sample is collected by holding stick in urine stream.	Colloidal Gold Particle Immunoassay
Fact Plus	Test cube, displays (+) or (-).	5 minutes	Advanced Care Products	Test control window turns red to inform user the test is functioning.	ELISA
First Response Pregnancy Test	Test stick, with control window.	3 minutes	Carter Products	Sample is collected by holding stick in urine stream.	Colloidal Gold Particle Immunoassay
Q-test Pregnancy Test	Stick; blue color positive, White or pale blue negative	9-16 minutes	Becton Dickinson	Has error control pad.	ELISA
Precise	Test cube displays blue check if positive	1 minute	Becton Dickinson	Test turns pink to inform user the test is functioning.	ELISA

* All test kits listed except the Answer Quick & Simple can be used on the day of the missed period.

OVULATION PREDICTION[21]

Home Ovulation Prediction Kits

In women desiring to become pregnant, 80-90% will succeed within a 12 month period. If pregnancy does not occur within a year, frequently a woman will use a home ovulation prediction kit whether upon their own initiative or upon a recommendation from their physician. Women wishing to plan a pregnancy may also use a home ovulation prediction kit to identify the preovulatory LH surge in the urine.

Ovulatory Phase

The ovulatory phase ideally occurs during days 14-15 of a 28-day cycle. During this time, sustained estrogen levels cause the pituitary gland to initiate the surge of serum LH. This LH surge is responsible for maturation of the follicle, ovulation, and formation of the corpus luteum (ruptured follicle).

Prior to the serum LH surge, urinary LH levels fall in the range of 5-20 mIU/ml. As the actual peak concentration of LH is difficult to precisely determine, the LH surge is more predictive of ovulation. The onset of the LH surge is an easier reference point to identify and in some studies has arbitrarily been defined as 35, 40 or 60 mIU/ml.[37,38] Another author has defined the LH surge to occur at urinary concentrations of 30mIU/ml or greater.[39] Ovulation is thought to occur between 24-38 hours after the abrupt rise in the level of serum LH.[38,39] Concentrations of LH in the urine, however, are not seen for a number of hours after the serum LH surge.

Mechanism of Action of Ovulation Prediction Kits

Monoclonal antibodies are used to detect the onset of LH surge by selectively binding to LH in the urine. LH is a glucoprotein composed of two polypeptide subunits (alpha and beta). The alpha subunit is common to other hormones such as FSH, HCG, and TSH. As with the home pregnancy test kits, an enzyme-linked immunoassay or rapid assay technology[29] indicates the amount of LH bound to a monoclonal antibody via a change in color intensity. A test that is a darker shade than the reference chart/dot, or the presence of a colored line in the test window indicates the surge of LH. Radioimmunoassay (RAI) is considered the standard in testing LH concentrations in plasma or urine but is costly and impractical for home use as the test must be conducted in a laboratory.

Selecting an Ovulation Prediction Kit

The correct use of home urinary LH kits is thought to have advantages over other methods of identifying ovulation such as basal body temperature (BBT) measurements, cycle-averaging, and cervical mucous examination. An increase in BBT and thickening of the cervical mucous occurs after ovulation, making these methods less desirable. Also, factors such as stress, physical body movement, and fever can all affect the BBT.

Ovulation prediction kits are also useful in predicting the timing of artificial insemination, postcoital examinations, endometrial biopsy for luteal phase defect, and in some instances egg retrieval for in-vitro fertilization. Following ovulation, the ovum remains viable for 12-24 hours. Because sperm can survive up to 72 hours after intercourse, the optimal days for fertilization include the two days preceding ovulation, the day of ovulation and the day following ovulation.

The ovulation prediction test kits are not indicated for use in contraception because sperm are viable for up to 72 hours after intercourse. Also, the fertile phase of the menstrual cycle is one day before and two days after the LH surge. Therefore, this overlap can mean the difference between contraception and conception.

The majority of ovulation prediction kits are designed to detect urinary LH concentrations at or above the range of 20-50 mIU/ml.[39,41,42]

Proper Testing Techniques

Ovulation prediction test kits contain series of 5-10 urine tests that take from 3-60 minutes to perform depending on the specific test. A woman must first determine how many days are in her menstrual cycle, day one being the first day of menses even if she is only spotting. Once the number of days are calculated, the woman can then determine which day she needs to start urine testing by using a table provided in the instruction booklet of the kit.

During the testing period, a daily collection of urine is tested. Depending on the test kit, the results may be interpreted in one of two ways. The daily result may be compared to a baseline control (OvuGen, OvuQuick, OvuKit). If there is a color change or if the color is darker than the control, then the LH surge has been detected.

Other kits (e.g., ClearPlan Easy,[42] Conceive,[43] First Response[44]) require that a test line be compared to a reference line or the daily result to be kept over the course of the testing period and compared for a change in color or intensity. The LH surge is indicated if either of these occur.

Test users should note that the LH surge does not occur at the same time during each menstrual cycle. Additionally, one study examined the possibility that there might also be seasonal variation in the time of onset of the LH surge.[45] Therefore, if a patient does not conceive during the first month of using an ovulation prediction kit, she may have to purchase a new kit each month to predict her fertile period. Also, if a woman does not have an LH surge during a given month, inappropriate timing or the possibility that she did not ovulate that month may be the cause.

Ovulation is thought to occur in the early morning hours, and after detection in serum, it takes several hours before LH can be detected in the urine. For this reason some kits, such as OvuKit and OvuQuick require urine collection to occur between 10:00 AM and 8:00 PM. Other kits, such as OvuGen allow the urine to be collected at anytime of the day except the first-morning urine. The manufacturer of OvuGen suggests first-morning urine should be avoided since unusually high concentrations of LH may be present which may produce a false-positive result. Other kits which allow the woman to test the urine at anytime of the day include ClearPlan Easy, Conceive, and Q-Test.

The timing of urine collection is important in whatever time the first urine sample is collected and tested, subsequent samples and tests should be performed at the same time of day for the duration of the testing period. Additionally, it is important to refrain from fluid intake 2-4 hours before urine collection to avoid the possibility of producing dilute urine, which could yield a false result. Because fluid intake is usually minimized during sleeping hours, many tests generally require morning urine since it contains the greatest concentration of LH.

After urine collection, the specimen should be tested within eight hours. If this is not possible, the urine can be stored in the refrigerator for up to 24 hours and then allowed to reach room temperature (over 20-30 minutes) before testing occurs.

Timing of the various steps is critical for accurate results when using an ovulation prediction test that requires multiple steps. An area with running water, good light, and a watch or timer with a second hand is essential for most test kits.

Drug Interference

Several drugs and conditions may potentially affect test results. Drugs such as menotropins, danazol, steroids, and oral contraceptives can produce a false-positive result with the ovulation prediction test since LH levels are artificially elevated or can cross-react with the assay for LH. Patients receiving clomiphene therapy, which also elevates LH levels, can use a home kit for detecting a LH surge. However, home testing should not begin until three days after discontinuation of clomiphene therapy. Additionally, medical conditions such as endometriosis, ovarian cysts, hyperthyroidism, tumors, and the onset of menopause can cause abnormally high levels of LH that are not due to the onset of ovulation.

Errors when using ovulation prediction test kits may occur due to patient confusion. In one study where 27 women evaluated the OvuQuick test, 26% stated they had problems reading the results, although 93% stated they believed the test to be simple.[46] Frustrations often occur from inexact timing of the various steps, not holding the test stick with absorbent tip facing down, mixing or rinsing inappropriately, inaccurate interpretation of results, and the expense of the tests. In some instances where there is ambiguity in reading the result, the patient should be urged to collect a urine sample later in the day and retest for urinary LH surge.

Some kits (OvuQuick, OvuKit, OvuGen, and Conceive) produce results that are reproducible at a latter time. These may be used when the patient would like the pharmacist or physician to confirm results. Other kits, such as First Response, produce test results that darken in color over time. For this reason, a patient should be informed to compare results with the color reference provided in the kit and not with a test result taken on a previous day.

Refills are also available for some ovulation prediction test kits. Refills can increase the ability to predict the LH surge by increasing the number of days of the month a woman can test.

Although written on a tenth to twelfth grade education level,[47] patient instructions can be confusing. All of these factors make it important for the consumer to be properly educated on the proper use and interpretation of the test results.

A comparison of currently available ovulation prediction test kits can be found in Table 12-6.

Table 12-6 Ovulation Prediction Test Kits

Product	Results	Total Assay Time	Ease of Use	Manufacturer	Comments
Answer	Test well; Positive result if pink color on test well membrane, negative if white color.	3 minutes	Moderate	Carter Products	
Clearplan Easy	Absence or presence of a line in large window indicates LH. Small window to confirm test is working correctly.	5 minutes	Easy	Whitehall Laboratories	One piece stick test. Tip of test stick must be held pointing toward ground for accurate results. Accuracy of 98% in lab.
Conceive	Built in reference line, compare test line to reference.	3 minutes	Easy	Quidel	One piece stick test. Accuracy of 88.9% in consumer home studies (98% in lab).
First Response Ovulation Predictor Test	Test well; positive results if pink color on test well membrane, negative if white color on test well membrane.	3 minutes	Moderate	Carter Products	Reference color is included.
Fortel Home Ovulation Test	Test tube mixing after waiting periods. Blue color in tube indicates positive.	40 minutes	Moderate	Biomerica	
OvuGen	Mixing and incubation times. Results are compared daily to a reference dot on pad.	3 minutes	Moderate	Biogenex Labs	Visual 2-dot system indicates test is working properly; the color intensity distinguishes low levels of LH from actual surge. Do not use first morning urine.
OvuKit	Test tube mixing after waiting periods. Blue color on paddle indicates positive.	60 minutes	Moderate	Quidel	Surge guide is used. Accuracy of 96% in consumer studies (96% in lab).
OvuQuick	Test pads are used and results are compared daily to a reference dot on pad.	4 minutes	Moderate	Quidel	Accuracy of 94% in consumer home studies (98% in lab).
Q-Test	Test strip turns from pale blue color to dark blue color if positive result. Error control pad present.	3 minutes	Moderate	Becton Dickinson	

FECAL OCCULT BLOOD DETECTION KITS

One of the most widely used in-home detection kits are the occult blood detection kits. These kits are used to detect small amounts of occult (hidden) blood in stool. Fecal occult blood can be an indicator of colorectal bleeding due to various causes including bleeding hemorrhoids, diverticulitis, or an adverse reaction to medications that can cause gastrointestinal irritation (i.e., non-steroidal anti-inflammatory drugs) or drugs that can increase the risk of bleeding (i.e., warfarin). However, one of the most publicized uses of fecal occult blood tests (FOBT) is as a screening tool for the early detection of colorectal cancer.

Colorectal cancer is the second leading cause of death due to cancer in the United States.[48] It is responsible for an estimated 60,000 deaths in 1992.[48] Early detection and treatment of colorectal cancers are thought to increase survival. In one review, the limitations and inefficiencies of using FOBT's for colorectal cancer screening are outlined.[49] This review notes that "approximately 2-10% of all screeners have positive test results. Of these, 88-98% will not have colorectal cancer".[50-53] These false-positives are attributed to other sources of blood in stool such as bleeding hemorrhoids, fissures, gastrointestinal bleeding brought on by direct mucosal irritants (i.e., medications), or interactions with the test itself. The author also contends that the sensitivity of FOBT's "for colorectal cancer during screening probably will not exceed 30%", or that FOBT's will produce a false-negative rate of 70%.[49]

When early colorectal cancers bleed, they bleed intermittently, reducing the chances of detecting blood in the stool. It should also be noted that most premalignant colorectal adenomas may not bleed and are missed with FOBT's.[54] In a recent prospective, blinded, multi-center study subjects were asked to mail in stool samples that would be checked for occult blood using a guaiac paper slide (Hemoccult II) and a newer quantitative test for occult blood (HemoQuant). Although many studies to date document the insensitivity of FOBT's to detect colorectal cancer, until recently none have shown that these tests can decrease mortality through early detection. In May of 1993, Mandel and associates published the results of a 13 year study that demonstrated a 33% decrease in mortality in a study group that tested fecal samples annually versus a control group.[56] This study followed 46,551 participants that were randomized into three groups: those who had FOBT's every year, every two years, and a control. Mortality data from the three groups indicated that per 1000 participants, the annual screening group had 5.88 deaths, the biannual group, 8.33; and the control group, 8.83. The difference between the annual testing group, and the control group is statistically significant. Patients in the testing groups were asked to smear two samples of each of three consecutive stools onto a guaiac impregnated paper slide and submit these for testing. In most cases the paper slides were rehydrated before testing, to improve sensitively of the test. If one or more of the six samples were found to be positive for blood, the patient was contacted and urged to return to the hospital for further evaluation. Evaluation of a positive FOBT included medical history and physical examination, rigid proctosigmoidoscopy or colonoscopy, barium enema, and routine blood and urine tests. Authors of this study concluded that the use of FOBT's may increase the number of diagnostic procedures by fourfold, possibly increasing cost of care. This cost of care will have to be weighed against the possible benefit of reducing mortality of colorectal cancer by 33%. The results of this study demonstrated that both tests had a sensitivity for cancers of 26%, and for polyps 1.0 cm or larger of 13% and 11% by Hemoccult II and HemoQuant, respectively. It was the conclusion of these researchers that fecal occult blood appears to be a poor marker for colorectal neoplasia.[55] The results of this study will be either confirmed or denied when the results of four other randomized, controlled trials that are evaluating the efficacy of FOBT's as a screening tool are published.[50-53]

The National Cancer Institute and the American Cancer Society currently recommend the following for colorectal screening: 1) During a regular physical examination, a digital rectal examination is performed annually after age 40; 2) after age 50 years, annual FOBT and sigmoidoscopy, preferably flexible, are done every 3-5 years; and 3) the physician should give special attention to patients at high risk. These patients include those with a familial history of colorectal cancer, or a personal history of colon polyps, colorectal, breast, endometrial or ovarian cancer, or inflammatory bowel disease.[56] Although none of these procedures have had a definitive evaluation as to their ability to increase detection of early colorectal cancer, they are based in facts. Approximately 10% of colorectal cancers are found within 7-10 cm of the anus, within reach of a digital rectal examination. After age 50, the risk of colorectal cancer doubles every ten years until age 70.[58,59]

The earliest FOBT detected blood by using the guaiac reaction (Hemoccult II, SmithKline Diagnostics). This reaction utilizes hemoglobin and hydrogen peroxide to convert a colorless compound (alphaguaiaconic acid) to a quinone compound that is blue.[59] Other tests that are based on this oxidation reaction include the guaiacol and tetramethylbenzidine (EZ Detect, Biomerica) tests.[61] An advantage to using these tests is that they do not react with vegetable peroxidases. Newer tests that detect blood in stool include immunochemical tests (e.g., HemeSelect, SmithKline Diagnostics) and the heme-porphyrin assay (e.g., HemoQuant, SmithKline Bioscience). The immunochemical test detects human hemoglobin by reacting with globin. This selectivity for human red blood cells reduces the need for dietary restrictions before and during stool testing.[49] The heme-porphyrin test measures the amount of hemoglobin and fecal heme altered by bacteria, and quantifies this amount as fecal hemoglobin equivalents.[62] Guaiac and guaiacol tests are only available for physician or lab use, or for mass screening programs. The immunochemical and heme-porphyrin tests are more costly and are used only in reference laboratories.[62] As of this writing, only the tetramethylbenzidine test is currently available for in-home use.[61] However, because of Mandel and colleagues' report of lower mortality rates due to early detection, other manufacturers may release FOBTs in the future.[56]

Paper guaiac slides require retrieval of a stool sample that is applied to the paper. In an attempt to make in-home testing more appealing, the current in-home product (EZ Detect, Biomerica) allows for the patient to simply float a reagent-treated pad face up in the toilet after a bowel movement. The toilet is flushed twice before the patient has a bowel movement. A reagent pad is floated in the toilet with the specimen. If there are significant amounts of blood present in the water (2.0 mg hemoglobin/100 ml water)[63] the pad indicates this with a blue cross within two minutes. Ideally, this tests for blood that has dissipated from the surface of the stool, on to the surface of the water rather than stool matrix blood. After the test results are recorded, the pad and the specimen are flushed away.[63] Checking three consecutive bowel movements is recommended, as with most occult blood tests. This is to decrease the chance of missing an intermittently bleeding lesion. Another toilet bowl test kit, ColoCARE (Helena Laboratories. Beaumont, TX), is only marketed for professional use and is not directly available to the public.

Although dietary restrictions are not recommended with the tetramethylbenzidine test, certain dietary measures have been recommended to increase the probability of an accurate result. Patients should be encouraged to eat a diet high in fiber two days before the testing period to increase the possibility of gastrointestinal bleeding. By eating moderate amounts of fruits, cooked and raw vegetables, peanuts and popcorn, polyps and other cancerous growths within the bowel will be induced to bleed by the increased bulk scraping the interior of the gut.[64] A false negative result with guaiac tests has been attributed to diets containing more than 250 mg of vitamin C per day. Large doses of vitamin C may interfere with the oxidation process resulting in inhibition of color reaction even though blood is present. Manufacturer information available for the tetramethylbenzidine test indicates that up to 1000 mg of vitamin C did not interfere with the test.[61]

Certain medications should be avoided during the testing period because of a potential false positive test result. Gastrointestinal irritants such as aspirin products, corticosteroids, dipyridamole, iron-containing products, nonsteroidal anti-inflammatory agents, povidone-iodine, and reserpine should be avoided at least two days before and during the test period.[65] The use of rectal dosage forms should also be avoided.[65]

In addition to medications, dietary factors can lead to false-positive results with the guaiac tests and should be avoided at least three days before and during the test period. Foods to be avoided include: red meats (beef, lamb), certain vegetables (broccoli, carrots, cauliflower, mushrooms, radishes, turnips), fruits (cantaloupe, grapefruit) and horseradish. Animal source hemoglobin and peroxidase contained in vegetables and fruits can react with the guaiac based occult blood tests resulting in a false positive reading.[66] The tetramethylbenzidine reagent used in EZ Detect is not affected by dietary peroxidase, or by the consumption of rare beef.[61]

Other sources of false readings include the fact that hemoglobin is converted by bacteria in the gut to porphoryins. Porphoryins do not react with guaiac and, therefore, upper gastrointestinal bleeding may not test positive by the guaiac method.[67] In addition, dehydrated stools, constipation and diarrhea may give false results.[65] Non-gastrointestinal sources of blood may also give false positive results. These can include testing during menstruation, swallowed blood from nosebleeds, or testing toilet water with hematuria in it.

In addition to the basic patient education for these products outlined above, instructions for physician follow-up is essential. Positive results may not always indicate colorectal cancer, however they need to be evaluated. As indicated earlier, negative results need to be followed because they do not indicate the absolute absence of cancer.

Other important patient education tips for FOBT's that have not been mentioned include: 1) Protect the testing kit from direct sunlight, 2) if required, accurately time test as specified, and 3) check the expiration date of the test. For a complete summary list of patient education tips for the FOBT's see Table 12-7.

CHOLESTEROL MONITORING

Hypercholesterolemia, along with hypertension and smoking, are known risk factors for the development of cardiovascular disease. Coronary heart disease (CHD), a manifestation of cardiovascular disease, is the leading cause of death in the U.S. Early detection of elevated serum lipid levels and subsequent treatment, among other factors have led to a decline in the number of deaths due to CHD in recent years.[68]

The National Cholesterol Education Program

Table 12-7 Patient Education Tips for the FOBT's

I. DIET

1. Two days before, and during the test period eat high fiber foods (raw, cooked vegetables, some fruits, peanuts, popcorn, etc.)
2. If guaiac tests (e.g.., Hemoccult II) are to be used, avoid eating: broccoli, carrots, cauliflower, mushrooms, radishes, turnips, cantaloupe, grapefruit, and horseradish prior to and during the testing period.

II. MEDICATIONS

1. Two days before, and during the test period avoid taking medications listed in Table 12-1. (i.e., aspirin, corticosteroids, non-steroidal anti-inflammatory drugs, etc.) Patients should check with their pharmacist or physician before stopping any medication.
2. Do not use rectal suppositories, creams, or enemas during testing period.
3. If guaiac tests are to be used, do not take more than 250 mg of Vitamin C per day during the testing period.

III. THE TEST

1. Read all instructions carefully before proceeding with test.
2. Check test's expiration date.
3. Protect test kit from direct sunlight and extreme temperatures.
4. Remove toilet sanitizers from toilet, and flush toilet before defecating.
5. Do not test if you are menstruating, constipated, or have bleeding hemorrhoids.
6. Test three consecutive bowel movements.
7. Time test accurately as outlined by directions.
8. Report all results to physician (positive and negative results).

(NCEP) in 1988 published its recommendations on the detection, evaluation, and treatment of increased blood cholesterol levels.[69] The NCEP recommended that desirable levels of total cholesterol and low density lipoprotein (LDL) cholesterol should be < 200 mg/dl and < 130 mg/dl, respectively. Total cholesterol and LDL cholesterol levels greater than these put the patient at risk for developing CHD. An additional factor was identified when the results of the Framingham Heart Study were analyzed.[70] In this study it was found that a strong, inverse relationship was found between high density lipoprotein (HDL) cholesterol and CHD. Since that time a number of clinical trials have confirmed the finding that even if total cholesterol levels are below the NCEP suggested level of 200 mg/dl, if the HDL cholesterol level is also reduced the patient is at risk of developing CHD.[71,72,73] In June of 1993, the Second Report of the National Cholesterol Education Program (NCEP) Expert Panel on Detection, Evaluation, and Treatment of High Blood Cholesterol in Adults was published.[74] The panel identified positive and negative risk factors for coronary heart disease (CHD). See Table 12-8. Desirable levels of total cholesterol remained less than 200 mg/dl, and a desirable level of HDL was determined to be greater than 35 mg/dl. Desirable LDL levels, however, are dependent on whether or not the patient has CHD and if one or more of the risk factors are present. Treatment decisions as to how to treat patients are determined by the total cholesterol, HDL, and LDL levels, and the presence or absence of risk factors. See Table 12 -9. It is currently recognized that total cholesterol, HDL, and LDL levels, as well as the presence or absence of risk factors such as male sex, family history of premature CHD, cigarette smoking, hypertension, diabetes mellitus, definite cerebrovascular or peripheral vascular disease, or severe obesity should be taken into account when assessing a patient's risk of developing CHD.

In March 1993, the Food and Drug Administration approved for marketing to the general public the first home cholesterol test. Produced by Chem Trak, Inc. (Sunnyvale, CA), the AccuMeter Cholesterol Self-Test kit measures total cholesterol using a fingerstick sample of blood. A fixed quantity

Table 12-8 Coronary Heart Disease Risk Factors (NCEP)[74]

Positive Risk Factors

Age: Male ≥ 45 years
Female ≥ 55 or premature menopause without estrogen replacement therapy
Current cigarette smoking
Diabetes Mellitus
Family history of premature CHD (Definite myocardial infarction or sudden death before 55 years old in father or other male first-degree relative, or before 65 years old in mother or other female first-degree relative.)
Hypertension (blood pressure ≥ 140/90 mm Hg, or taking antihypertensive medication.)
Low HDL cholesterol (< 35 mg/dl)

Negative Risk Factor

High HDL cholesterol (≥ 60 mg/dl)

Table 12-9 Treatment Decisions As Recommended by NCEP[73]

1.	IF Blood Cholesterol ≥ 240 mg/dl, or HDL < 35 mg/dl, then check LDL.	
2.	Treat with diet if patient is:	<u>and LDL level is</u>:
	without CHD and with < 2 risk factors	≥ 160 MG/DL
	without CHD and with > 2 risk factors	≥ 130 MG/DL
	with CHD	> 100 MG/DL
3.	Treat with medications if patient is:	<u>and LDL level is</u>:
	without CHD and with < 2 risk factors	≥ 190 MG/DL
	without CHD and with > 2 risk factors	≥ 160 MG/DL
	with CHD	> 130 MG/DL

(five microliters) of serum reacts with cholesterol esterase and cholesterol oxidase where the cholesterol contained in the sample is converted to hydrogen peroxide. The hydrogen peroxide reacts with horseradish peroxidase and a substrate that is fixed uniformly to chromatographic paper. This results in a color change in the form of a stripe, the length of which is an indication of the amount of cholesterol in the fingerstick sample of blood.[75]

Although the principles of this test are similar to other reagent strip tests used in the home, the enzymes, wicking reagent, and fingerstick sample separating and measuring devices are all self-contained in a cassette system. The cassette system has a sample well on one end, a tab that when pulled starts the test, and a window that runs the length of the cassette where the color band can be read. On each end of this window are indicator spots, at the bottom of the window one is marked "Test Working" and at the top of the window another labelled "Complete".[75]

In order to perform the test the patient will have to prick her/his finger and apply 2 to 3 drops of blood into the sample well. Once the third drop of blood is in the well the patient waits two minutes. During this two minutes the erythrocytes are separated from the plasma and 5 microliters of plasma is deposited onto a sample pad. After the two minutes have elapsed the tab is pulled to start the reaction. Pulling the tab brings the sample pad into contact with the wicking reagent, which draws the sample through the enzyme reagent pad and on to the measurement region of the strip. The test will take 10 to 12 minutes until the "Complete" indicator window turns green. When the "Complete" window turns green, a color band is read from the measurement region. The calibrations along this region are then checked against a chart to determine the cholesterol reading.[76]

In one study, the AccuMeter Cholesterol test was found to be comparable to the Boehringer Mannheim High Performance reference assay with a correlation coefficient of 0.97.[75] The AccuMeter Cholesterol test appears to be an innovative approach to total cholesterol monitoring. Possible roles that it may be used for include screening programs, and monitoring of cholesterol-lowering diets or drug therapy. It should be kept in mind, however, that this test only measures total cholesterol. As presented earlier, recent data supports the interpretation of total cholesterol levels along with an HDL level. Therefore, the lay public should be counselled on the correct use of the test, as well as the meaning of the results. That is, a total cholesterol level of < 200 mg/dl may not indicate a CHD risk-free level, that HDL and LDL levels are also needed in order to adequately assess a patient's risk for dyslipidemias.

RENAL SCREENING

Kidney disease affects 12 million Americans. Renal problems can arise from unknown etiology, an acute disease state such as an infection, or a complication due to chronic disease states such as hypertension or diabetes. Two common urinary manifestations of renal diseases include hematuria and proteinuria. Reagent strips that tested for these conditions have been used in laboratories and physician offices for years. Currently, in-home tests are now available to detect these two conditions.

Products That Detect Hematuria

Hematuria, although usually a sign of a kidney or urinary tract abnormality, is not a specific sign of any one disorder.[77] There are several reasons for blood to appear in urine including glomerular diseases, neoplasms, inflammatory or infectious disorders of the kidneys, ureter, or lower urinary tract, and systemic disorders. Blood may appear in the urine for non-pathological reasons as well, including after severe exercise, and in a condition known as benign recurrent hematuria of childhood.[77] These are usually the exception, not the rule.

In-home reagent strips that are marketed directly to the consumer and detect hematuria include the EZ Detect (Biomerica, Inc., Newport Beach, CA) and Biotel Kidney (Biotel, Corp., New York, NY). Other urine screening products that are available through wholesale distributors, but are not directly marketed for in-home use include the Multistix product line (Miles Diagnostics, Elkhart IN), and the Chemstrip 4 through 10 product line (Boehringer Mannheim Diagnostics, Indianapolis, IN). EZ Detect and Biotel Kidney utilize the pseudoperoxidative activity of hemoglobin which catalyzes oxidation of tetramethylbenzidine by oxygen released by hydrogen peroxide.[78,79] The reaction results in a color change of a reagent pad. A comparison of these products are summarized on Table 12-10.

Antioxidants can potentially render false-negative results with these tests. A common dietary antioxidant that is excreted renally is ascorbic acid, or Vitamin C. Patient instructions for both products warn patients against consuming Vitamin C containing foods and products two days prior to testing. One product, EZ Detect, actually tests for the presence of ascorbic acid in the urine. Patients are instructed to disregard the results of the test if the Vitamin C reagent pad changes color after exposure to urine. EZ Detect also warns against testing during menstruation.[78] Biotel Kidney's package insert includes instructions on how to run a quality control check on the reagent strips using household chlorine bleach and baking soda.[79]

Products That Detect Proteinuria

Unlike blood, there is a daily urinary loss of protein. Urinary protein is normally made up of albumin, tissue proteins from renal and other urogenital tissues, immunoglobulins and other plasma proteins. Normal protein excretion rates are less than 150 mg per 24 hours, although up to 300 mg per 24 hours has been seen in apparently normal healthy adolescents.[80] Chronic proteinuria of greater than 750 mg per 24 hours is considered a specific indica-

Table 12-10 Comparison of Urine Occult Blood Tests[77,78]

	EZ Detect	Biotel Kidney
Dip time	5-10 sec.	1 sec.
Read results after	1 min.	30 sec.
Interactions	Vitamin C	Vitamin C
Sensitivity	<3 RBC's per1/100 of a drop of urine	5-10 RBC's/microliter of urine
Number of tests/kit:	6	12
Also tests for	Vitamin C	Proteinuria

tor of kidney disease such as interstitial or glomerular damage. Accelerated hypertension and severe congestive heart failure has been known to produce massive proteinuria.

Diabetic nephropathy is a complication of diabetes mellitus that affects up to 40% of persons who have insulin dependent diabetes mellitus (IDDM) for 20 years or longer. Non-insulin dependent diabetes (NIDDM) patients may also develop this complication but it is seen less frequently than in IDDM.[81] Hypertension along with diabetes increases the risk of developing this complication, which accounts for approximately one third of all new cases of end stage renal disease (ESRD). Among its earliest signs is persistent microalbuminuria, or small amounts of albumin lost through the urine (20 to 300 mg per 24 hours).[81] Microalbuminuria is seen 10 to 15 years after the original diagnosis of diabetes is made. A rule of thumb is that the albuminuria excretion rate is about three quarters of the urinary protein excretion rate.[81]

Biotel Kidney (Biotel Corp., New York, NY) is currently the only product that is marketed directly to consumers for renal screening and proteinuria detection. As with other products mentioned including the Multistix product line, Uristix, Albustix (all produced by Miles Diagnostics, Elkhart, IN) and the Chemstrip 4 through 10 product line (Boehringer Mannheim, Indianapolis, IN) these products are available through wholesale distributors; however, these companies do not market these products for in-home use.

Proteinuria reagent strip tests utilize the "protein error of indicators" principle.[81] The reagent pad contains a buffered indicator that changes color when exposed to albumin. Biotel Kidney's proteinuria reagent pad uses tetrabromphenol blue. When the indicator is exposed to albumin, the yellow, protonated form of the indicator, shifts to the anionic form producing a greenish blue color change. The greater the amount of albumin in the urine, the darker the color change. The minimum sensitivity of Biotel Kidney for protein is 10 mg protein/dl urine.[79] It has been suggested that with the proteinuria reagent strips the first morning urine should be tested since it is more concentrated and not affected by postural factors,[83] however the manufacturer of Biotel Kidney does not note this in its package insert.[79]

Possible sources of test interferences and errors are noted on Table 12-11. Alkaline urines can result in a false positive result. Possible causes of an increased urine pH include ingestion of sodium bicarbonate, acetazolamide, and potassium citrate.[83] Also vegetarian diets, citrus fruits, milk and other dairy products can produce alkaline urine and affect this test.[83] Patients should be warned against ingesting these prior to testing.

As with other screening tests, patients should be instructed to tell their physician the results of these tests regardless of the results. A negative finding may not rule out an active disease state, and a positive result may not indicate active renal disease.

URINARY TRACT INFECTION DETECTION

Urinary tract infections (UTI) are consid-

Table 12-11 Sources of Interferences with Proteinuria Dipstick Tests [78,80]

FALSE POSITIVE RESULTS
Prolonged dipping of strip in urine
Highly alkaline urine
Testing after infusion of a blood substitute
Testing during menstruation, or with urinary tract infection
Drugs: Quinine
FALSE NEGATIVE RESULTS
Very dilute urine
OTHER SOURCES OF TEST ERROR
Inaccurate matching of reagent pad color to color chart

ered to be one of the most common infections. Women experience UTI more frequently than men, until late in the fifth decade of life when the prevalence increases in men. One third of women will have a UTI before the age of 65. Populations at risk for developing a UTI include the new born, prepubertal girls, young boys, sexually active young women, and the elderly. The severity of these infections can range from simple, localized infections that are easily treated with a single dose of antibiotic, to major bacteremia resulting in death.[83]

Reagent strips that detect various signs of a UTI have been available for use in physicians' offices for years. These test strips check the urine for the presence of, among other things, nitrite. Nitrite is derived from the reduction of nitrates by some gram negative bacteria. Escherichia coli is found to be the causative bacteria in almost 80% of uncomplicated urinary tract infections and is a known nitrite producer.[84] Bacteria that do not convert nitrate to nitrite will not be detected. These include gram positive organisms, and Pseudomonas.

Biotel u.t.i. (Biotel Corp.) is the only product available that is marketed for in-home screening of urinary tract infections. The package contains a canister of twelve test strips, a foil wrapped Positive Control strip used to run a quality control on any unused strips, and a patient package insert. The test is run by wetting the test strip with urine. The test strip can be either dipped in urine collected in a clean, dry container, or passed through a stream of urine. The urine used should be first morning urine. The overnight delay allows time for bacteria to produce more nitrite. After wetting with urine, the strip is tapped to remove any excess urine. If nitrite is present in the urine, the sensor pad changes to a shade of pink after 30 seconds. Any color change after 1 minute is invalid and the patient is told to disregard this result. The test will detect 0.05 to 0.1 mg/dl of nitrite in urine. False negative results may be produced if ascorbic acid is present in the urine. The package insert warns the patient to avoid using vitamin C or eating foods high in vitamin C prior testing. Other causes of false negative results include low nitrate diets, antibiotic therapy, and very dilute urine. Patients are instructed to call their physician in case of a positive result.[85] However, it may be prudent to have the patient report any result to their physician since nitrite is not produce by all urinary tract pathogens.

Some of the Chemstrip (Boehringer Mannheim) and Multistix (Miles Diagnostics) urine products check for nitrite in urine as well. These products can be ordered through distributors, but are not packaged or marketed for in-home use.

FUTURE

The future is promising for the home test kit market. Kits have been streamlined and made easier to use over the past couple of years. Kits such as the pregnancy and ovulation tests are now one piece devices. This is an important feature since the easier the product is to use the more likely a consumer will be able to follow directions and produce accurate results.

In the next few years, a new generation of products will be available for the consumer to use at home. Tests currently waiting for FDA approval include a home strep throat kit and a home HIV test.[86-89] Other areas that are promising include a test to detect fertility with saliva, and tests for chlamydia, gonorrhea, and trichomonas.[90-93]

The willingness of consumers to become involved in monitoring and assessing their own health care will bring about more products that can be beneficial in the home environment.

REFERENCES

1. Lewis R. Biotech devices-replacing test animals, improving diagnosis. FDA Consumer. 1992-1993; 27(1):15-18.
2. Young F E. A doctor's advice on self-care. FDA Consumer. 1988-1989; 22(1):6-7.
3. Tanouye E. Home medical test past healthy sales. Wall Street Journal. November 12, 1992.
4. The Joint National Committee. The fifth report of the Joint National Committee on the Detection, Evaluation, and Treatment of High Blood Pressure. (JNC V). Arch Intern Med. 1993; 153:154-183.
5. Soghikian K, Casper SM, Fireman BH, et al. Home blood pressure monitoring. Effect on use of medical services and medical care costs. Medical Care. 1992; 30(9):855-865.
6. American Society of Hypertension. Recommendations for routine blood pressure measurement by indirect cuff sphygmomanometry. Am J Hypertension. 1992; 5:207-209.
7. Veerman DP, Van Montrans GA, Wieling W. Effects of cuff inflation on self-recorded blood pressure. Lancet. 1990; 335:451-453.
8. Schmidt GR, Wenig JH. An evaluation of home blood-pressure monitoring devices. American Pharmacy. 1989; NS29:25-30.
9. Latman NS. Evaluation of finger blood pressure monitoring instruments. Biomedical Instrumentation and Technology. 1992; 26(1):52-57.
10. Hunt JC, Frohlich ED, Moser M, et al. Devices used for self-measurement of blood pressure. Revised statement of the national high blood pressure education program. Archives of Internal Medicine. 1985; 145:2231-2234.
11. Nykamp D, Barnett CW, Lorys RA, Miyahara RK. Accuracy of stationary automated blood pressure monitoring devices in the community setting. Consultant Pharmacist. 1992; 7(10):1074-1079.
12. Nykamp D, Barnett,CW. Use of stationary automated blood pressure devices in pharmacies. American Pharmacy. 1992; NS32:33-36.
13. Anonymous. Report assess use of blood pressure monitoring devices for ambulatory patients. Clinical American Pharmacy. 1991; 10(3):175.
14. Smith MM. Home blood pressure monitoring. American Pharmacy. 1985; NS 25:46-48.
15. Anonymous. Blood pressure monitors. Consumer Reports. 1987; 5:314-319.
16. Anonymous. Blood pressure monitors. Consumer Reports. 1992; 5:295-302.
17. McNeil Consumer Products. Health Advisor Tylenol. Fort Washington, PA 19034.
18. Marshall Electronics, Inc. Lincolnshire, IL. Guide To Understanding And Recording Your Ovulation Cycle.
19. Thermoscan, San Diego, CA 92121.
20. Hallcrest Products, Glenview, IL 60025.
21. Nykamp D. Pregnancy detection and ovulation prediction: home monitoring with monoclonal antibody technology. Accepted for publication, U.S. Pharmacist. 1992.
22. Braunstein G, Grodin J, Vaitukaitis J, Ross G. Secretory rates of human chorionic gonadotropin by normal trophoblast. Am J Obstet Gynecol. 1973; 115:447.
23. Chard T. Pregnancy tests: a review. Human Reproduction. 1992; 7(5):701-710.
24. Sagraves R, Letassy NA. Obstetrics. In Koda-Kimble Ma, Young LY: Applied Therapeutics, The Clinical Use Of Drugs, 5th ed. Vancouver, WA: Applied Therapeutics, Inc. 1992; 68/2-68/3.
25. Tami JA, Parr MD, Brown SA, et al. Monoclonal antibody technology. Amer J Hosp Pharm. 1986; 43:2817-24.
26. Drug information for the health care professional, 12th ed. Rockville, MD: United States Pharmacopeial Convention, Inc. 1992; 2317-19.
27. Policar MS. New pregnancy test technology & clinical applications. Outlook, 2-6,1986.
28. May K. Home tests to monitor fertility. Am J Obstet Gynecol. 1991; 165:2000-2002.
29. Whitehall Laboratories Clearblue Easy® Package insert. New York, NY, 1989.
30. Fields SA, Toffler WL. Pregnancy testing-home and office. Western Journal of Medicine. 1991; 154(3):327-328.
31. Advice for the Patient, 12th ed. Rockville, MD: United States Pharmacopeial Convention, Inc. 1992; 1051-52.
32. Miyahara RK, Nykamp D. On the shelf and in the future. US Pharm. 1990; 9(12):50-61.
33. Lee C, Hart LL. Accuracy of home pregnancy tests. DICP Ann. Pharmacother. 1990; 24:712-713.
34. Valanis B, Perlman S. Home pregnancy testing kits: prevalence of use, false-positive rates, and compliance with instructions. Am J Public Health. 1982; 72:1034-1036.
35. Hicks JM, Losefsohn M. Reliability of home pregnancy test kits in the hands of laypersons. N Engl J Med. 1989; (Letter)320:320-321.
36. Coons SJ, Churchill l, Brinkman ML. The use of pregnancy test kits by college students. 1990; 38:171-175.
37. Rebar RW. Practical applications of home diagnostic products - a symposium. Journ Reproductive Medicine. 1987; 32 (9):705-727.
38. Garcia JE, Jones GS, Wright GL. Prediction of the time of ovulation. Fertil Steril. 1981; 36(3):308-315.
39. Corsan GH, Gahzi D, Kemmann E. Home urinary

luteinizing hormone immunoassay: clinical applications. Fertil Steril. 1990; 50:591-601.
40. Elkind-Hirsh K, Goldzeieher JW, Gibbons WE, Besch PK. Evaluation of the ovustick urinary luteinizing hormone kit in normal and stimulated menstrual cycles. Obstet Gynecol. 1986; 67:450-453.
41. Quidel Ovustick Package Insert. San Diego, CA.
42. Whitehall Laboratories ClearPlan Easy Product Information, New York, NY.
43. Conceive Product Information, Quidel, 10165, McKellar Court, San Diego, CA 92121.
44. Carter Products First Response Ovulation Prediction Production Information, New York, NY.
45. Testart J, Frydman R, Roger M. Seasonal influence of diurnal rhythms in theonset of the plasma luteinizing hormone surge in women. J. Clin. Endocrinol. Metab. 1982; 55:374-377.
46. Bieglmayer C, Fischl F, Janisch H. Evaluation of a simple and fast self-test for urine luteinizing hormone. Fertil Steril. 1990; 53:842-846.
47. Catania PN, Rosner MM. Self monitoring aids for the home care patient. In: Home Health Care Practice. Palo Alto, CA, Health Markets Research. 1987; 19:159-161.
48. American Cancer Society. Cancer facts and figures: 1991; New York: The Society. 1992; 1-10.
49. Ahlquist DA. Occult blood screening. Cancer 1992; 70(5):1259-65.
50. Gilbertsen VA, Church TR, Drewe FJ, et al. The design of the study to assess occult blood screening for colon cancer. J Chron Dis. 1980; 33:107-114.
51. Hardcastle JD, Thomas WM, Chamberlain J, et al. Randomized controlled trial of fecal occult blood screening for colorectal cancer: the results of the first 107,349 subjects. Lancet. 1989; 1:1160-4.
52. Kewenter J, Bjork S, Haglind E, et al. Screening and rescreening for colorectalcancer: a controlled trial of fecal occult blood testing in 27,000 subjects. Cancer. 1988; 62:645-51.
53. Kronborg O, Fenger C, Olsen J, et al. Repeated screening for colorectal cancer with fecal occult blood test: a prospective randomized study at Funen, Denmark. Scand J Gastroenterol. 1989; 24:599-606.
54. Ransohoff DF, Lang CA. Small adenomas detected during fecal occult blood test screening for colorectal cancer: the impact of serendipity. JAMA. 1990; 264:76-8.
55. Ahlquist DA, Wieand HS, Moertel CG, et al. Accuracy of fecal occult blood screening for colorectal neoplasia. JAMA 1993; 269:1262-1267.
56. Mandel JS, Bond JH, Church TR, et.al. Reducing mortality from colorectal cancer by screening for fecal occult blood. N Engl J Med. 1993; 328:1366-71.
57. Levin B, Murphy GP. Revision in American Cancer Society recommendations for the early det ection of colorectal cancer. CA 1992; 42(5):296-9.
58. Winawer SJ, Miller PG, Sherlock P. Risk and screening for colo-rectal cancer. Adv Intern Med. 1984; 35:33-48.
59. Fath RB, Winawer SJ. Early diagnosis of colo-rectal cancer. Ann Rev Med. 1983; 34:501-517.
60. Knight KK, Fielding JE, Battista RN. Occult blood screening for colo-rectal cancer. JAMA. 1989; 261:587-93.
61. Gray SL. Fecal occult blood testing for colorectal cancer. Am Pharm. 1992; NS32(10):50-53.
62. Ahlquist DA, McGill DB, Schwartz S, et al. Hemoquant, a new quantitative assay for fecal hemoglobin: comparison with hemoccult. Ann Intern Med. 1984; 101:297-302.
63. EZ Detect Product Information. Newport Beach, CA: Biomerica Inc.
64. Gossel T. Over-the-Counter Fecal Occult Blood Testing Kits. U.S. Pharmacist. 1984; 9:10.
65. Engle JP, Donnelly AJ, Lewis RK. Fecal occult blood tests: potential drug interactions. Consultant Pharm. 1988; 7-8:356-358.
66. Gnauck R, Macrae FA, Fleisher M. How to perform the fecal occult blood test. CA. 1984; 34:134-47.
67. Burton RM, Landreth KS, Barrows GH, et.al. Appearance, properties, and origin of altered human hemoglobin in feces. Lab Invest. 1976; 35:3-5.
68. National Center for Health Statistics. Vital Statistics of the United States, 1968-1988. Washington, D.C., Government Printing Office, 1968-1988.
69. The Expert Panel. Report of the National Cholesterol Education Program Expert Panel on Detection, Evaluation and Treatment of High Blood Cholesterol in Adults. Arch Intern Med. 1988; 148:36-69.
70. Castelli WP, Garrison RJ, Wilson PWF, et al. Incidence of coronary heart disease and lipoprotein cholesterol levels: the Framingham Study. JAMA. 1986; 256:2835-8.
71. Miller NE. Associations of high-density lipoprotein subclasses and apolipoproeins with ischemic heart disease and coronary atherosclerosis. Am Heart J. 1987; 113:587-97.
72. Gordon DJ, Probstfield JL, Garrison RJ, et al. High-density lipoprotein cholesterol and cardiovascular disease: four prospective american studies. Circulation. 1989; 79:8-15.
73. Stampfer MJ, Sacks FM, Salvini S, et al. A prospective study of cholesterol apolipoproteins, and the risk of myocardial infarction. N Engl J Med. 1991; 325:373-81.
74. Cardinale V. New cholesterol guidelines to factor in age, women. Drug Topics 1993; 137:40-3.
75. Allen MP, DeLizza A, Ramel U, et. Al. A noninstrumented quantitative test system and its application for determining cholesterol concentration in whole blood. Clin Chem. 1990; 36:1591-7.
76. Accumeter Cholesterol Test Kit. Product information, Chem Trak, Sunnyvale, CA.
77. Andreoli TE. Approach to the patient with renal disease. In: Wyngarden JB, Smith LH, Eds. Cecil Textbook of Medicine, 17th Edition. Philadelphia, PA: W.B. Saunders CO.1985; 483-90.
78. EZ Detect Product Information. Newport Beach, CA: Biomerica Inc.
79. Biotel Kidney Product Information. New York, NY: Biotel, Corp.
80. Dennis VW. Investigations of renal function. In: Wyngarden JB, Smith LH, Eds.Cecil Textbook of

Medicine, 17th Edition. Philadelphia, PA: W.B. Saunders Co. 1985; 507-515.

81. The prevention and treatment of complications of diabetes. Department of Health and Human Services. CDC. 1991; 52-57.
82. Silverman LM, Christenson RH, Grant GH. Amino acids and proteins. In: Tietz NW, ed. Textbook of Clinical Chemistry. Philadelphia, PA: W.B. Saunders Co. 1986; 519-618.
83. Anonymous. Urine Studies, in: Fischback FT. A manual of laboratory diagnostic tests, 2nd ed. Philadelphia, PA: J.B. Lippincott Co. 1984; 105-186.
84. Neu HC. Urinary tract Infections. Am J Med. 1992; 92(suppl 4a):4a-63s to 4a-70s.
85. Biotel U.T.I. Product information. Biotel Corp., New York, NY.
86. Buchta R.M. Use of a rapid strep test (first response) by parents for detection of streptococcal pharyngitis. Pediatr Infec Dis J. 1989; 8:829-833.
87. Fraguso MA, Manning L, Frenkel LD. Can parents do a throat culture? Pediatr Infec Dis J. 1989; 8:845-847.
88. Walker AM. Evaluating the impact of a home screening test for streptococcal pharyngitis. Pediatr Infec Dis J. 1989; 8:834-837.
89. Gannon K. New home testing kits bursting onto market soon. Drug Topics. 1990; 24-26.
90. Starr C. From aids to strep throat: home kits to face big test. Drug topics. 1987; 27-28.
91. Jellin J. Pharmacist's Letter - Aids. American Pharmacy. 1992; NS32:27.
92. Gannon K. Self-monitoring drives diabetes devise sales. Drug Topics. 1993; 24-25.
93. Lewis R. Biotech Devices - Helping Sick Kids, Tracing Drugs. FDA Consumer. 1993; 27(2):23-25.

13 The Urinary Incontinent Patient

Todd A. Brown, R.Ph.

Urinary Incontinence (UI) is defined by the International Continence Society (ICS) as a "condition in which involuntary urine loss is a social or hygienic problem and is objectively demonstrable."[1] The cause of urinary incontinence may involve physiologic, psychologic and social factors.

The prevalence of UI varies by age and gender. Approximately 20% of children experience episodes of incontinence through the midteenage years. Among the population age 15-64 years, the prevalence of UI ranges from 1.5-15% in men and 10-25% in women.[2] In older adults (age greater than 60), the prevalence is between 15-30%, with women having twice the prevalence as men.[3] Institutionalized elderly have UI prevalence rates between 35% (for those in acute care hospitals) to 50% (for those in long term care facilities).[4] Women in general experience more UI due to a shorter urethra, childbirth and menopause. Other factors play a role but the significance has not been determined.

The social and psychological consequences combined with high prevalence rates make UI a major health problem in the elderly. Untreated urinary incontinence often becomes progressively worse and can lead to secondary problems such as skin rashes, decubitus ulcers and urinary tract infections. In addition to the physical problems, patients with UI may be afraid to socialize and thus become depressed.[5] More than 50% of admissions to nursing homes are prompted by problems with incontinence. It is estimated that the cost of caring for patients with incontinence is $10.3 billion annually.[6]

One of the most disturbing problems associated with UI is the misconceptions of the public and health professionals. Many people who experience UI do not seek treatment because of the belief that it is a normal part of aging or they were unaware treatment was available. Those that do seek help often receive inappropriate advice.[7] Pharmacists can have a significant role in the treatment of UI. The trust from the public and the availability of the pharmacist can stimulate questions about incontinence. If pharmacists focused on supplying information to dispel the myths associated with this condition and referring patients to appropriate medical personnel when indicated, this would be a significant step in treating this health problem.

ANATOMY AND PHYSIOLOGY OF THE URINARY TRACT

The production of urine begins in the kidneys. Urine flows from the kidneys through the ureter to the bladder where it is stored. Urine is eliminated by traveling out of the bladder and through the urethra. Control of the flow of urine is dependent on smooth muscles that are present in the lower urinary tract. These muscles control the flow of urine by increasing (contraction) or decreasing (relaxation) pressure in specific areas. The bladder contains three interlacing sets of smooth muscle fibers called the detrusor muscle. Contraction of the detrusor increases the pressure inside the bladder and facilitates the flow of urine out of the bladder and into the urethra. The urethra contains two muscles that control the flow of urine. At the base of the bladder where it connects to the urethra is a muscle called the internal sphincter. Farther down the urethra is the external sphincter.

There are some important differences between the male and female urinary tract. The female has a shorter urethra (1.5 inches vs 9 inches) and a less defined external sphincter. The female external sphincter lacks muscle thickness and does not provide significant pressure (urethral resistance). The pressure from the urethra is supplied primarily by the internal sphincter. In premenopausal women, estrogen is beneficial in preventing incontinence by increasing the tone of the muscles in the pelvic floor. In the male, the prostate gland plays a major role in causing incontinence due to its proximity to the urethra. Enlargement of this gland as in benign prostatic hyperplasia can increase urethral resistance.

In the normal adult, micturition is a voluntary activity. As the bladder fills with urine, the stretch and pain receptors located in the bladder wall send impulses to the spinal cord and the cerebral cortex of the brain causing the urge to urinate. This usually occurs when 300-400 ml of urine has been accumulated. If it is an inconvenient time the cerebral cortex can inhibit this stimulation and cause the bladder to distend and continue to collect urine. If it is an appropriate time, the cerebral cortex will send signals to increase detrusor contractions and relax the internal and external sphincters.

Neurologic control involves several nervous systems. The parasympathetic system provides stimulation into the bladder. The sympathetic system can affect bladder storage through alpha and beta adrenergic stimulation. Alpha stimulation increases urethral resistance by stimulating the internal sphincter. Beta stimulation increases bladder storage by indirectly affecting the parasympathetic nerves in the body of the bladder. The somatic system plays a part by increasing the external sphincter tone.

CAUSES OF INCONTINENCE

Incontinence is frequently categorized by the predisposing factor(s) associated with the condition. These are grouped into two categories: transient and established incontinence. Transient incontinence is precipitated by a specific condition and is usually treated by resolving the causal factor. Causes of transient incontinence can be recalled by the mnemonic **DIAPPERS** (Table 13-1).[4]

Table 13-1 Causes of Transient Incontinence[4]

Delirium/confusion
Infection, urinary
Atrophic urethritis/vaginitis
Pharmaceuticals
Psychological
Excessive excretion (e.g., CHF, hyperglycemia)
Restricted mobility
Stool impaction

Psychological factors may play a role in causing incontinence. Medications and other conditions that impair mental functioning should be considered. Depression has also been linked to incontinence.[5] In the postmenopausal woman, the lack of estrogen causes atrophic urethritis. This decreases the urethral mucosal coaptation and urethral muscle tone. Incontinence that is caused by medication or surgery is sometimes called iatrogenic incontinence. Many commonly used medications can cause incontinence (Table 13-2). Since the elderly consume more medications and they have a higher incidence of UI, diagnosis can become critical even though it can be complicated. A complete medication history should be taken for all patients that suddenly develop UI.

Incontinence that is a result of mobility limitations is termed functional incontinence. Constipation can also affect incontinence as the control is on the same location of the spinal cord and the proximity of the location. Often treatment for incontinence will include bulk laxatives to ensure regular stool movement. Patients experiencing UI may attempt to decrease their fluid intake throughout the day to resolve incontinence problems. This should be discouraged as a more concentrated urine can cause irritation to the urinary tract. A decrease in fluids during the evening is sometimes used in patients who have incontinence problems during the night.

Established incontinence involves a disorder of the lower urinary tract or damage to the nerves that control the functions. Once the disorder is diagnosed, treatment can be individualized. Common causes of established incontinence include: stroke, Alzheimer's disease, multiple sclerosis, prostatic hypertrophy, diabetes and parkinson's disease.

Table 13-2 Medications That Can Cause Urinary Incontinence[9]

Medication	Effect
Sedative Hypnotics	Reduce mobility and impair mental functioning
Diuretics	Increase volume and frequency of urination
Anticholinergics	Urinary retention
Alpha-adrenergics	Increase sphincter tone
Alpha blockers	Decrease sphincter tone
Calcium blockers	Decrease detrusor tone

TYPES OF INCONTINENCE

UI is classified by the area or function of the urinary tract that is affected. The classifications are not mutually exclusive and frequently patients will have more than one type (mixed incontinence).

Urge incontinence is characterized by a loss of urine immediately after a strong desire to void. It is caused by involuntary detrusor contractions. Detrusor hyperactivity is a common cause of urge incontinence. If the hyperactivity inhibits the ability to contract, this condition is called detrusor hyperactivity with impaired contractility (DHIC). Incontinence occurs when these individuals are unable to stop the flow of urine by contracting the external urinary sphincter. The amount of urine leakage can vary greatly as the detrusor contractions are not dependent on the volume of urine in the bladder.

Stress incontinence is characterized by the loss of a small amount of urine during activities such as coughing, laughing or sneezing. These activities cause an increase in the abdominal pressure which causes the urine leakage. This type of incontinence is caused by sphincter incompetence or urethral instability.

Overflow incontinence is characterized by difficulty in starting urination combined with frequent desires to void and dribbling of urine. This is caused by an obstruction in the bladder or urethra. As the bladder becomes increasingly distended it can become atonic. This type is most common in men and is caused by prostate hypertrophy.

DIAGNOSIS

The diagnosis of UI requires a comprehensive medical work-up due to the number of factors that can affect this condition. The evaluation of urinary incontinence should include the following components:

History - A complete medical history will assist in identifying possible causes and contributing factors. A neurologic history will indicate if the patient has contributing neurologic problems. A urologic history can detect damage to the urinary tract. A history of medical conditions and treatments may detect conditions or medications that could precipitate or aggravate urinary incontinence. The presentation of the incontinence (presence of the urge, frequency and volume) can suggest the type of UI. The loss of large amounts of urine immediately after a strong urge to void may suggest the urge incontinence is present. Symptoms of incontinence while laughing or coughing may indicate stress incontinence is likely. The constant loss of small amounts of urine would be an indication that overflow incontinence should be suspect. It is important to remember that the presentation of incontinence is only one piece of information and can often be misleading due to similar symptoms and the possibility of mixed incontinence.

Physical exam - The physical exam will test for neurologic problems and may provide additional information to identify the type of incontinence. Evaluation of the sacral and perineal nerves will detect nerve damage. Assessment of mental status will indicate if psychological problems are part of the condition. In the female patient a pelvic exam is completed to evaluate the vaginal and urethral mucosa, look for structural problems and estimate post-void residual (PVR) volume. PVR volume is a measure to assess the contractile strength of the detrusor. In the male patient a rectal exam is used to measure the size of the prostate and measure PVR volume.

Additional tests - The following tests, in addition to the history and physical exam, may assist in identifying the type and cause of the UI. They may also assist in determining proper treatment.

- Urinalysis - To detect hematuria, pyuria, bacteriuria, glycosuria and proteinuria.
- Urine cytology - To screen for malignancy in patients with hematuria.
- Voiding diary - A record kept by the patient for a few days to document the frequency of voiding, incontinence and the volume of urine.
- Urethral pressure profilometry - Measures the pressure of the urethra and its ability to function.
- Cystourethroscopy - Visual inspection of the urinary tract with a cystoscope inserted through the urethra.

Urodynamic tests are used to assess the status of the lower urinary tract. These include uroflowmetry, a measure of the urine flow rate and generation of a flow curve; and cystometry, a measure of the capacity of the bladder and the detrusor activity, sensation and compliance.

TREATMENT

Options available for the treatment of UI fall into three categories: behavioral techniques, pharmacologic agents and surgery. Research on the effectiveness of these options is not complete and more studies are needed that compare treatment options. The Agency for Health Care Policy And Research has compiled the existing research and developed "Urinary Incontinence in Adults: Clinical Practice Guideline". [9] This publication contains outcome tables for treatment options and treatment algorithms for each type of UI.

Behavioral Techniques

Behavioral techniques are often the treatment of choice due to their low risk, low cost and absence of adverse effects. They are most effective in motivated patients.[8] Behavioral techniques include:

Bladder training - Consists of education, scheduled voiding and positive reinforcement. Once the patient is educated about their condition and a history of voiding frequency is obtained, a schedule of voiding is developed. The schedule is changed to increase the time interval between voiding. This develops the ability to delay voiding to a schedule instead of responding to the urge to void.

Habit training - Similar to bladder training is the development of a voiding schedule that matches their natural voiding interval. During habit training the interval between voiding remains constant and the patient is encouraged to adhere to the schedule.

Prompted voiding - Used for cognitively or mobility impaired patients in nursing homes. In prompted voiding the patient is asked on a regular basis if they are wet or dry. They are also asked (prompted) to try to use the toilet and praised if they attempt to use the toilet or remain continent.

Pelvic muscle exercises - Also called Kegel exercises. They increase urethral resistance by strengthening the pelvic floor muscles. During these exercises the patients are instructed to sustain contractions of the muscles for 10 seconds followed by a period of relaxation. These exercises are performed 30 - 80 times a day for at least 6 weeks and sometimes indefinitely.

Vaginal cones - These devices are used as an adjunct or an alternative to pelvic muscle exercises. Patients insert a weighted cone intravaginally and attempt to retain it for 15 minutes. The weight of the cone is gradually increased to strengthen the pelvic muscles.

Biofeedback - This is used in conjunction with other behavioral techniques to assist the patient in relearning control of the urinary tract. It demonstrates that a response has occurred through visual or auditory displays. Biofeedback is used to assist patients in inhibiting detrusor contractions and contracting the urethral sphincters.

Electrical stimulation - Stimulation of the nerves and muscles of the urinary tract may help some patients in regaining continence. Electrical stimulation is administered through electrodes that are implanted under the skin. Further research is needed to determine its effectiveness and evaluate different methods of use.[9]

Pharmacologic Agents

There are several medications used in the treatment of urge and stress incontinence. The use of these products usually results in improvement of incontinence symptoms but rarely resolve all complaints.[9] In addition most agents have significant adverse effects. These adverse effects are often not tolerated well and can interact with other diseases or medications that the patient is taking. Since no single agent has been proven to be superior, they are usually selected to avoid certain adverse effects or because of past experience of the prescriber. Pharmacists can have input in the use of these agents by providing information to prescribers about interactions with concurrent medications or conditions and assisting patients in avoiding or treating adverse effects. Medications used in the treatment of incontinence include:

Propantheline - This anticholinergic agent is used to block bladder contractions. The dose is typically 15 - 30 mg three or four times a day. Many patients cannot tolerate this dose or have conditions that prohibit the use of anticholinergic agents.

Oxybutynin - Primarily used for urge incontinence due to its anticholinergic and smooth muscle relaxant activity. A typical dose is 2.5 - 5 mg three or four times a day. Adverse effects are common and many patients cannot tolerate them.

Dicyclomine - This is an anticholinergic agent with smooth muscle relaxant activity. It is an alternative to a pure anticholinergic agent. A typical dose is 10 - 20 mg three times a day.

Flavoxate - A smooth muscle relaxant that has been commonly used for urge incontinence. The efficacy of this agent has not been proven.

Calcium channel blockers - These agents inhibit detrusor contractions by blocking the influx of calcium. The high rate of adverse effects limit the usefulness of these agents.

Tricyclic antidepressants The central alpha-adrenergic and anticholinergic properties make these agents one of the most commonly used medications for urge incontinence. The long half-life allows for a single dose at bedtime to reduce adverse effects. Imipramine is the most common agent used but desipramine and nortriptyline have also been used. A typical dose of imipramine is 25 - 100 mg daily.

Phenylpropanolamine (PPA) - This alpha-adrenergic agonist is used in the sustained release form in stress incontinence to increase sphincter tone. Adverse effects are usually minimal and blood pressure is not significantly increased. A typical dose is 25 - 75 mg twice daily.

Estrogen - Administration of estrogen restores urethral mucosal coaptation and muscle tone in post menopausal women. It is used in stress incontinence with or without an alpha adrenergic agonist. A typical dose of conjugated estrogen is 0.3 - 1.25 mg per day orally or two grams per day vaginally. Progestin (usually medroxyprogesterone) should be administered when giving estrogen to inhibit stimulation of the endometrium if the uterus is present. A typical dose of medroxyprogesterone is 2.5 - 10 mg per day continuously or intermittently (one week out of every four weeks).

SURGERY

Surgery should be considered when other less invasive treatments have failed or when an anatomic problem has been objectively confirmed and the procedure will have a significant impact the patient's quality of life. Surgery is usually the treatment of choice for overflow incontinence caused by obstruction. Surgical procedures fall into three categories:[10] procedures for stress incontinence due to an anatomic problem; procedures for stress incontinence due to sphincter dysfunction; and procedures for incontinence due to bladder dysfunction.

URINARY INCONTINENCE MANAGEMENT DEVICES

The following devices are used as an adjunct to the treatments described above. These products are typically available in community pharmacies that specialize in home health care and represent an area where pharmacists can assist patients in managing their condition. These products include:

Penile clamp or compression cuff - These are devices that apply pressure to the penis to compress the urethra. These devices must be removed every 3 hours to allow for voiding and decrease tissue damage. They should be used with caution due to the propensity for complications.[9]

Pessary - A soft donut shaped device that is inserted into the vagina to support the soft tissue structures in the pelvis. Patients need to be taught proper insertion and removal techniques. Due to the pressure these exert, patients should use them intermittently.

Intermittent catheter - They are used several times a day for patients who have difficulties voiding. A clean non-sterile catheter is inserted through the urethra and into the bladder. This facilitates the flow of urine. Patients of all ages can be trained to use intermittent catheters. They are preferable to indwelling catheters as less complications (infection, damage and formation of stones) are seen.[11] Antibiotic prophylaxis is not required with these products.[9]

Indwelling catheter - Also called a foley catheter, is inserted through the urethra and into the bladder. Once the sterile catheter is inside the bladder, a balloon located at the tip is inflated to keep the catheter secure. The size of the catheter is designated by the french scale (FR) with various size balloons available. A standard size would be a 16 FR or 18 FR catheter with a 5 cc or 10 cc balloon. An indwelling catheter is made of various material (silicone, latex and teflon) to inhibit the formation of encrustation and reduce friction during insertion and removal.[12]

Male external catheter - Also called a condom catheter because of its appearance. Male external catheters are connected to collection devices such as a leg bag (for ambulatory patients) or a bedside drainage bag via plastic tubing. Male external catheters may have adhesive or an adhesive strap that is wrapped around the penis to keep it secure. Some patients change the catheter on a regular basis and others use one catheter as long as it remains secure (several days). Complications can occur if the catheter becomes twisted or kinked and the penis is exposed to urine. Some catheters have reinforced tips to prevent this problem.

Female external collection system - This device fits snugly in the vagina and may have adhesive to help keep it secure. It is attached to a drainage system like a male external catheter. These devices are worn for 24 hours and then removed and cleaned. The efficacy of the female external collection system has not yet been determined and adverse effects have been reported.[13]

Urinal - Designed for patients confined to a bed or chair. Used to collect and measure the volume of urine. Both male and female urinals are available. The male urinal has a round opening and the female urinal has a concave opening to facilitate urine collection. Urinals are made out of plastic or autoclavable enamel.

Bedpan - Used to collect urine and feces from a patient confined to a bed. They are also made of plastic or enamel. A fracture bedpan is shaped like a wedge to limit the movement of the patient.

Nocturnal enuresis alarm. Used in children to treat bedwetting. It modifies behavior to encourage the child to awaken from the urge to void. This alarm is attached to a pad that is placed in the underwear. The pad contains electrodes that when wet complete an electric circuit and cause the alarm to sound. The alarm awakens the child so they can void. After repeated use the child will awaken themselves and not require the alarm. There are different protocols for use, although none has been proven to be superior.

Waterproof sheeting - Vinyl or plastic sheets that may be lined with flannel for added comfort. They are designed to protect the mattress in a UI patient. Waterproof sheets come in different sized to fit all sizes of beds.

Proper skin care is important in UI patients as repeated exposure to urine can irritate the skin and sores and infections can develop. After each exposure to urine the skin should be cleaned and dried. Moisturizers can also be used to soften and lubricate the skin. Many moisturizers specifically designed for incontinence are commercially available. If the skin becomes irritated protective barrier ointments can be used to protect the skin from future exposure. Often patients will want to control the odor associated with UI. There are two types of deodorizers, external or internal. External deodorizers can be applied to the skin or to equipment that comes into contact with urine (i.e., collection devices). Some moisturizing creams contain deodorizers. Internal deodorizers that contain chlorophyll can be ingested to decrease the odor of the urine.

In addition to the devices listed above, absorbent products are available to help UI patients manage their condition. The availability and use of these products have increased dramatically over the past decade due to educational and promotional efforts of the manufacturers of these products. The positive aspect of these changes is the increased awareness of UI but there is some concern that some patients might become dependent on disposable products without considering other treatment options.[14] Absorbent products need to be changed regularly to minimize the contact with urine. Disposable absorbent products are made from pulp or a synthetic polymer. Pulp has an advantage of being less expensive but is bulky and can be noisy for active patients. The synthetic polymer is less bulky and less noisy and has the capacity to absorb greater amounts of urine but is also more expensive. Absorbent products include the following:

Shield - A disposable absorbent pad that is placed in the underwear and held in place with a adhesive strip on the back of the pad. Shields are used for light incontinence problems.

Undergarment - A disposable garment used for moderate incontinence problems. They are secured with reusable elastic straps that are placed around the hips. Undergarments are available in one size that fits most people.

Brief - Looks like an adult diaper. It is used for heavy incontinence problems or non-ambulatory patients. They are secured with adhesive strips similar to a disposable diaper. Briefs are available in different sizes depending on the patient's hip size.

Underpad - A disposable absorbent pad with a waterproof back that is placed under an incontinent patient confined to a bed. They are used to protect the bed linens and mattress.

Drip collector - An absorbent disposable pouch

that fits around the penis and scrotum to absorb small amounts of urine.

Incontinence system - A garment that is designed to look like traditional underwear that contains a pocket in which a disposable or reusable pad is inserted. Incontinence systems are designed for long-term use and look like traditional underwear to minimize the psychological stigmas associated with this condition.

CONCLUSION

With a complete understanding of urinary incontinence there are several ways the pharmacist can be involved in the treatment of this condition. The pharmacist is an underutilized resource and represents a way to increase awareness and decrease costs associated with this common condition. The "Clinical Practice Guideline: Urinary Incontinence In Adults" is available from the Agency for Health Policy and Research, and is an excellent resource for pharmacists who want more information. There are also advocacy groups for patients with UI which can provide support and services to patients. These include: The Simon Foundation for Continence, PO Box 815, Wilmette, IL 60091, and Help for Incontinent People Inc., PO Box 544, Union, SC 29379.

REFERENCES

1. Abrams P, Blaivas JG, Stanton SL, et al. The standardization of terminology of lower urinary tract function. Scandinavian Journal of Urology and Nephrology. 1988; 114(suppl):5-19.
2. Thomas TM, Plymat KR, Blannin J, et al. Prevalence of urinary incontinence. British Medical Journal. 1980; 281(6250):1243-1245.
3. Diokno AC, Brock BM, Brown MB, et al. Prevalence of urinary incontinence and other urological symptoms in the noninstitutional elderly. Journal of Urology. 1986; 136(5):1022-1025.
4. Resnick NM. Urinary Incontinence in older adults. Hospital Practice. 1992; 10,15:139-184.
5. Mitteness LS. Social aspects of urinary incontinence in the elderly. AORN Journal. 1992; 56(4):731-737.
6. Hu TW. Impact of urinary incontinence on health-care costs. Journal of the American Geriatrics Society. 1990; 38(3):292-295.
7. Goldstein M, Hawthorne ME, Engeberg S, et al. Urinary incontinence: Why people do not seek help. Journal of Gerontological Nursing. 1992; 4:15-20.
8. Battcock TM, Castleden CM. Pharmacological treatment of urinary incontinence. British Medical Bulletin. 1990; 46(1):147-155.
9. Urinary Incontinence Guideline Panel. Urinary Incontinence in Adults: Clinical Practice Guideline. AHCPR Pub. No. 92-0038. Rockville, MD: Agency for Health Care Policy and Research, Public Health Service, U.S. Department of Healthand Human Services. March 1992.
10. Urinary incontinence. In Doughty D. Ed: Urinary and fecal incontinence: Nursing management. 1991 Mosby-Year Book Inc. St. Louis MO.
11. Webb RJ, Lawson AL, Neal DE. Clean intermittent self-catheterization in 172 adults. British Journal of Urology. 1990; 65(1):20-23.
12. Liedberg H, Lundeberg T, Ekman P. Refinements in the coating of urethral catheters reduces the incidence of catheter-associated bacteriuria: An experimental and clinical study. European Urology. 1990; 17(3):236-240.
13. Johnson DE, Muncie HL, O'Reilly JL, et al. An external urine collection device for incontinent women: Evaluation of long-term use. Journal of the American Geriatrics Society. 1990; 38(9):1016-1022.
14. Starer P, Libow LS. Obscuring urinary incontinence: Diapering of the elderly. Journal of the American Geriatrics Society. 1985; 33(12):842-846.

14 The Diabetes Patient

Beverly Yachmetz, Pharm.D., CDE

Diabetes mellitus (DM) is one of the most common chronic diseases in the United States today. Approximately 7 million individuals have been diagnosed with the disease and an additional 5 million may unknowingly have the disease. Each year, more than 650,000 new cases of diabetes are identified.[1] In addition, DM is associated with an increased incidence in an aging population with a prevalence of 18% of those between the ages of 65 to 75[2], and an estimated prevalence of more than 40% in individuals over 80 years old.[3]

Diabetes is characterized by abnormal metabolism of carbohydrates, proteins and fats. The disease is diagnosed through detection of elevated blood glucose levels (hyperglycemia) with or without symptoms. In addition, long-standing diabetes is associated with specific microvascular, macrovascular and neuropathic complications. Due to the prevalence, pharmacists encounter diabetes and the resultant complications frequently. There are multiple areas for the pharmacist's intervention in the prevention, education, treatment, management, and supportive services which improve patient care and the individual's quality of life. To fully explore the pharmacist's role in the care of the individual with diabetes, a brief review of important issues and recent developments is presented first.

DIABETES: FOCUSING CARE

Diabetes is a whole life disease. The extensive nature of behavioral changes necessary for successful treatment coupled with the invasive long-term complications result in diabetes touching every aspect of the individual's life. Patients require an entire team of care providers whose efforts are coordinated, cooperative, and directed at individualized care. Paramount to individualized care are the needs, concerns and priorities of the patient, the patient's family and the patient's caregivers.

The health care team delivering services to these patients encompasses multiple specialties and subspecialties. Care must be directed at both the short-term management of symptoms and glycemic control as well as prevention and treatment of long-term complications. To address effectively the individual's needs, the care team could be divided into a "core team" which focuses on the day-to-day issues of management and the "adjunct team" which coordinates with the "core team" for specialty services. The core team consists of the patient, patient's family, primary care physician (in some cases this may be an endocrinologist or diabetologist), diabetes educator, dietitian and pharmacist. The adjunct team consists of ophthalmologist, dentist, and podiatrist. Other subspecialists which may be important, depending on the individual's specific complications, include a cardiologist, nephrologist, neurologist, and urologist. Psychologists, psychiatrists and social workers are also necessary, in certain cases.

Pharmacists have multiple opportunities to work with individuals with diabetes. It is estimated that these patients require the pharmacist's services for medication or diabetes-related products an average of two to three times per month.[4] Pharmacists have the advantages of medication knowledge, product knowledge, and ability to provide beneficial services. By interacting with the patient and other care providers, the pharmacist can facilitate care and overcome barriers to treatment goals.

DIABETES: THE DISEASE

It is now known that diabetes is a group of heterogenous disorders for which hyperglycemia is the common factor.[5] Hyperglycemia may produce the classic symptoms of diabetes termed the "polys"- polyuria, polydipsia, and polyphagia. In addition, symptoms may include extreme weight loss, blurry vision, fatigue, headache, slowed mentation, ketosis, slow wound healing and frequent infections, particularly urinary tract infections and vaginitis.

There are three clinical subclasses of diagnosis for diabetes. These subclasses are based on the underlying pathology for the hyperglycemia related to defects in insulin production, insulin sensitivity or combinations of both. The type of diabetes impacts on the clinical presentation and has implications for the treatment modalities which are successful in the management of the specific subclass. A summary of the features of the subclasses are presented in Table 14-1 and are briefly described as follows:

Type I diabetes, Insulin Dependent Diabetes Mellitus (IDDM), previously termed Juvenile Diabetes, occurs generally in non-obese, young individuals. Type I diabetes is associated with complete destruction of insulin-producing capacity through an autoimmune attack on the beta cells of the pancreas. While the development of hyperglycemia appears acute, with rapid progression, new research indicates the destructive process may take months to years in individuals at risk.[6] Risk factors for the development of this subclass of

Table 14-1 Types of Diabetes Mellitus and Characteristics[5]

<table>
<tr><th>Type of Diabetes</th><th colspan="2">Characteristics</th></tr>
<tr><td rowspan="3">Type I</td><td colspan="2">Insulin Dependent Diabetes Mellitus (IDDM)</td></tr>
<tr><td colspan="2">May present at any age, usually thin, usually have abrupt onset of signs and symptoms with lack of insulin, and prior to the age of 30. The major peak of onset occurs at 11 to 12 years of age.</td></tr>
<tr><td colspan="2">More common in the white population and associated with genetic markers indicating a genetic component, and the presence of specific antibodies indicating an autoimmune process.</td></tr>
<tr><td rowspan="4">Type II</td><td colspan="2">Non-Insulin Dependent Diabetes Mellitus (NIDDM)</td></tr>
<tr><td colspan="2">Usually older than 30 years at diagnosis, obese, and present with relatively few symptoms of hyperglycemia. Ketosis is rare, except in times of extreme stress.</td></tr>
<tr><td colspan="2">More common in minority populations such as African-American, Hispanic and Native Americans. Strong genetic component.</td></tr>
<tr><td colspan="2">Associated with insulin resistance.</td></tr>
<tr><td rowspan="16">Other types of diabetes mellitus</td><td colspan="2">Have certain associated conditions or syndromes such as:</td></tr>
<tr><td rowspan="4">Pancreatic disease</td><td>Pancreatectomy</td></tr>
<tr><td>Hemochromatosis</td></tr>
<tr><td>Cystic fibrosis</td></tr>
<tr><td>Chronic pancreatitis</td></tr>
<tr><td rowspan="5">Endocrinopathies</td><td>Acromegaly</td></tr>
<tr><td>Pheochromocytoma</td></tr>
<tr><td>Cushing's syndrome</td></tr>
<tr><td>Primary aldosteronism</td></tr>
<tr><td>Glucagonoma</td></tr>
<tr><td rowspan="5">Drug/chemical</td><td>Glucocorticoids</td></tr>
<tr><td>Related Estrogen products</td></tr>
<tr><td>Psychoactive agents</td></tr>
<tr><td>Thiazide diuretics</td></tr>
<tr><td>Catecholamines</td></tr>
<tr><td colspan="2">Pregnancy</td></tr>
</table>

diabetes include genetic markers and still unidentified environmental factors or stressors. Due to the total lack of insulin, these individuals are unable to control lipolysis when in an insulin deficient state and are then prone to ketoacidosis. This life-threatening complication may represent the initial clinical presentation for previously undetected diabetes. Approximately 10% of known cases of diabetes are type I.[5]

Type II diabetes mellitus, Non-Insulin Dependent Diabetes Mellitus (NIDDM), formerly termed adult onset diabetes, is by far the most common diabetes accounting for nearly 90% of all known cases of diabetes.[5] The same symptoms of hyperglycemia may occur in individuals with type II diabetes, however, ketosis is rare and symptoms generally appear gradually. The risk factors identified are increasing age, obesity, heredity, and gestational history. Women with a history of large babies (greater than 9 lbs), stillbirths, and/or diagnosed gestational diabetes are at increased risk. In addition, minority populations, specifically African-American, Hispanics, and Native Americans have a disproportionately higher incidence of diabetes ranging for two- to five-fold the rate of the non-Hispanic white population.[1] Type II diabetes is characterized by a relative lack of insulin, that is, inadequate insulin to handle the glucose level. This concept has been emphasized to account for the hyperinsulinemia and insulin resistance which are common in type II.

The third class of diabetes mellitus, grouped together as "other types of diabetes mellitus", represents diabetes which has an identified cause or is part of a specific condition or syndrome. Included in this category are pancreatic diseases, endocrinopathies, drug/chemically-induced, insulin receptor abnormalities, genetic syndromes and miscellaneous conditions such as malnutrition.[5] In theory, if the primary cause is treated, the diabetes is eliminated. Other causes for hyperglycemia must be eliminated whenever possible.

TREATING DIABETES

Since the discovery of insulin in 1921, the emphasis on treatment has become more and more directed at normalized blood glucose patterns (euglycemia). Treatment must include an assessment to determine the therapeutic goals for the individual and the resources necessary to obtain these goals. Goals must be precise, realistic, and mutually agreeable to the patient and the health care providers. There are varying degrees of control listed in Table 14-2 which are defined by blood glucose values. Monitoring parameters for therapeutic effect and toxicity, advantages, and disadvantages are listed in Table 14-3. It is important to realize that diabetes is a dynamic disease. Physiological, psychological, and socio-economic changes occurring over time require continual assessment of efficacy of treatment.

The decision of therapeutic intervention is first determined by the type of diabetes. Due to total lack of insulin, type I must be treated with insulin replacement. Individuals with type II diabetes have additional treatment options which should be initiated and given adequate opportunity for success prior to instituting insulin therapy. These options begin with nutrition and exercise, followed by oral hypoglycemic agents when treatment goals are not met. These treatments are addressed prior to insulin use because type II is seen in the overwhelming majority of patients.

Diet and exercise are the foundation of treatment of type II diabetes and critical in the management of individuals with type I. In addition, any successful management of diabetes, regardless of pharmacological intervention must include a properly designed nutrition plan which also considers weight reduction, if necessary, and treatment of concomitant diseases which are also amenable to diet therapy (high blood pressure, high cholesterol). Nutrition counseling is generally not in the scope of pharmacy practice, however, pharmacists can reinforce the importance of diet as a therapeutic intervention and

Table 14-2 Levels of Glycemic Control in Order of Strictness[7]

1. Before-meal and bedtime snack glucose concentrations of <180 mg/dl.
2. Before-meal and bedtime snack glucose concentrations of <150 mg/dl.
3. Before-meal and bedtime snack glucose concentrations of <120 mg/dl.
4. One to 2 hour postmeal glucose concentrations of <210 mg/dl (<210 mg/dl for individuals using home blood glucose monitor.)
5. One to 2 hour postmeal glucose concentration of <150 mg/dl.

Table 14-3 Monitoring Therapeutic and Toxic Effects of Diabetes Treatment [5,8]

Monitoring Therapeutic Effect		
Subjective/Objective Outcomes	**Advantages**	**Disadvantages**
Symptoms of hyperglycemia	Reflects individual's quality of life. Educates patient to the relationship between disease and symptoms.	Subjective. Not all individuals experience symptoms; Blood glucose levels which produce symptoms higher than desired for prevention of long-term complications.
Fasting plasma glucose level	Easily obtained. Relatively inexpensive. Traditional method of assessing DM control.	Possibly painful to patient. Does not reflex overall diabetes control. Affected by personal desire to please the clinician by focused attention shortly before appointment. Affected by inappropriate preparation for test i.e., not fasting.
Fructosamine	Reflects glycemic control over time period of approximately 2 weeks. Allows clinician to see a move toward improved glycemic control.	May be painful to patient. Not fully standardized for monitoring purposes. Test inferences. Relatively expensive.
Hemoglobin A1c	Reflects glycemic control over approximately 6 to 8 weeks. Allows clinician to see a move toward improved glycemic control.	May be painful to patient. Not fully standardized between laboratories. Reports an average blood glucose reading over the time frame but does not reflect wide fluctuations in glucose values. Affected by hemo- globinapathies such as sickle cell anemia.
Urine testing	Relatively inexpensive. Not painful. Detects urine glucose.	Messy. Objectionable to patient/caregiver. Not quantitative. Does not indicate hypoglycemia. Renal threshold for glucose varies between individuals and increase with age.
Home blood glucose monitoring	Allow individual to participate in treatment. Provides instant feedback to patient with diet/medication change. Quantitative. Detects hypoglycemia. Reflects daily patterns of glycemic control.	Painful to some individuals. Costly if not covered by insurances. Must be performed according to machine directions.
Indices of Toxic Effects		
Symptoms of hypoglycemia	same as above	Hypoglycemic unawareness. Acute onset. May be fatal if undetected. Demoralizing to patient.
Fructosamine	same as above	same as above
Hemoglobin A1c	same as above	same as above
Home blood glucose monitoring	same as above	same as above

refer individuals to community-based resources such as Registered Dietitians/Certified Nutritionists, diabetes education programs, or a Certified Diabetes Educator. When properly instituted, diet has dramatic impact on glycemic control.

Individuals not responding to diet alone or those with extremely elevated blood glucose readings may need additional intervention with the use of oral hypoglycemic agents, the sulfonylurea class. However, it is important to assess continually for the symptoms of hypoglycemia as the individual becomes more knowledgeable and capable of dietary control.

Selection of a specific sulfonylurea agent is based on characteristics of the medication and the patient's unique profile of concomitant chronic diseases and medications. The pharmacist is critical in the assessment and monitoring of the treatment regimen to prevent or minimize the impact of drug interactions, toxicity, and therapeutic failure. Table 14-4 lists considerations in selecting a sulfonylurea agent.

Insulin is used for individuals who do not achieve glycemic control with the combination of diet/exercise and sulfonylurea or have a contraindication to sulfonylurea treatment (allergy, pregnancy). In addition, insulin must be used in all those with type I diabetes. Currently available insulins vary according to source (animal or human), onset and duration (short, intermediate, and long-acting). Commonly used insulins are U-100 meaning each ml contains 100 units of insulin. Various insulins can be combined based on duration of action and peak effects with dosing schedules designed to approximate endogenous insulin secretion. In addition, pre-mixed insulins are available with a set ratio of NPH and regular. However, due to individual sensitivity and rate of metabolism, treatment with insulin requires careful monitoring for adjustments aimed at achieving the predetermined treatment goals. Prior to the availability of home blood glucose monitoring, the risk of hypoglycemia prohibited strict control. Once daily NPH insulin was common therapy. Based on insulin kinetics and the multiple factors determining the resulting blood glucose, strict control was rarely achieved with this regimen. Regimens designed to obtain strict control, generally requiring the mixing or combined use of two insulins with different durations, onset, and peaks, are outlined in Table 14-5.

Several important points must be observed when mixing insulins. First, individuals must be taught proper technique for mixing insulins. Short-acting insulin becomes contaminated and patients experience blunted peak action when the mixture is prepared improperly. The technique for extemporaneously mixing insulins is outlined in Table 14-6. Secondly, not all insulins retain the desired peaks characterized by the individual insulins when mixed. Therefore, only certain combinations are useful. Lente insulins can be mixed in any ratio, at any time. Regular mixed with NPH insulin seems to be the preferred type because this combination retains the same rapid and intermediate action as if the insulins were administered separately. Combinations of regular with lente insulins has a binding action which

Table 14-4 Considerations in Sulfonylurea Treatment[9]

1. Age of patient
2. Renal function
3. Hepatic function
4. Medication half-life, duration of action
5. Cost of therapy and generic availability
6. Treatment with drug interactions:
    - Salicylates
    - Sulfonamide antibiotics (i.e., Bactrim)
    - Warfarin
    - Ethanol use
7. History of allergic reaction to sulfonylurea agents
8. Pregnancy or planning pregnancy

Table 14-5 Insulin Regimens for Achieving Strict Control[7]

Regimen	Before Breakfast	Before Lunch	Before Supper	Before Bedtime
A	NPH/Regular		NPH/Regular	
B	NPH/Regular		Regular	NPH
C	Regular	Regular	NPH/Regular	
D	Regular	Regular	Regular	NPH
E	Ultralente/Regular (separate injections)	Regular	Regular	
F	Insulin pump therapy (small amount of continuous, basal regular insulin with boluses of regular given prior to each meal.			

Note: Regular insulin should be injected 30 minutes before designated meal.

begins immediately, remains in a state of flux for 24 hours, and delays the rapid onset on the regular insulin.[11]

Individuals needing insulin include visually-impaired, individuals with poor manual dexterity, arthritis victims, and elderly. Devices available which aid in syringe filling range from simple plastic cards which create a contrast to elaborate devices which hold the syringe, insulin and have a counting mechanism to accurately measure the dose. Due to the multiple products available, pharmacists are referred to American Diabetes Association (ADA) to obtain copies of the "Buyer's Guide to Diabetes Products" which provides the name and source of currently available products. This list is compiled and updated annually.

In addition, pharmacists can provide a valuable service by preparing prefilled syringes for use by the patient at a later time. Recent studies indicate premixed NPH and regular insulins retained response of the regular insulin for a three-week period when stored under refrigeration. When considering sterility, prefilled syringes should be provided in supplies of three weeks at a time. Patients must be educated to adequately resuspend the insulin preparation through shaking or rolling when an NPH or lente is used.[11]

Pharmacists can also supply individuals with multiple devices available to aid in the injection of insulin. Major syringe manufacturers have aided the patient by developing finer and sharper needles to reduce the pain. Proper technique aids in reducing fear and pain. Pharmacists must assess individuals for proper injection technique to enhance the desired insulin action and reduce the risk such as infection. Steps for injection are outlined in Table 14-7. Proper injection includes education about the appropriate site for injection and appropriate site rotation. The action of insulin is affected by the site of injection. Therefore, the ADA now recommends rotation on insulin injections within the same anatomical region.[12] Recent studies indicate the abdomen is least affected by exercise and is currently the preferred site.[13]

Multiple aids are available to assist the individual in the injection step. Automatic injectors are spring loaded devices which quickly insert the needle through the flesh. The needle is hidden from the view of the patient. However, the plunger must still be manually pushed to expel the insulin. Individuals who cannot self inject may benefit from automatic, needleless injectors, such as Medi-Jector EZ, which uses air pressure to deliver the insulin through the skin. The Freedom Jet has features of a click-count dosing wheel to determine the amount of units to administer. While these devices may be beneficial to those who cannot self-inject, the cost is high, usually more than $700.00, and the delivery system alters the insulin action which then requires a dosage adjustment. Changes from syringes to the air injection techniques require supervision by a clinician.[14]

Table 14-6 Technique for Mixing Two Types of Insulin[10]

1. Work in clean area. Wash hands.
2. Roll intermediate-acting insulin bottle to gently resuspend the particles.
3. Cleanse rubber stoppers.
4. Pull plunger of syringe to equal the number of intermediate-acting insulin units to be injected.
5. Insert the needle in the intermediate-acting insulin bottle and inject the air into the bottle.
6. Pull plunger of syringe to equal the number of units of short-acting insulin to be injected.
7. Inject the air into the short-acting insulin bottle and withdraw the same number of units of short-acting insulin.
8. Check for air bubbles.
9. Insert the needle into the intermediate-acting insulin bottle and slowly draw the plunger to the TOTAL amount (Intermediate-acting and short-acting insulins) to be injected.

Table 14-7 Technique of Insulin Injection[10]

1. Select site for injection.
2. Cleanse area with soap and water. If using alcohol, allow the skin to dry prior to injection.
3. Pinch the skin between the thumb and fingers.
4. Hold the syringe like an pencil and insert the needle, quickly, at a 90 degree angle (straight down) or 60 degree angle.
5. Push the plunger slowly.
6. Remove the needle quickly. Do not massage the site of injection.
7. Dispose of syringe with needle attached in a properly designed container. Do not break or cut the needle from the syringe.

Note: Waste disposal companies have programs to dispose of home medical waste through approved, environmentally safe methods. Contact local waste disposal companies for local and regional regulations.

An additional option to obtain glycemic control are insulin pump devices. Pumps available are both external and implantable but at present are not practical for all individuals requiring insulin therapy. Highly motivated individuals with good knowledge about diabetes are the best candidates.

An additional option for the treatment of diabetes, particularly for individuals with type II, has been the combination use of a sulfonylurea agent with insulin. The combination use has been studied intensely over the past three years, however, the results remain controversial. Considering the mechanism of action of the oral agents to enhance the peripheral utilization of insulin, it was hoped that combining this effect with insulin would enhance control and lower the daily requirement of insulin. By lowering the daily insulin requirement, it was hoped to decrease the hyperinsulinemia which has been linked to accelerated coronary artery disease. A review of available literature reports combined therapy does not achieve euglycemia in NIDDM individuals. In addition, studies which indicated a small decrease in exogenous insulin requirements in combined therapy, also detected an increase in endogenous insulin secretion. The net effect is little difference in the peripheral insulin levels. Therefore, there was no benefit to the patient. The addition of a second agent to the regimen increases the cost considerably over the use of insulin alone. Finally, individuals treated by both agents have increased risk of adverse drug reactions which may be unnecessary.[15] Careful consideration concerning the risk versus the benefit must be addressed prior to the institution or continuation of this treatment.

HOME MONITORING

Individuals with diabetes can home monitor using both urine and blood. Urine testing for glucose has few advantages, and multiple disadvantages which make this testing unacceptable. Urine testing for ketones, most significant in individuals with type I diabetes, must accompany glucose monitoring to truly assess the severity of the high glucose readings. Positive urine ketones in the presence of hyperglycemia is the forerunner to diabetic ketoacidosis and must be attended to immediately to prevent further deterioration.

Home blood glucose monitoring has revolutionized the treatment of diabetes. Blood glucose monitoring can take the form of visual reading of color change after glucose reacts with a reagent-impregnated pad or through the use of a mechanical meter which detects changes in color or reaction energy to determine glucose concentration. Visual blood glucose readings are more accurate than urine; however, these readings are influenced by the individual's ability to distinguish shades of blues and greens. In addition, the reading scales are too wide to use for adjusting doses. Blood glucose meters are currently the most valuable tool available for home monitoring. Individuals with diabetes, and those caring for them, can now see the effects of diet, exercise, and medication on the blood glucose levels. A major advantage is the ability to detect and document episodes of hypoglycemia. Through home monitoring the patient and the clinician can see the patterns of blood glucose and can more readily determine when dosage adjustments are necessary.

Proper meter selection is critical to the success of home use. The emphasis on glucose control has created a market for innovative meters to meet the needs of individuals with diabetes. As a result, multiple meters are available with differences which make product selection difficult for the user. Pharmacists are ideally situated to provide the guidance necessary to match the patient with an appropriate meter. In addition, pharmacists supply the necessary equipment to maintain blood glucose monitoring such as strips, lancets, and machine batteries.

It is important to realize that all blood glucose meters meet required standards for accuracy. All meters are priced within a fairly narrow range and are often accompanied with rebates, trade-in promotions and specials which lower the price. However, meters vary tremendously in the ease of use. Accuracy is dependent on correct performance of the necessary procedure. Some machines require wiping and blotting steps which may be difficult for individuals with poor manual dexterity. In addition, visually-impaired individuals (diabetes is the leading cause of new-onset blindness) may have difficulty inserting the prepared strips into small slots for the actual test reading.

The most common source of error in home blood glucose monitoring is user technique.[16] Therefore, the user (whether this is the patient, the caregiver, or the clinician) must be teachable on the selected machine. All machines have precise procedures. Some require exact timing to perform certain steps. Deviations for the test procedure alter the results. Inaccurate results may lead to inappropriate dosage changes or a false sense of security about the level of control.

Table 14-8 compares the currently available meters and provides notes about their functional use. Other areas deserve attention as the effect may be significant in certain populations.

- Sample size. The amount of blood necessary to perform a test varies from 7 microliters for the Glucometer-3 to 50 microliters for the Accu-Chek III. This may be important for individuals with poor circulation or difficulty with painful lancing.
- Interfering substances. Some machines are affected by high levels of ascorbic acid, uric acid and some results are invalid with extremely elevated lipid and triglyceride levels which are common in individuals with uncontrolled diabetes.
- Hematocrit. Home blood glucose monitors use whole blood versus plasma. Therefore, the hematocrit plays a role in the accuracy of the results. This is particularly important in populations prone to anemia, such as those which chronic renal failure.
- Visual impairment. Some meters have small, hard to read display areas. One Touch by Lifescan has an attachable "Talk and Touch" and Boehringer Mannheim has the Freedom

Table 14-8a Comparison of Home Blood Glucose Monitors[17,18]

PRODUCT/MANUFACTURER	METER PRICE	STRIP PRICES	WARRANTY	RANGE (mg/dl)
Accu-Chek III Boehringer Mannheim Corp. 1-800-858-8072	$70	$30-40 per 50 strips	2 years	20-500
Accu-Chek EASY Boehringer Mannheim Corp. 1-800-858-8072	$60	$30-35 per 50 strips	3 years	20-500
Tracer II Boehringer Mannheim Corp. 1-800-858-8072	Under $50	$26-27 per 50 strips	2 years	40-400
Diascan-S Home Diagnostics, Inc. 1-800-342-7226	$85-125 minus rebates	$31-33 per 50 strips	2 years	10-600
Ultra Home Diagnostics, Inc. 1-800-342-7226	$135-150	$40 per 50 strips	2 years	0-600
One Touch II LifeScan, Inc. 1-800-227-8862	$100-160 rebates available	$35-40 per 50 strips	3 years	0-600
One Touch Basic LifeScan, Inc. 1-800-227-8862	$50-60 rebates available	$35-40 per 50 strips	3 years	0-600
Exactech Companion MediSense, Inc 1-800-537-3775	$85-100	$35-40 per 50 strips	4 years	40-450
Exactech Pen MediSense, Inc. 1-800-537-3775	$85-100	$35-40 per 50 strips	4 years	40-450
Glucometer-3 Miles, Inc. Diagnostic Division 1-800-348-8100	$40-50 minus rebates	$30-35 per 50 strips	3 years	20-500
Glucometer M+ Miles, Inc. Diagnostic Division 1-800-348-8100	$150-160	$30-35 per 50 strips	3 years	20-500
CheckMate Cascade Medical 1-800-525-6718	$160-175	$30-35 per 50 foil wrapped strips	2 years	40-400
Supreme British American Medical 1-800-866-1187	$79.95	$28.95 per 50 strips	2 years	40-400

Table 14-8b Comparison of Home Blood Glucose Monitors[17,18]

NAME OF TEST STRIP	VISUAL READ CAPACITY	TEST TIME	MEMORY	SPECIAL FEATURES/SPECIALS CONSIDERATIONS
Chemstrip bG	Strip can be read visually	120 seconds	Stores date, time and 20 test results	Rejects inadequate sample. Must wipe and time. Requires large blood sample which may be difficult for some patients. Hematocrit range of 25 to 60%. Displays date and time. Has an audio component available titled Accu-check Freedom which is used for visually impaired. Much improved calibration technique than previous model. Information stored in memory bank can be down loaded through the Merlin System to be graphically displayed and analyzed.
Easy Test Strips	Visual verification	15-60 seconds Varies according to the glucose concentration	Stores 30 test results	No timing or wiping. Easy calibration. Rejects inadequate samples. Has computer capabilities through the Merlin System.
Tracer bG	Visual verification	120 seconds	Recalls last 10 tests results	Must wipe and time. Visual cues given to aid in preforming procedure. Strips are durable and requires small blood sample. However small strips may be difficult for individuals with arthritis are peripheral neuropathy due to small slot for insertion. Independent testing indicates this machine requires cleaning more often than indicated in product literature. Testing indicated cleaning was required every 10 to 15 test due to build up of fibers and cotton on the optical window .
Diascan Strips	Strips can be read visually or used to verify meter reading	90 seconds	10 tests	Use can smear sample and still get clinically acceptable test results. Must wipe and time. Large, easy to read display area. Results may be displayed in mg/dl or mmol/L. Temperature compensation range 41-98 F, adjusts to 73 . Change code to read whole blood or venous blood. No updated information of the effects of hematocrit on reading.
Ultra non-wipe	Can be read visually for verification	45 seconds	2 tests	No timing, wiping or blotting. Automatic temperature correction. Large easy to read display . Results in mg/dl or mmol/L. Due to strip design, there is a delay between the time the sample is placed and the beginning of the testing process. User should be warned because they become concerned machine is not functioning properly. Results are affected by light. Visual cues are displayed to indicate interference.
One Touch test strips	No visual check	45 seconds	Storage capacity for 250 tests. Memory includes date and time of the test, and can distinguish between blood samples and control solutions	No timing, wiping or blotting. Display messages indicate when machine needs cleaning or check strip procedure. Rejects inadequate sample size. However, users should be instructed to verify sample size by checking the reverse side of strip for a full circle of blue indicating reaction area totally filled. Machine uses countdown timing. Can be programmed to display commands in 7 languages, including English and Spanish, as well as universal symbolic codes. Communicates with Data Manager unit to display and analyze data through the use of IBM compatible personal computers. Has an audio component, TALK 'n TOUCH, available through the American Federation of the Blind, which talks the individual through the test procedure.
One Touch Strips	No visual reading	45 seconds	Stores last test result.	Contains all the great basic features of home monitoring of the One Touch II, however none of the "frills" of additional languages, computer capabilities or audio components. This is reflected in the economical price.
ExacTech test strips (foil wrapped)	No visual reading	30 seconds	Last test reading	One button operation. No wiping, blotting or timing. Has small slot for insertion of strip. Has had poor accuracy results on independent testing . Has non-replaceable battery.
ExacTech test strips (foil wrapped)	No visual reading	30 seconds	Last test reading	One button operation. No wiping, blotting or timing. Very small slot for insertion. May be difficult for someone with poor manual dexterity to operate this model.
Glucofilm test strips	Visual verification up to 240mg/dl	60 seconds	Recalls last 10 test results	Must wipe and time. Durable strip. Has short time frame from wiping to insertion of strip of 20 seconds. Elderly and those with poor manual dexterity may have difficulty getting strip inserted with the allotted time. Has non-replaceable battery. More accurate with hematocrit in 20-60% range.
Glucofilm test strips	Visual verification up to 240mg/dl	60 seconds	Stores blood glucose test results with date and time (up to 300 events)	Has alarm clock. Meter and log book combined. Allows input of insulin, diet, exercise and other diabetes-related events. Meter functions are accurate with hematocrit in 20-60% range. Has computer linking capacities.
CheckMate test strips (foil wrapped)	No visual reading	90 seconds	40-test storage capacity	Has built-in lancet device. No wiping, blotting, or timing. Automatic check for adequate sample. Automatic rejection of used or damaged test strip. Corrects for hematocrit. Results in mg/dl or mmol/L. Test procedure can be difficult to follow due to sequence of the button manipulations.
Supreme test strips	Visual verification	50 seconds	14 tests	No wiping. Test strips are more economical than others currently available. Currently has limited distribution in the United States.

meter which are audio components which verbalize the test procedure steps.

Because technique is so critical in obtaining accurate, clinically valuable results, proper training is essential. Poor training may result in noncompliance with home testing. When instructing the user (be it the patient, the caregiver, or another health care provider) the following should be included:

- Explain preparation for the test procedure.
- Inform the user of all necessary additional supplies such as cotton balls, gauze, etc.
- Explain and demonstrate proper methods to obtain blood sample. Hands should be clean and dry. It is unnecessary to use alcohol as this dries and toughens the skin when used repeatedly (some individuals may have to test multiple times daily depending on level of control).
- Instruct individuals to use the "heel" (or side) of the finger to minimize pain and calluses which form when the fingertip is used.
- Demonstrate the actual test procedure. Observe the individual performing the test to validate comprehension.
- Demonstrate calibration procedures, maintenance procedures, and any systems check procedures.
- Show individual where and how to replace the battery.
- Inform them about company toll-free numbers, trouble-shooting procedures and error codes.
- Inform patient about obtaining replacement supplies such as batteries, strips, and lancets.
- Explain the importance of the relationship between blood glucose, interpretation of results, results in relationship to food intake, and the relationship between the results and symptoms of hypo- and hyperglycemia.
- Reinforce the "monitoring prescription" given by the clinician. The timing of blood glucose readings reflect the activity of the various components of the insulin regimen and guide the clinician to adjust the appropriate insulin. Table 14-9 outlines the relationship between the time of injection and the test time. Often the individual must intensify monitoring around dosage changes and during times of illness and infection.
- Emphasize the importance of recording the results and assist in determining when to contact the physician.

To properly assess a meter, the pharmacist must personally perform the test procedure, with a critical approach, evaluating for populations which will have barriers to the particular meter as well as populations who will benefit from special features. Recording these observations leads to an organized summary for quick reference. A form such as the one in Table 14-10 can serve as a guide.

DIABETES EDUCATION

Pharmacists have the knowledge and skills to participate also in formal educational

Table 14-9 Timing of Home Blood Glucose Tests and the Insulin Dose Reflected by the Test[7]

Insulin	Time Injected	Period of Activity	Test Reflecting Insulin Action
Regular	Before a meal	Between that meal and either the subsequent meal or snack, if insulin is taken before supper	Both following meal before which insulin is injected and before next meal or bedtime snack, if insulin is taken before supper
NPH	Before breakfast	Between lunch and supper	Before supper
NPH	Before supper or before bedtime	Overnight	Before breakfast
Ultralente	Before breakfast or before supper	Mostly overnight because regular over-rides its effect over the day	Before breakfast

Table 14-10 Evaluation of a Blood Glucose Monitor[17,18]

NAME OF MONITOR	
Manufacturer	
Toll-Free Number	
Cost of Meter	
Cost of Strips	
Source of Distribution	
Rebate Offer	
PROCEDURE	
Ease of Use	
Timing Features	
Blotting/Wiping	
Sample Size	
Accuracy Data	
Visual Back-Up	
Memory	
LIMITATIONS	
Interfering substances	
Temperature	
Humidity	
Ranges Covered	
MAINTENANCE	
Battery	
Replacement	
Cleaning procedure	
Systems Check	
Features	
SPECIAL FEATURES	

programs which empower patients to manage their disease. Patient education programs vary; however, key topics are essential to a comprehensive program. Essential topics are:

- Disease process
- Signs and symptoms of hyper- and hypoglycemia
- Psychological adjustment to disease
- Behavioral modification
- Diet instruction
- Exercise benefits and effects
- Medication treatment of DM (Oral Agents and Insulin)
- Monitoring of DM
- Complications of DM
- Sick day management
- Personal hygiene and preventive care (i.e., foot care)

Excellent educational materials are available through national organizations such as the American Diabetes Association and the Juvenile Diabetes Foundation. In addition, manufacturers of products used by individuals with diabetes have helpful written materials. Prior to using printed materials, the pharmacist should review the content and determine if the reading level matches that of the patient population. Teaching Patients with Low Literacy Skills by Doak, Doak, and Root is an excellent guide in working with this special population.

Throughout this chapter, concepts of diabetes education have been inserted. However, it is critical to emphasize that education must be emphasized throughout the interactions between the pharmacist and individuals with diabetes, the family and the caregivers. In addition to formal education, the pharmacist must take every opportunity to reinforce, clarify, and assess the comprehension of instructions.

Education for the pharmacist may need to extend beyond traditional programs. Pharmacists who meet the requirements are eligible to seek certification in diabetes education through the American Association of Diabetes Educators. This certification demonstrates a high level of commitment to serving those with diabetes.

CONCLUSION

Diabetes is a common, chronic disease that gives the patient tremendous responsibility for self management. Successful self management requires the focused efforts of the health care providers, the patient, the patient's family and caregivers. These efforts must be directed at knowledge and skills to overcome barriers to treatment success. Pharmacists are ideally situated to provide products and services which aid in these efforts, improve treatment outcomes and individual's quality of life.

REFERENCES

1. U.S. Department of Health and Human Services, Public Health Services. Diabetes and chronic disability conditions. Healthy People 2000: National Health Promotion and Disease Prevention Objectives. 1990; 460.
2. Harris MI, Hadden WC, Knowler WC, et al. Prevalence of diabetes and impaired glucose tolerance and plasma glucose levels in US population, ages 20-74 years. Diabetes. 1987; 36:523-534.
3. Morley JE, Mooradian AD, Rosenthal MJ, et al. Diabetes in the elderly patients: Is it different? Am J Med. 1987; 83:533-544.
4. Campbell RH, Garrelts L. Developing a diabetes care specialty practice. US Pharm. 1992; 11(suppl)5-16.
5. American Diabetes Association. Diagnosis and classification of diabetes mellitus. Physician's Guide to Non-Insulin Dependent (Type II) Diabetes: Diagnosis and Treatment. 2nd Ed. 1988; 3.
6. Thai AC, Eisenbarth GS. Natural History of IDDM. Diabetes Reviews. 1993; 1(1):1-14.
7. Davidson MB. How to get the most out of insulin therapy. Clinical Diabetes. 1990; 8(5):67-73.
8. Gebhart SSP, Wheaton RN, Mullins RE, Austin GE. A comparison of home glucose monitoring with determinations of hemoglobin A1c, fructosamine, and random glucose in diabetic patients. Arch Intern Med. 1991; 151:1133-37.
9. Gerich JE. Oral hypoglycemic agents. N Eng J Med. 1989; 21:1231-9.
10. Milchovich SK, Dunn-Long B. Injection technique. Diabetes mellitus: a practical handbook. Bull Publishing Co. 1990; 115-118.
11. Anderson JH, Campbell RK. Mixing insulins in 1990. The Diabetes Educator. 1990; 16(5):380-7.
12. ADA Position Statement. Insulin Administration. Diabetes Care. 1991; 14(Suppl.2):30.
13. Zehrer C, Hansen R, Battle J. Reducing blood glucose variability by use of abdominal insulin injection sites. The Diabetes Educator. 1990; 16(6):474-7.
14. Fine N. Injecting insulin. Diabetes Self-Management. 1992; 3,4:10-16.
15. Peters AL, Davidson MB. Does insulin + sulfonylureas = effective treatment of NIDDM? Clinical Diabetes. 1992; 10(2):19-21.
16. Gadsden RH. Sources of variation in blood glucose testing. Challenges in Diabetes Management/Milestone in Monitoring. Health Education Technologies. New York. 1988; 63-6.
17. Yachmetz B. Prescribing a blood glucose monitor for your patient. Pharmacy Times. 1992; 10:134-40.
18. ECRI. Portable blood glucose monitors. Health Devices. 1992; 21(2):43-78.

15 Home Respiratory Care

Rene F. Steffen, B.S., RRT, RCP

The number of chronic pulmonary disease patients in the United States continues to increase due to improved care of acute respiratory illness, increased longevity of the population and exposure to pollutants.[1] Continuation of these trends will further increase the demand for chronic care of respiratory diseases, as evidenced by a projected compound annual growth rate of 9.9 percent for U.S. home respiratory care between 1991 and 1996.[2] As with other types of chronic care at home, home respiratory care is a multi-billion dollar industry in the U.S.[2,3]

Table 15-1 Devices for Home Respiratory Care

HME used for chronic respiratory care is discussed according to function. The major uses and associated device types are:

USE	DEVICE TYPES
Environmental conditioning	Purifiers, Air Cleaners, Humidifiers,
Physical therapy	Percussors, Incentive spirometers
Delivering drug therapy	Atomizers, Nebulizers, Metered dose inhalers, MDI extenders
Delivering oxygen	Tanks, Regulators, Enhancers, Concentrators

Most patients with chronic pulmonary disease receive drug therapy, either for underlying related disease (e.g., cardiovascular conditions) or for direct therapy of respiratory illness. A variety of devices are used to deliver pharmacologic agents to the lung, and other devices are used to provide physical therapy or to modify the patient's environment. The home health care (HHC) pharmacist is in a unique position to provide both drugs and devices to these patients, counsel them regarding their use, and aid in coordinating drug therapy with other therapeutic modalities.(See Table 15-1)

This chapter provides an introduction to the home care of patients with chronic respiratory insufficiency, and emphasizes drugs and home medical equipment (HME). The disease states associated with chronic pulmonary dysfunction are briefly reviewed, as well as the means used to identify the patient and test for the dysfunction. (The use of home parenteral antibiotic therapy for respiratory infections is discussed in Chapter 24.)

Because an important part of chronic respiratory therapy is home oxygen therapy, a discussion of oxygen's physical properties and medical uses is included. Finally, the chapter discusses the organization and provision of home respiratory services, with emphasis on the pharmacist's role in home oxygen therapy.

DISEASE STATES REQUIRING HOME RESPIRATORY CARE

Patients requiring home respiratory care are individuals whose pulmonary function is compromised such that they cannot adequately control concentrations of oxygen and carbon dioxide in their blood, or whose acid-base balance is impaired. Before discussing the diseases which may impair pulmonary function, it is useful to review pulmonary function tests.

Functional and Diagnostic Tests

Tests that aid in the diagnosis of lung disease include examination of sputum, pleural fluid, and tissue. These specimens are obtained by lavage, endoscopy, and/or biopsy, and are subjected to bacteriologic, cytologic, and biochemical testing. Blood is sampled for hematologic as well as acid-base and blood gas studies. Tests of pulmonary physiologic function are also performed. These measure changes in compartments of the lung which may be indicative of lung function changes or disease.

Pulmonary Function Tests

Some of the physiologic tests that pharmacists should be familiar with are:

1. Forced vital capacity (FVC): the maximum volume of exhaled air after maximal inspiration. Vital capacity will vary with height and chest expansion, and inversely with age.
2. Forced expiratory volume (FEV): the volume of maximally fast expiration starting at full inspiration and measured over time. When measured over one second, this value is identified as FEVl. Typically, 70% of the total FVC is exhaled in the first second, so FEV/FVC should normally equal 0.7 or above.
3. Residual volume: the volume remaining after a maximum expiration. This cannot be measured directly by spirometry.
4. Functional residual capacity (FRC): the amount of air in the lungs at the end of a quiet expiration. This is a buffer to prevent wide fluctuations in alveolar oxygen and carbon dioxide tensions during respiration.
5. Tidal volume: the amount of air inspired or expired during the respiratory cycle.
6. Total lung capacity: the volume of air in lungs at the end of a full inspiration. This is equal to FVC plus residual volume.

While these do not represent all of the physiologic tests, they are ordered for the majority of patients experiencing breathing difficulty. More complete discussions of pulmonary function testing and tables for calculating normal values are available in standard textbooks.[3,4]

Blood Gas Studies

Blood gas studies include oxygen saturation and pressure, and carbon dioxide content and pressure. Oxygen is carried in the blood either in solution or chemically combined with hemoglobin (as oxyhemoglobin). The partial pressure of oxygen in arterial blood (PaO_2) is approximately 100 mmHg. To determine the volume percent of dissolved oxygen, one multiplies the PaO_2 by the solubility constant of oxygen (0.003 ml/100 ml/mmHg) to yield a normal 0.3 vol% dissolved oxygen. The partial pressure of oxygen in venous blood in 40 mmHg with 0.1 vol% in solution.

The remaining oxygen is combined with hemoglobin and it is readily apparent that the oxygen carrying capacity of blood is heavily dependent on the amount of hemoglobin present. One gram of hemoglobin combines with 1.34 ml of oxygen, and if one assumes a normal hemoglobin concentration of 15 g/100 ml, approximately 20 ml of oxygen can be combined with the hemoglobin in 100 ml of blood (20 vol%).

The amount of oxygen that is actually combined with hemoglobin is expressed as percent saturation. A healthy individual with normal lung function and a PaO_2 of 100 mmHg will have an oxygen saturation of 95% or greater in arterial blood. Venous blood will be only 70% saturated.

The transport of carbon dioxide in the blood is more complex. A small portion is bound to plasma proteins, and about 5% is dissolved in the plasma water. About 20% of $C0_2$ released into the lung is transported by hemoglobin, and the remaining gas is transported as carbonic acid and bicarbonate ion. Thus, carbon dioxide exchange is important in regulating the acid base balance of the blood.

At an actual blood pH of 7.4, a bicarbonate ion-carbonic acid ratio of 20:1 must exist. Any alterations in this ratio will result in a change of pH. As the denominator in the Henderson-Hasselbalch equation, carbon dioxide pressures provide specific information on ventilation. A higher partial pressure of carbon dioxide ($PC0_2$) means inadequate ventilation and low pH. A low $PC0_2$ results in an increase in pH with hyperventilation. Normal $PC0_2$ levels are 38-44 mmHg. Because carbon dioxide is very soluble in blood, a small change in the partial pressure of carbon dioxide is related to large changes in carbon dioxide content. Table 15-2 shows some expected changes in blood gas values for various respiratory conditions.

Respiratory failure occurs when the lungs fail to adequately exchange oxygen and carbon dioxide for body needs. Laboratory values showing a pH of 7.3 or less, a PaO_2 less than 50 mmHg, or a $PC0_2$ greater than 50 mmHg all suggest respiratory failure. Normally, blood returning to the left atrium and left ventricle has an oxygen saturation of 94 to 98% and a partial pressure of 95 to 97 mmHg. The oxygen saturation of blood entering the pulmonary alveoli is 70%.

Presenting Symptoms

Patients with respiratory difficulty may

Table 15-2 Blood Gas Patterns in Compromised Lungs[7]

CONDITION	PaO2	PaC02	pH
Hyperventilation	N	D	I
Metabolic Acidosis	N	D	D
Hypoventilation	N	I	D
Diffusion/Perfusion Problem	D	D	I
Impaired Diffusion	D	D	D
Bronchial Asthma, Emphysema, Cardiac Failure, Pneumonia	D	N	N

Key: N=Normal, D=Decreased, I=Increased

experience varying degrees of symptoms in a variety of combinations. Common major symptoms are cough, increased sputum production, hemoptysis, chest pain, dyspnea, and wheezing. Other symptoms that may be present are headache, anxiety and restlessness, somnolence, hoarseness, calf pain and tenderness, erythema nodosum of lower legs, facial edema, arm and shoulder pain, polyarthralgia, and cold and allergy symptoms.

Cor pulmonale is a symptom complex commonly associated with respiratory disease. The term itself means "pulmonary heart disease." The complex includes dyspnea, chest pain, syncope, tachypnea, and wheezing associated with right heart enlargement.

Diagnosis

Assigning a diagnosis by the physician to a symptom complex will require the diagnostic and pulmonary function tests described above, plus additional physical examinations, x-rays, and a detailed history including family and environmental factors. Diagnostic categories are not always precise and a diagnosis of chronic obstructive pulmonary disease (COPD) instead of asthma or bronchitis may hinge largely on semantics.

Conditions Predisposing To Chronic Pulmonary Insufficiency

Chronic respiratory failure often follows a history of prior disease. It is hoped that prevention or early treatment of predisposing conditions can forestall later respiratory failure. Early detection is important and the pharmacist should encourage patients with predisposing conditions to seek early appropriate care. The most common conditions resulting in chronic respiratory care are smoking, acute bronchitis, pneumonia, asthma, and environmental diseases.[5]

Chronic Diseases Requiring Respiratory Care

Because proper exchange of gases is dependent on both ventilation and perfusion, it can be seen that respiratory care is necessary for those diseases that interfere with airflow in and out of the alveoli and bronchi, with pulmonary muscular function, or with pulmonary circulation. Perhaps the most important group of diseases are those that interfere with air flow, or the obstructive diseases.

Chronic Obstructive Pulmonary Disease

There are many respiratory conditions that may be classified as chronic obstructive pulmonary disease (COPD). Other terms and acronyms that may be used in place of COPD are chronic obstructive lung disease (COLD), chronic airway disease (CAD) and chronic airway obstruction (CAO).

COPD is commonly seen in urban areas, in the socio-economically disadvantaged, and in men. It is progressive if not treated, presents as episodic worsening with sudden onset of dyspnea, and may be misdiagnosed as pneumonia. Primary symptoms are cough, dyspnea, and bronchoconstriction. There is impaired air flow (primarily outflow) associated with increased airway resistance.

The principal complication is congestive heart failure (CHF), the leading cause of death for patients with COPD. Other causes of death, in descending order of frequency, are respiratory failure, pneumonia, bronchiolitis, pulmonary thromboembolism, hemorrhage from a peptic ulcer, and spontaneous pneumothorax.

Emphysema and chronic bronchitis are the two forms of COPD most commonly encountered by the HHC pharmacist. Emphysema is characterized by abnormal increases in the size of the alveoli with destructive changes in alveolar walls. Fibrosis may or may not be present. The enlarged airspaces reduce the amount of surface area available for gas exchange. The damaged tissue may form lesions which block airflow or weaken the bronchiolar walls. This may allow inspired air to leak out, or the walls may collapse, trapping air on expiration. Patients with emphysema have been called "pink puffers" as they are well aerated when relatively sedentary, but become quite breathless upon exertion.

Chronic bronchitis has a different underlying defect, but similar end results. In bronchitis the pulmonary tissue responds to a stimulus with an increase in mucus production and accompanying swelling of the mucosal tissue. Increased mucus production may encourage bacterial growth and subsequent breakdown of lung tissue. Excess mucus may form complete or partial lung plugs which diminish air flow. Patients with bronchitis have been called "blue bloaters," and are generally cyanotic at rest. Any activity will cause breathlessness and wheezing. Because trapped air can cause tissue breakdown, a patient with chronic bronchitis may show symptoms and changes identical to those exhibited by a patient with emphysema.

Conditions Affecting Ventilation

A variety of diseases can affect respiratory function by impairing muscular function or limiting chest wall expansion. Included in this category are multiple sclerosis, muscular dystrophy, amyotrophic lateral sclerosis, paralysis, scleroderma, lupus erythematosus, and non-respiratory cancers. The pharmacist who provides drug therapy to treat the primary disorder should be alerted to the possibility that the patient is receiving respiratory care, possibly from another source.

Cardiovascular Disease

Changes in blood flow and pressure can directly affect the respiratory system. Respiratory insufficiency with dyspnea, orthopnea, congestion, and pain are common symptoms of congestive heart failure and hypertension. Other related illnesses that can affect the respiratory system are angina pectoris, myocardial infarction, polycythemia, arrhythmias, and stroke.

Cancer

Carcinomas of the respiratory system are primarily associated with smoking, or exposure to industrial toxins, heavy metals, or radiation. Initial symptoms include cough, dyspnea, and pain. While the majority of respiratory carcinomas are treatable if detected early, progression of the disease usually leads to a variety of symptoms and locations, and can compromise other body systems.

Additional Resources

The preceding discussion is of necessity a general review. The reader is referred elsewhere for more complete discussions.[6,7]

HOME MANAGEMENT OF RESPIRATORY DISEASE

The home management of a patient with chronic respiratory disease includes four major modalities, often used in combination: environmental conditioning, exercise and pulmonary drainage, pharmacologic agents, and home oxygen. Each of these therapies is aided by a variety of medical devices that the HHC pharmacist may provide.

Environmental Conditioning

Increased bronchoreactivity to inhaled irritants is common among patients with long-standing respiratory disease. In addition, adequate moisture in inspired air can minimize drying of the bronchial tree and aid in liquefying sputum so that it may be cleared more easily. Inhaled irritants can be removed from the home environment by air cleaners and purifiers, and patients going outdoors can use masks to reduce exposure to pollens and dusts. Humidifiers and vaporizers are used to add water vapor to the room air.

Air Cleaners

To "clean" air, one would like to remove offensive odors, noxious gases, infectious agents, and particulate matter. Most air cleaners concentrate on the removal of particulate matter, and in doing so reduce odors and infectious agents that adhere to the particles being removed. Three common approaches to removal of particles in the air are filters, electrostatic precipitators, and negative ion generators.

High efficiency particulate air (HEPA) filters can effectively remove particles as small as 0.1 microns in diameter, the size of the smallest particles in cigarette smoke. These filters are used in laminar flow hoods to create an aseptic environment for sterile product production, but require large motors and air volumes. Lower efficiency filters are used in smaller devices to remove particles from room air, but they cannot be expected to be as effective as HEPA filters.

Electrostatic precipitators can be used to remove particles from a larger volume of air, and have been widely adopted for use as part of home heating and air conditioning systems. These devices consist of one or more frames supporting a matrix of electrical discharge points, placed in the stream of air. They may be combined with prefilters to remove gross particulate matter. Electricity is discharged at the points, and particles passing by are given a negative charge. A set of collecting grids are given a positive charge, to which the negatively charged particles are attracted. The collecting grids are periodically removed and washed.

Negative ion generators use a point discharge method, like the electrostatic precipitators, but air molecules, not particles, are the recipients of the negative charge. These negative ions attach to dust particles, causing them to aggregate. The aggregates are heavy enough to fall to the floor or other surfaces, where they are removed by dusting. A variety of claims have been made for the beneficial health effects of the negative ions generated by these devices, few, if any, of which are proven.[8] As noted below, however, these devices are effective in removing particles from the air.

A series of tests were made of the effectiveness of small air cleaners.[8] Cigarette smoke was generated in a room that was approximately 11 x 13 x 5 feet, and the density was measured over the ensuing four hours. Filter cleaners, negative ion generators, and one brand of a filter/negative ion generator combination were compared against three control procedures: no device at all, a large room fan, and a large room air cleaner that used a HEPA filter. With no device at all, 17% of the smoke cleared in 4 hours. A large room fan alone cleared 54% of particles in the same time, presumably by forcing the particles to collide with the floor, ceiling, and walls. The HEPA filter device removed 100% of the smoke in less than 3 hours. The small fan-filter devices were inefficient; none removed more than 45% of the particles in 4 hours (less than a large room fan alone), and most averaged a 22% reduction in particles. By contrast, most of the negative ion generators removed more than 95% of the particles in 4 hours or less. The combination of a negative ion generator plus a fan-filter unit removed 100% of the smoke in less than 2 hours.

When recommending an air cleaning device, the pharmacist should consider whether a single room or an entire home must be treated. A filter/electrostatic precipitator unit installed in the central heating system is likely to be the most efficient and cost effective method for an entire home. For a single room, however, a negative ion generator with or without a filter is quiet, but causes a buildup of dust on exposed surfaces. All units should meet EPA requirements for maximum ozone production. Patients particularly sensitive to the low levels of ozone produced by precipitators and ion generators will be better served by a room sized HEPA filter device.

Masks

Filter masks can be used outside the home to reduce exposure to pollens, dust, and other airborne particulate matter. Foam masks can be worn that cause inspired air to be mixed with some of the patient's own exhaled air, thus warming the incoming air in cold weather. Several varieties of "pollen masks" and "cold weather" masks are commercially available.

Devices designed to prevent exposure to industrial dusts, toxic particles, and gases must meet standards set by the Occupational Safety and Health Administration (OSHA). These regulations refer to "masks" as devices designed to reduce exposure to relatively nontoxic agents, and set higher standards for "respirators," devices for use around toxic substances. Two of the officially described masks are a Nontoxic Particle Mask and a Nuisance Odor Mask. Specific respirator standards have been developed for asbestos, acid gas, dust, hydrofluoric acid, mercury vapor, and organic vapor, among others. State agencies charged with industrial safety enforcement may set more stringent standards, and the pharmacist supplying masks for industrial use should verify that the product meets the standards in his or her locale.

Humidifiers And Vaporizers

Room humidifiers and vaporizers are

designed to increase the water content of the ambient air. They are widely used in acute respiratory illness, particularly in treatment of upper tract symptoms. They may also be recommended for patients with chronic disease. Specific devices are used to humidify oxygen from tanks or concentrators, and other devices provide a breathable mist; these are discussed later.

Vaporizers produce steam. Older models were actually fashioned after tea kettles, with a heating element that caused water in the unit to boil and be expelled through a small opening. These have been abandoned due to the inherent dangers of boiling water and steam pressure. Modern vaporizers consist of a water reservoir into which is inserted a heating unit. A small hole in the base of the unit allows water to enter a chamber containing two electrodes. Current flowing through the water heats the water in the chamber only, producing steam. The water in the larger reservoir may become warm, but never hot. Because the heating chamber does not touch the bottom of the reservoir, the vaporizer never boils dry. As soon as the water level drops below the electrodes, the circuit is broken and steaming terminates.

Vaporizers are quiet and inexpensive. Users in areas with hard water must add distilled water to the unit to prevent excessively rapid steaming. In areas with soft water, electrolyte must be added to allow electricity to flow. Weak electrolytes (e.g., baking soda) should be used; table salt (NaCl) will produce excessive steaming, as well as corrosion. The electrodes must be periodically removed and cleaned. A danger of electric shock exists whenever the unit is plugged in, even if it has "turned itself off" due to low water. Water spilled around the top may be electrically live, for example.

Humidifiers use a motor driven impeller to create vapor. Water is drawn from the reservoir into the unit, where the rapidly rotating impeller forces the water against a baffle, creating minute droplets. These are expelled into the room. The humidifier does not pose the danger of electric shock or burns that a vaporizer does, and does not heat up the room. However, the units are noisier and more costly. In areas with hard water, the humidifier may cause a fine residue of minerals to build up in the room. In addition, because no heat is produced, mold and bacterial growth in the reservoir and unit is more likely. Users should be cautioned to clean the unit after storage and before use with detergent and/or a mild hypochlorite solution.

For the intended purpose of adding humidity to the room air, either device is effective. The water vapor is the important element, and vaporizer additives are unnecessary, expensive, and may require more frequent cleaning of vaporizers. No additives should be used with humidifiers.

Physical Therapy

Physical therapy for the patient with respiratory problems is directed towards improving ventilation and mobilizing secretions. Physical therapy is often combined with other forms of treatment such as humidification and medication.

Improvements in ventilation are obtained through exercise and retraining in proper breathing technique. Exercise consists of timed patterns of forced inspirations and expirations. Patients with compromised lung function often must be retrained in breathing techniques to eliminate inefficient (rapid, shallow breathing) patterns developed as a result of respiratory insufficiency. Physical exercise programs are developed to gradually recondition a patient to function somewhat normally despite a reduced pulmonary capacity.

An important device used in training is the incentive spirometer. A transparent tube contains a light weight ball, similar to a ping pong ball. As the patient blows through a mouthpiece and tube connected to the spirometer, the air flow will cause the ball to rise. The patient works to make the ball reach a given level, and also to keep the ball at the level for progressively longer periods of time. The incentive spirometer provides the patient with a measurable goal and monitors progress.

Thick mucus can be liquefied by improving fluid intake, by humidifying the inspired air, or by inhalation of liquefying vapor. The particle size of the liquefaction agent (usually sterile water or sterile normal saline) is important. Smaller sized particles tend to travel deeper into the bronchial tree where secretions are most difficult to reach. The devices used to provide this vapor are discussed below under nebulizers.

Gentle clapping techniques may be applied to the chest and back to physically break up secretions. Manual clapping is effective, but percussors, powered by motors or compressed air, may be used to relieve fatigue on the part of the caregiver. Sometimes hand held vibrators are used in addition to percussion to provide a different frequency of vibration that may assist in mobilizing secretions.

Gravity and body positioning also play a major role in physical therapy as they enhance breathing and range of motion, as well as promote drainage. Postural drainage is accomplished by placing the patient with the head lower than the thighs. Depending on which lung segments are to be drained, the patient may lie on the back or side. Postural draining couches are available for use in intermittent postural drainage. Adjustable hospital beds are also used.

Drug Therapy

The principal classes of drugs used in treating chronic respiratory disease are antibiotics, xanthine derivatives, corticosteroids, sympathomimetics, bronchodilators, and medical oxygen. The pharmacology and therapeutic considerations of the first four groups are well covered in other texts. This section will focus on devices used to provide medical oxygen or other agents directly to the respiratory system.

Atomizers

Atomizers produce a spray of fairly large droplets, and are used primarily for application of drugs to the nasal mucosa or to the throat. The droplets are produced by a two-piece nozzle called a venturi, which takes advantage of the Bernoulli effect. (When a gas passes over a surface, the pressure is inversely proportional to the velocity of the gas). One part of a venturi is a siphon tube placed into the liquid to be atomized and the other is a tube connected to a gas supply. The outlet of the second tube is placed adjacent and at an angle to the upper end of the siphon tube. When the gas flows through its tube, a partial vacuum is created at the top of the siphon tube, and liquid is drawn from the reservoir into the stream of gas, where it is dispersed as a spray.

Nebulizers

Nebulizers are used to create a much finer mist which is inhaled into the lungs. They operate on the same principle as atomizers, except that the venturi is placed within a larger chamber. The mist created by the venturi is trapped in the larger chamber, and when the patient breathes in, air flowing through the larger chamber picks up only the finest droplets; heavier droplets return to the solution in the reservoir.

Hand held nebulizers have been largely replaced by metered-dose inhalers (MDIs), particularly for acute administration of bronchodilators in asthma patients. Compressor driven nebulizers are widely used in conjunction with other respiratory therapy equipment, particularly in the home setting. Normal saline or distilled water alone may be inhaled to aid in liquefying mucus, and bronchodilators or acetyl cysteine may be added to the nebulizer reservoir for inhalation.

Administration of bronchodilators via nebulizer can be performed using continuous or intermittent flow nebulization. In either case, air flow from the compressor is constant, but continuous flow means that drug is constantly mixed with the air flow. With intermittent flow nebulization, the patient can control nebulization by covering or uncovering a valve on the nebulizer. Intermittent flow is preferred if the patient has sufficient coordination, because with continuous flow drug is lost to the atmosphere between breaths.

When drugs are administered by nebulizer, it should be remembered that there will always be a small amount of fluid left in the reservoir after nebulization. This residual volume varies with different nebulizers, but is approximately 0.5 ml. The percentage of the total dose which remains in the nebulizer can be determined by the following formula:

$$\text{Percent Dose Remaining} = \frac{\text{Residual Volume}}{\text{Total Volume}} \times 100$$

As an illustration of the trade-offs involved in choosing a dilution rate and total volume of solution used in a nebulizer, consider the following order:

Bronkosol 30 ml
N.S. qs ad 270 ml
Sig: 3 ml in nebulizer q.i.d.

Bronkosol® contains 1% isoetharine, and a 1:9 solution will provide 3.3 mg in 3 ml. With a typical nebulizer, it will take between 20 to 30 minutes of intermittent flow nebulization to deliver the dose. Could nebulization time be reduced by using a more concentrated solution and smaller total volume? Table 15-3 demonstrates the effect of different combinations of dilution and volume, all of which place the same amount of isoetharine in the nebulizer at the beginning of nebulization, assuming the residual volume is constant at 0.5 ml.

In most situations where intermittent flow is

Table 15-3 Dilutiom and Volume Effects on Dose

Dose in Nebulizer	Dilution Used	Volume in Nebulizer	Volume Actually Given	Drug Actually Administered
3.3 mg	1:9	3 ml	2.5 ml	2.7 mg
3.3 mg	1:6	2 ml	1.5 ml	2.5 mg
3.3 mg	1:3	1 ml	0.5 ml	1.7 mg

used, a 3 ml volume in the nebulizer represents a reasonable compromise between time needed to administer the dose and drug lost to residual volume. With continuous nebulization, a larger total volume (about double) is given to compensate for drug lost between inhalations.

Ultrasonic Nebulizers

Ultrasonic nebulizers produce an exceptionally fine mist, and penetration of the mist to the lungs may be greater than with standard nebulizers. The mist is generated in the nebulizer chamber by vibrations from a piezoelectric crystal oscillating at approximately 1.3 MHz. The vibrations are transmitted through a coupling chamber containing pure water to a diaphragm at the base of the nebulizer reservoir. The mist generated above the surface of the nebulizer solution is picked up by carrier gas flow generated by an external blower or from the oxygen line.

As with other nebulizers, either constant or intermittent flow may be used. The nebulization rate with the ultrasonic nebulizer may be as great as 3 ml per minute, and the reservoir holds to up 200 ml. The nebulization rate varies with the temperature of the solution, and is inversely related to the viscosity of the nebulizer solution. If surfactants remain in the reservoir from prior cleaning, nebulization may be inhibited, so thorough rinsing is essential. Some therapeutic agents with surfactant properties may be unsuitable for delivery by the ultrasonic nebulizer.

Cleaning and Sterilization

Inhalation devices are potential sources of infection, particularly in patients with compromised host defenses. Sterilization of nebulizers, tubing, cannulas, and other equipment is not essential for most ambulatory patients, but thorough cleaning prior to use is important. Equipment that is cleaned but not dried completely prior to storage is prone to mold and bacterial growth. Each manufacturer provides specific cleaning instructions for its products, and the HHC pharmacist should review these carefully with the patient.

Metered Dose Inhalers and Extender Devices

Inhaled corticosteroids and bronchodilators are now commonly administered by MDIs, which combine the drug and fluorocarbon propellant in a canister and control the dose via a metering valve. MDI are advantageous because they are convenient, portable, and provide an accurate dose. However, the accuracy of the dose delivered to the lungs depends upon the patient's ability to coordinate release of the dose with inhalation. Up to 89% of initial users of MDI are unable to use them properly, and between 15 and 30% of all users exhibit improper inhalation technique after repeated instruction.[10] Thus, for nearly two-thirds of patients using these devices, pharmacists have an important role in training them to use the device properly. For the remaining patients, a variety of extender devices have been developed.

Spacer type extenders are tubes that attach to the canister and provide a longer pathway between the aerosol valve and the mouth. The patient clears the drug from the chamber with a single slow inhalation. Chamber type extenders allow the mist to enter a large accumulation chamber. The chamber is cleared by multiple inhalations. With all extenders, close timing between pressing the cartridge and inhalation is less essential than with MDI alone and some devices actuate the cartridge automatically on inspiration.

Several studies have been performed to examine the effect of different extender designs on drug delivery. Comparisons have been made between MDI alone, MDI with extenders, nebulizers, and intermittent positive pressure breathing (IPPB) aerosolization. Self and Fuentes concluded that pharmacists should make every effort to teach patients the correct use of MDI alone.[9] They further recommend that for patients who cannot properly use an MDI alone, an extender should be recommended before trying nebulizer machines, because extenders were less expensive and more convenient.[9]

OXYGEN THERAPY

The use of oxygen in the home was considered dangerous and of questionable value until recently. Controlled low flow oxygen therapy has been demonstrated effective and safe in the ambulatory setting,[5] and clinicians have become more comfortable prescribing this therapy for hospital and home use. The primary purpose of controlled low flow supplemental oxygen is to increase the amount of oxygen available for exchange, thereby increasing the arterial tension levels to normal range.

Medical Oxygen

Medical oxygen can be provided as compressed gas, liquid oxygen, or by oxygen concentrator. Medical oxygen must meet all USP requirements including those for quality control testing. Containers which store compressed gas must also meet stringent standards for quality and safety as set forth by the Compressed Gas Association of America (CGA).

The respiratory drive in most individuals derives from a combination of elevated $C0_2$ and decreased 0_2 levels in arterial blood, with the $C0_2$ levels exerting the greatest influence. Patients with chronic respiratory insufficiency gradually adapt to elevated $C0_2$ levels, however, and are driven to breathe primarily by diminished 0_2 tension. When exogenous oxygen administration raises arterial tension, the respiratory drive is lost and the patient may experience respiratory arrest. In addition, uncontrolled use of oxygen can present alveoli with too much gas for exchange, creating continuous high pressures that initiate irreversible damage to the lungs. Because of its possible fatal side effects, medical oxygen is classified as a legend drug.

Delivery of oxygen can be accomplished by nasal cannula, by face mask, or through a tube placed in the trachea. Nasal cannulas tend to stay in place longer, allow the use of the oral cavity while receiving therapy, and enable the patient to communicate and move about more freely. Face masks allow delivery of heated humidified oxygen and certain pharmacologic agents. The primary use of a trachea tube is with a ventilator, and to bypass the area from the mouth to the esophagus if needed.

Physical Characteristics of Oxygen

Oxygen is combustible, not explosive, and its combustion requires the presence of a flame or spark. The mixture of oxygen with petroleum products creates the likelihood of spontaneous combustion.

At the pressure of 50 atmospheres and a temperature of -119° C (-182° F), oxygen becomes liquid. Therefore, by changing temperature and pressure, oxygen can be readily converted from gas to liquid. Liquid oxygen is available in insulated containers at a temperature of -183° C (-297° F). Compressed gas is available in cylinders under pressures of 2,000 to 2,400 pounds per square inch (psi).

Safety and Legal Requirements

The CGA has published guidelines for handling of all gases, including medical oxygen. The U.S. Department of Transportation also has specific requirements for the transportation and storage of hazardous materials, including gases. Intrastate shipment of compressed gases from dealer to patient does not require registration with the DOT, but shipment between dealers or interstate deliveries can only be undertaken by carriers that are registered. Local fire departments have additional policies regarding physical plant, storage, and in-home use of gases. All three agencies are willing to assist dealers in complying with locally active regulations.

Compressed Gas Systems

Completely filled oxygen cylinders are pressurized between 1,800 and 2,400 psi. As the gas is drawn off, the pressures drop accordingly. Precautions must be taken to insure against leakage or trauma to the cylinders. The refill valve on the neck of the cylinder also serves as the regulator attachment site. In the unlikely event that a valve breaks off, the cylinder turns into a rocket. Cylinders that must be connected together for use should be done so only using approved manifolds or tubing, and only where permitted by law. Steel cylinders can withstand pressures of up to 6,000 psi, and aluminum cylinders are rated at up to 3,500 psi. Filled cylinders fall well within the safety margin provided.

A regulator must be used to reduce the

cylinder pressure to a level safe for patient use. Regulators are set to allow a minimum delivery pressure and an adjustable constant rate of flow. Also attached to the regulator is a pressure gauge which monitors the volume remaining in the cylinder. The pressure gauges are calibrated in psi, and may indicate safe ranges for full and refill pressures on the face. The flow meter is usually calibrated in 0.25 L increments and will allow a flow rate between 0.25 and 15 L/min.

Liquid Oxygen

Liquid oxygen systems represent a unique form of oxygen delivery. Because liquid oxygen is at a temperature of -183° C(-297° F), the home reservoir units resemble a sophisticated Thermos® bottle. A typical liquid oxygen container consists of an inner stainless steel reservoir tank that is wrapped in an insulating material, and suspended inside another stainless steel tank. The inner tank is cushioned at the bottom with insulation and is under a vacuum to insure temperature protection. At the top of the container is a heat exchange coil attached to an exit port. The coil is approximately 30 feet long and provides a region where the cold liquid warms, converting to gaseous oxygen for delivery to the patient. Contents are usually held at 20 to 25 psi. After passing through the heat exchange coil, the gas is released to the patient through a regulator set at 10 psi delivery pressure. As with gaseous oxygen, a flow meter is used to control delivery at rates between 0. 25 and 15 L/min.

Pressure relief and venting valves may be placed between the storage container and the heat exchanger, and also between the heat exchanger and the regulator. These valves are designed to open if pressures exceed 22 to 25 psi. The reservoir unit also contains an electronic or a float type contents gauge. The entire assembly is encased in a durable plastic/synthetic casing. Mobile bases are available for the reservoirs.

Portable reservoirs are available that allow patients to move from room to room or to travel outdoors. Portable liquid units are scaled down versions of the larger reservoir, and operate at lower pressure. The units may be refilled from the reservoir unit as needed. An average size portable unit (1.5 - 2 L of liquid oxygen) will provide 8 to 10 hours of continuous use at a gaseous oxygen flow rate of 2 L/min.

Liquid oxygen reservoirs must be kept in an upright position, since liquid oxygen, like any liquid, can be spilled from an upended container. Reasonable care must be exercised to avoid spilling the liquid on one's skin; the resulting burn can be severe.

Oxygen Concentrators

Oxygen concentrators provide a third means of oxygen delivery. In the past, the reliability and service reputation of concentrators limited their use for home oxygen patients. Their size and noisiness also detracted from their appeal. The advent of computerization, microcircuitry, and the use of plastics has revitalized the use of concentrators in many patient settings. Current models are light weight, compact, mobile, attractive, and quiet enough for home use.

Concentrators remove nitrogen from room air, leaving "purified" oxygen. Room air is forced into a sieve bed under pressure. The pressurized material has a high affinity for nitrogen which is trapped in the bed. The free oxygen is forced out of the sieve bed and into a holding tank. After the oxygen is removed, the sieve bed depressurizes, releasing the nitrogen into the room. Most concentrators contain two sieve beds which cycle back and forth trapping and releasing nitrogen.

To protect the valve systems and sieve beds from airborne matter, the room air is passed through several filters prior to entering the sieve bed. Both gross particulate matter and fine particulates are removed from ambient air. The sieve beds are sealed to prevent moisture from entering and inactivating the sieve material, and the filters help remove moisture from the air as well. The process of forcing air into the sieve beds creates heat which further helps dry the air. Oxygen which passes through the concentrator valves and tubing will be 2° to 5° warmer than room temperature. Because the oxygen has been dried by the filtering and extraction process, it usually passes through a bubble humidifier before it reaches the patient.

Output and efficiency of concentrators vary with manufacturers and specifications. There is an inverse relationship between flow rates and oxygen concentration. At high flow rates room air flows more rapidly through the sieve bed material and less nitrogen is removed. The majority of concentrators can deliver oxygen at flow rates between 0.5 and 6 L/min with corresponding purity levels of 80 to 98%.

Most concentrators can detect problems, illuminate an indicator, and sound an alarm. Typical alarm conditions include plugged filters or inadequate pressure in the system. Many units include self-diagnostic circuitry to further pinpoint problem areas. For serious problems, an automatic shut-off is activated to protect the machine from damage.

Typical power consumption ranges from 200 to 420 watts, depending on manufacturer. Noise levels range from 43 dBas to 53 dBas. Excess noise is the most common complaint of concentrator users. It may be wise to provide a noise and vibration absorbing pad to patients using these devices.

Maintenance of oxygen concentrators is easy, and should be performed routinely as outlined by the manufacturer to prevent serious malfunctions. Instruction manuals provide patients with basic maintenance and troubleshooting instructions to guide them in the use of the machine. Dealers will provide more extensive monthly maintenance and will assist and follow up on patient concerns. Oxygen purity levels should be checked at least once a month, and more frequently if required by the manufacturer. Active patient participation and instruction will help reduce anxiety, build patient confidence, and eliminate needless maintenance calls.

Oxygen Enrichers

Oxygen enrichers provide an alternative to concentrators for patients requiring high humidity but lower oxygen purity. They may be operated at higher flow rates, which is psychologically reassuring to some patients. Although they are as expensive as concentrators, they are quieter and use less power.

Oxygen enrichers force room air and water vapor first through a gross particle filter and then through a selectively permeable synthetic membrane. This membrane allows oxygen and water to pass through rapidly and completely, but inhibits the passing of nitrogen, particulates, and bacteria. This enriched, high humidity oxygen mixes with room air in the patient's nasal passages and is inhaled. Enrichers typically yield an oxygen purity of 40% to 60% or higher. Humidity or water saturation levels can be adjusted on some models. Some models allow simultaneous use of aerosol medications by simply changing a mouthpiece.

Enrichers also have alarm systems similar to those found on oxygen concentrators. Typical power consumption is 200 watts and the devices are relatively quiet (45 dBas). Maintenance is similar to that of oxygen concentrators.

Choice of Delivery System

Although there are clear differences in types of oxygen and delivery systems, and also in the medical conditions that may require oxygen use, selection of a delivery system for a particular patient may be primarily determined by nonmedical criteria. Some of these considerations are the patient's insurance coverage and financial status, physical condition, emotional state, lifestyle and physical environment, anticipated usage rate, and economic and operational considerations that impinge on the dealer.

Insurance Related Issues

Of the considerations listed above, the most influential factors are often insurance coverage and financial status. Many third party payers have explicit criteria that individual patients must meet to qualify for oxygen therapy. Insurers may view the provision of oxygen therapy as a product that requires little or no service, and incomplete coverage may result.

Medicare currently has the most stringent limitations on home oxygen services. To qualify, patients must demonstrate low blood oxygen levels and must also suffer from one of several specific medical conditions. Currently, a PaO_2 of 55 mmHg or less is considered a documented physiological need. An arterial saturation level of 88% or less would qualify. For patients with a PaO_2 of 56-59 or SaO_2 of 89%, with a diagnosis of congestive heart failure, or pulmonale, or polycythemia, Medicare has established additional requirements for reimbursement. The major requirement is that the patient must be retested and recertified between day 61 and 90 of home oxygen therapy. Documentation must be provided by an approved facility or practitioner as outlined in the Medicare oxygen guidelines. Only an approved laboratory, a physician, a respiratory therapist, or a trained employee of a physician can document this need by oximetry. A proper diagnosis must also be indicated (e.g., COPD, lung cancer, diffuse parenchymal disease, diffuse interstitial lung disease, CHF with evidence of edema, etc.). Documentation must be supported by appropriate records if requested, and some patients will be audited.

Physical Condition

The physical condition of the patient and caregiver can affect the type of oxygen delivery system selected. Arthritis, visual or hearing problems, and other physical infirmities must be considered when selecting a delivery system. A patient unable to turn a valve on a compressed gas cylinder may be quite adept at adjusting a liquid oxygen system, or at operating an oxygen concentrator.

Mental Status

The psychological makeup and mental acumen of patients may have a bearing on the type of system chosen. Many patients become psychologically attached to their oxygen, and develop dependent behavior. These patients are often anxious about their therapy, equipment and instructions, and may overuse oxygen. Flow restriction devices may be placed on their systems to assure proper therapy and compliance.

All patients should receive written and verbal instructions that they can understand. Patients who receive oxygen therapy are somewhat intimidated by the equipment, and are anxious about the conversion to the home setting. When patients are allowed to actively participate in their training and instruction, their anxiety may be reduced, which can result in fewer calls for the dealer. All patients should sign a form indicating that they understand them. A copy should be kept in the patient's file.

Patients also may feel stigmatized by being on oxygen therapy. They must make significant lifestyle changes, and the equipment may intimidate family and friends, and cause others to stare. Some patients end up in a self imposed exile, feel handicapped and embarrassed, are withdrawn, and are afraid to leave the "safety" of their homes. The equipment chosen for these patients should be as inconspicuous as possible to allow for as normal a lifestyle as possible.

Physical Environment

Many homes present unique mobility, health and fire hazards. Portable electric heaters, wood burning stoves, and overloaded electrical circuits are some of the problems that may be present. Patients who live considerable distances from the dealer, or who live in remote locations present challenges for dealers as well.

Patient Lifestyle

Patients who must exercise, or who are continuing to work will require portable delivery systems, and this may be best accomplished by a liquid oxygen system. Again, documentation by a physician may enable these patients to qualify for this type of delivery system. Patients with acute short term needs also require the use of systems that allow for mobility.

Anticipated Usage

The prescription provides a general guideline for anticipated use, and along with the patient prognosis, anticipated psychological need, and potential emergency use, should give the HHC pharmacist an estimate of daily consumption. Continuous use or "prn" use is not acceptable for reimbursement by the insurance company, nor should such instructions be accepted as adequate by the HHC pharmacist. New Medicare guidelines for the prescribing of oxygen indicate that an exact number of hours per day, or hours and times of day, be stated along with the flow rate on each prescription or certificate of need. The anticipated duration of therapy in months must also be specified to assure reimbursement. Specific usage guidelines for patients must be provided by the physician, and transmitted to the patient by the provider of oxygen services. The pharmacist must select a system that meets the patient's needs, the financial resources available, and his own ability to install and service the system.

Economic and Operational Considerations

A compressed gas system is the most costly system for the pharmacist to deliver and maintain. Compressed gas cylinders are heavy (large tanks can weigh 170 lbs), bulky, and require frequent replacement by delivery technicians. They are most appropriate for intermittent use at low flow rates for a few hours per day. Although they have the highest handling costs, they require the least investment. The large cylinders are usually rented from the oxygen wholesaler on a monthly basis (the demurrage charge is simply passed on to the consumer). Components owned by the pharmacist are a cylinder stand (or cart), cylinder wrench, and a regulator with contents gauge. These are also rented to the consumer. A humidifier may be rented to the patient, or like tubing and cannula, may be disposable and sold, as is the oxygen itself. Additional costs when more than one tank is used are cylinder stands for each additional tank, and a manifold or piggyback tubing (CGA approved) with "T" valve.

Gaseous oxygen is usually sold in multiples of 100 cubic feet. By providing multiple tanks at the house, less frequent deliveries are required. The amount of oxygen available to the patient is increased, and delivery costs are decreased with a minimal increase in capital investment. To accommodate such a system, more space is required in the patient's home. A typical liquid oxygen system includes a 30 L reservoir and stand, a 1.5 L portable reservoir and stroller cart, humidifier, tubing, and cannula or mask.

Liquid oxygen systems involve lower delivery expenses, and delivery can be accomplished in several ways. If a pharmacist has enough patients who require liquid oxygen, refills of the liquid system take place at the patient's home, using a specially outfitted vehicle with a reservoir sufficient for multiple refills. These vehicles are often modified to deliver compressed gas and other forms of home medical equipment (HME) as well. This approach reduces handling and trips to the warehouse, so drivers can be routed to make more stops per day providing an overall greater efficiency. If a pharmacist has few liquid oxygen patients, deliveries can be made on an exchange basis. When patients call for a refill, the dealer fills a reservoir at the warehouse, and exchanges a full system for an empty one. This requires additional liquid systems, enough to cover the possibility of many patients requiring a refill the same day, and results in increased handling costs as well.

Associated equipment costs for liquid systems are the highest of all oxygen systems. Vehicles used for delivering liquid oxygen may require significant modifications to meet the standards for handling hazardous materials. Home reservoir units (including a stand, a portable liquid unit and stroller type cart) can cost over $2,000, depending on size of the reservoir unit, size of the portable unit, and quantities ordered. Additional equipment includes a filling hose, pressure testing gauges, repair tools, venting wrenches, and selected spare parts. Traditionally, however, reimbursement rates for liquid oxygen and equipment have been sufficient to make liquid oxygen systems more profitable than other systems. Recent changes by Medicare and other private insurance carriers have severely reduced the reimbursement levels, and concurrent increases in cost and liability insurance have acted to dramatically erode this profit level.[11]

Aside from profitability considerations, liquid oxygen systems are preferred for patients who need high flow rates over long periods. They also are the preferred system for patients who need maximum mobility. Under changing insurance rules, documentation of these needs is essential.

A typical oxygen concentrator system consists of an oxygen concentrator, a humidifier, oxygen tubing, cannula, and a backup compressed gas system. Oxygen concentrators are the most cost effective means of delivering oxygen for patients who require continuous or near continuous use at low flow rates (0.5 L/min to 5 L/min). Dealer costs associated with this system are minimal because equipment costs are reasonable, and delivery with follow up maintenance consists of monthly visits on the average. The most frequently overlooked cost is the provision of a backup compressed gas system in case the concentrator fails, or in case there is a power outage. Additional costs include maintenance training for delivery technicians, replacement filters and miscellaneous parts, and the cost of an oxygen analyzer and repair kit.

Patient circumstances can often challenge a dealer's creativity in setting up home oxygen therapy. Severely ill patients, or those in unique geographical locations may require the unusual to assure proper oxygen therapy. It is not unheard of in black lung country to provide patients with a large number of compressed gas cylinders joined together by manifolds, or to provide multiple 200 L and 300 L liquid systems for patient's use at home. Unusual oxygen systems may require prior approval from third party payers to insure reimbursement. Whatever the situation, the dealer must be willing to coordinate all components associated with this type of therapy.

Emerging Trends

The use of oxygen in the home setting is well established and accepted by the medical community, the insurance industry, and other third party payers. Historically, coverage criteria for nonhospital oxygen therapy were loosely defined. To receive coverage, all that was needed was a prescription or certification by the physician that the patient required the use of oxygen in order to remain active and viable. Reimbursement limitations consisted of some kind of regional average of charges for similar equipment and services available to the patient. However, abuses of the system and rapidly rising charges for oxygen services have forced third party payers to reexamine coverages for HHC patients. The next few years will certainly test HHC pharmacists' abilities to adjust to a changing external environment, and their ability to work with referral sources.

Total Respiratory Support

Patients whose arterial partial oxygen pressures have not advanced beyond 50 mmHg and who are hypoxic with or without other complications (cardiac arrhythmias, hypotension and/ or pulmonary embolism) that may hasten respiratory failure, are candidates for total respiratory support.[1]

Total respiratory support consists of mechanical control of ventilation with the addition of supplemental oxygen through an endotracheal or tracheostomy tube. The devices used for total respiratory support are called respirators or ventilators. Patients requiring total respiratory support are severely ill, and require more intensive care than a normal home oxygen user. Extensive training of family members and caregivers is a necessity, and professional personnel who may assist in caring for the patient should be skilled in all facets of ventilator use and associated care.

A hospitalized ventilator patient may be discharged into a home setting if in fairly stable condition prior to leaving the hospital, and with a support system in place to assure a smooth transition into the home setting. Respiratory care dealers must work closely with supportive services and agencies, referring physicians, and the patient's family to assure that the support system is in place. Around-the-clock backup and emergency support must be available for these patients.[1]

Reimbursement for the use of ventilators in the home may be tied to supporting services (e.g., home health agencies), and may have to be billed through such an agency. Prior authorization for equipment, supplies, and services must usually be received before the start of home ventilator therapy. Often, national agencies will assist patients in paying for portions of care they must receive at home. Because of the nature of services provided to these critical care patients, liability insurance underwriters have been readjusting premiums to reflect the greater liabilities of respiratory care providers.

Equipment costs for total respiratory support patients are extremely high. Ventilator technology has changed dramatically over the past five years, and costs have kept pace with the changes. Supplies that patients require on a daily basis also add to the costs. The greatest single expenditure is for professional services. A detailed discussion of the variety of ventilator equipment available is beyond the scope of this chapter. The reader is advised to contact manufacturers or to visit a local hospital respiratory therapy department to obtain additional information.

Ventilators used in the home do not require the sophisticated monitoring and adjustments that hospital ventilators offer. All, however, should be easy to operate and service, have sufficient monitoring to provide for patient safety, provide humidification and a delivery method for pharmacologic agents, and should be easily transported. Some common features of ventilators suitable for home use include control of tidal volume, respiratory rate, inspiration/expiration ratio, inspiratory flow rate, and patient airway pressure. The device should detect and compensate for power fluctuations and low pressure. Additional features may include programming of periodic deep breaths (sighs), ability to deliver inspired oxygen at either constant or decelerating flow, adjustable pause between inspiration and expiration, monitoring of proximal airway or machine pressure, addition of positive end expiratory pressure (PEEP) and/or continuous positive airway pressure (CPAP), analysis of exhaled gas components, and calibrated oxygen enrichment, among many other.

It is important to remember that total respiratory support patients have a difficult time removing secretions and mucus from the lungs. Mechanical assistance in the form of a vacuum suction device is required to aid in fluid removal. There are many vacuum devices available, and proper suction catheters and connections must be provided.

THE RESPIRATORY CARE CENTER

A respiratory care center can be a stand alone operation, a subdivision of an existing pharmacy or HME business, or it can be a joint venture with referral sources, agencies, or hospitals. How one approaches this potential venture depends entirely on individual circumstances. It is especially important for the entrepreneur to make a comprehensive analysis of the situation to determine how it will be altered by the new venture. The entrepreneur must not underestimate the significant impact a new venture will have on preexisting professional and personal activities, e.g., family and lifestyle. It is important to examine all facets of the business before making a decision to enter or withdraw from a market. (See also Chapter 10.)

Preliminary Analysis of a New Business Venture

The preliminary analysis of a new business venture should examine several key areas, namely product/service mix, the market, business operations, financing, and risk. The pharmacist should prepare a written analysis, and may wish to obtain assistance from a management consultant in preparing the analysis. Pharmacy marketing and management texts cover this type of analysis in greater detail.[12,13]

Products and Services

Most home oxygen providers will stock the major types of delivery systems discussed earlier in the chapter, plus replacement parts and associated disposable supplies. They will also be prepared to repair the systems when field repair is possible. Only a few dealers are equipped to provide total respiratory support, which requires a significant capital investment, specialized knowledge, and for which market demand may be limited. Typical services offered by these firms are: free delivery, 24 hour emergency service, special weekend service, free patient guides and instructional materials, monthly or regularly scheduled visits by a respiratory nurse or respiratory therapist, automatic billing of third party payers, accept assignment on Medicare claims, automatic billing of secondary insurers, discounts on insurance copayments if made at time of service, free goods or convenience items at discounts, free setup and patient training, and inservice training to health care personnel and referral sources. Ancillary services such as those provided by a respiratory nurse or a respiratory therapist are generally not covered as separate expenses by third party payers. There may be instances where the same services are covered if the therapist or nurse is an employee of a home health agency. The home oxygen provider may be able to contract with a licensed home health agency for the services, allowing it to bill the third party payer, subject to possible local legal requirements and constraints.

A pharmacy that does not provide home oxygen therapy is nevertheless a natural source for disposable items needed by respiratory patients. An affiliation with an existing dealer who does not carry these items, or who is unwilling to provide a complete inventory could be beneficial to both parties.

Personnel and Operations

Typical personnel in a respiratory care center include a delivery technician, customer service representative, respiratory therapist, outside sales representative, and manager.

The delivery technician is the firm's direct representative in the patient's home, and must be knowledgeable about therapy and equipment, including setup, repair, maintenance, troubleshooting and safety. The delivery technician will participate in patient training and instructions. Because of the weight and bulk of the equipment, delivery technicians are usually males in excellent physical condition. He should have an unblemished driving record, be reliable, and willing to be on call for emergencies. The delivery technician must have a personality suitable for interaction with patients who have diminished physical abilities, debilitating illnesses, and limited education. He must be able to interface with grieving families and terminally ill patients. The ability to interact with clinical and home health personnel is essential. Other responsibilities include completing paperwork and verifying insurance information, maintenance of vehicles, repair and maintenance of equipment, and oxygen inventory control.

The customer service representative is an important key to the business and is often the person who gives referral sources and patients their first impression of the business. This position has many responsibilities and requires a person who is skilled in clerical work, insurance work, medical terminology, has knowledge of therapies and modalities of treatments, knows the equipment and can perform troubleshooting over the phone, can interact with clinicians and referral sources, and do light bookkeeping. The customer service representative will also handle patient complaints and problems and will work intimately with patients and their families or caregivers. Attention to detail is a must for this position which requires a great deal of tact and maturity.

A respiratory therapist or respiratory nurse lends credibility to the center in the eyes of referral sources. As a member of the HHC team, he/she visits patients on a scheduled basis and provides training, treatment evaluations and patient assessments. The respiratory nurse or therapist will monitor patient charts, instruct the patient and caregiver on how to assure good bronchial hygiene, and monitors the patient's progress via pulmonary functions tests and oximetry readings or blood gas studies. The respiratory nurse or therapist may also be actively involved in marketing activities, provides technical support, and assists in program development. In some cases this person may be "shared" with another agency. He must possess sound clinical skills, be professional in demeanor and dress, have good communication skills, and be able to interact with other clinicians and health care professionals.

Outside sales has long been overlooked as a marketing tool for pharmacy, but is an important component of the marketing effort of a respiratory care business. The sales representative must thoroughly understand the third party reimbursement system, the products and services available, business operations, disease states and treatment modalities, and be able to develop and implement marketing and sales strategies. A past history of working within the medical field is helpful. Since the primary method of promoting a home oxygen and respiratory care business is by direct selling, advertising and promoting, the importance of the sales representative should not be underestimated.

Although a respiratory care center may operate from an existing pharmacy or HHC pharmacy, a store front is not essential. The major physical requirements are an office, a workshop or repair area, storage facilities, and delivery equipment.

Open storage areas, such as fenced areas covered with gravel or concrete, may be as satisfactory as an enclosed warehouse. The Compressed Gas Association of America, local fire department, and oxygen wholesaler provide guidelines for storing compressed gases and liquid oxygen. Space needed to store compressed gas cylinders and liquid reservoirs varies depending upon frequency of delivery from the wholesaler, expected growth of the business, type of system and equipment mix required, and state and local storage regulations. As few as 200 square feet may be adequate. Additional space is required if delivery vehicles are stored in the same facility.

A step van with a heavy duty suspension, transmission cooler, heavy duty automatic transmission, power steering and brakes, tandem wheels, and power liftgate will provide an all-purpose delivery vehicle. Existing vehicles can also be modified to meet requirements for transporting compressed gas as well as liquid oxygen. Although it may vary considerably, total capital investment in a respiratory care business that provides a full range of services can be between $150,000 and $200,000.

Suppliers

Price, service, and support must all be considered when selecting an oxygen wholesaler. Prices for medical gases and cylinder rentals are not standardized throughout the industry, and depend greatly on a dealer's ability to negotiate. It is important to select a supplier who can meet expected needs, and provide support and training for personnel. Medical gasses represent a minor portion of the business for the majority of wholesalers, and they may not be able to support a respiratory care center with the training and services required. Equipment manufacturers can often direct a dealer to a reputable and competitive wholesaler.

Promotion

The respiratory care center is similar to other HHC pharmacies in the importance of professional referrals as a source of patronage. A survey of HHC pharmacies revealed that 70% of HHC patients are referred by health professionals, 22% are attracted by advertising, and 8% are referred by other patients.[14] The percentage of a respiratory care center's business generated by health professionals is likely to be even higher.

The primary marketing approach to professional referral sources is direct selling, which is the role of the outside sales representative. In order of importance, the representative will regularly call on hospital discharge planners, home health agencies, hospital respiratory therapy departments, visiting nurse services, and physicians. (Dentist and veterinarians will also be contacted, not as referral sources but as potential consumers of medical gases.) Sources with whom the dealer has a well established relationship may be contacted as often as weekly, and less prominent referral sources will be seen every four to eight weeks. In addition to the sales call, the pharmacist and respiratory nurse or therapist should maintain regular contact with referral sources for all active patients, including appropriate written follow up.

Promotion to consumers may include advertising in local newspapers, on radio, and in telephone advertising directories. Advertising generates 22% of the patients for HHC centers and over half of advertising referrals are generated by the directories. It is important to engender the good will of existing patients, who account for nearly one-third of all direct referrals and 8% of all new patients.[14]

Other avenues for promotion to consumers include articles or columns in newspapers, providing speakers for schools, civic clubs, and senior citizen organizations, sponsoring community health fairs, direct mail newsletters, and high visibility in the affairs of the local community. This last possibility is particularly important for small businesses: in the mind of the consumer, the owner's image is often synonymous with that of the firm.

In addition to a variety of brochures and aids from equipment manufacturers, more generalized references on promotion of home care business by pharmacists are two manuals prepared by Johnson & Johnson in cooperation with the National Association of Retail Druggists, Home Health Care Marketing, A Manual for Retail Pharmacies,[14] and Selling Skills: Home Health Care Marketing.[15]

CONCLUSION

This chapter has focused on the care of the respiratory patient in the home. The pharmacist dealing with patients who may have compromised respiratory function may not always be the supplier of home respiratory services, but should be aware of the nature of respiratory care. Many patients who obtain routine medications from one pharmacy will receive bronchodilators, liquefying agents, and medical oxygen from other sources. Ancillary products and supplies required by respiratory patients fit well in a pharmacy, and the pharmacist with a special interest in HHC is a likely source of information for the respiratory patient.

Some pharmacists may be sufficiently intrigued by the challenges of home respiratory care that they devote all or a major portion of their practice to it. These individuals must become thoroughly knowledgeable regarding reimbursement systems, legal guidelines, the nature of the market and competition, referral sources, and modes of therapy and the equipment needed to provide them.

REFERENCES

1. Weiner MP. Current Issues in Respiratory Therapy Home Care. Home Health Care Prac. 1989; 1:61.
2. Anon. Primer on In-Home Oxygen Therapy. HHC Pharm. June 1993; 6:3.
3. Petty TL. Intensive and Rehabilitative Respiratory Care, 3rd edition. Philadelphia Lea & Febiger. 1982.
4. Frost and Sullivan. Home Health Care Services and Products Markets. New York, Frost and Sullivan, Inc., 1983.
5. Petty TL. Ambulatory Oxygen. New York, Theime-Stratton, Inc., 1983.
6. Herfindal ET, et al. Eds. Clinical Pharmacy and Therapeutics, 5th edition. Baltimore, Williams & Wilkins. 1992.
7. Baum GL. Ed. Textbook of Pulmonary Diseases, 3rd ed. Boston, Little, Brown and Company. 1989.
8. Sherman M. Negative ion generators. U.S. Pharm. 1983; 6:57.
9. Anon. A test of small air cleaners. Rodale's New Shelter. 1982; 7:48.
10. Self TH and Fuentes RJ. Metered dose inhalers and extender devices. U.S. Pharm. 1985; 5:36.
11. Brown K. Home oxygen market; Changing with the tide. Homecare/Rehab. 1985; 10:35.
12. Smith HA. Principles and Methods of Pharmacy Management, 2nd ed. Philadelphia, Lea & Febiger. 1980.
13. Smith MC. Principles of Pharmaceutical Marketing, 3rd ed. Philadelphia, Lea & Febiger. 1983.
14. Anon. Home Health Care Marketing, A Manual for Retain Pharmacists. New Brunswick N.J. Johnson & Johnson Products, Inc., 1983.
15. Anon. Selling Skills: Home Health Care Marketing. New Brunswick, N. J. Johnson & Johnson Products, Inc., 1984.

16 The Ostomy Patient

Michael L. Kleinberg, M.S., FASHP

Ostomy, which literally means a surgically created opening, is the common term used when referring to a stoma from the gastrointestinal, or genitourinary tracts - such as a colostomy, ileostomy, or urostomy. Persons who have an ostomy are sometimes referred to, and refer to themselves, as "ostomates." The United Ostomy Association estimates that there are one million ostomates in North America.[1]

Some patients accept an abdominal stoma more easily than others. Some will view an ostomy as a relief; others will see it as a punishment or mutilation and may never be able to experience an acceptable quality of life.[2] Standard preoperative and postoperative protocols for other types of surgery do not provide sufficient psychological and technical support for persons who must sacrifice urinary or rectal continence and master mechanical methods of bladder or bowel control. Because of this, the United Ostomy Association has delineated a "Bill of Rights" specific to ostomates' unique requirements. An ostomate should have the right to preoperative counseling, an appropriately positioned stoma site, a well-constructed stoma, skilled postoperative nursing care, emotional support, individual instruction and information on the availability of supplies, information on community resources, post-hospital follow-up and life long supervision, benefit from the team efforts of health care professionals, and information and counsel from the ostomy association and its members.

When teaching, counseling, and discharge planning are tailored to the patient and initiated prior to surgery, the rehabilitative process for people with ostomies is more efficient. By the time patients are discharged from the hospital, they should have learned what type of ostomy they have, how to recognize stomal dysfunction, and how to care for themselves. They should know where to purchase supplies and how to pay for them if they do not have adequate insurance. Finally, they must know with whom to consult concerning general health problems as well as specific ostomy-related conditions. Written instructions should accompany patients when they are discharged from the hospital (see Appendix 16-A). It is not unusual for a patient with a new ostomy to leave the hospital without learning all of the details of ostomy care. Psychological recovery will be compromised and medical and surgical complications may be increased unless teaching is continued in the home by a home health nurse, a home health care (HHC) pharmacist, a surgical supplier, or a volunteer from the local Ostomy Association. It is important that the HHC members of the rehabilitation team have a clear understanding of ostomy function as well as the social and psychological hurdles that can be expected during the rehabilitative process. This chapter will focus on the special care of each of the most commonly performed ostomy operations to help pharmacists who provide ostomy supplies and services to assume their important role on the rehabilitation team.

COLOSTOMY

Colostomies are performed across the life span for varied reasons. During infancy and childhood, neonatal necrotizing enterocolitis (NEC), imperforate anus, Hirschsprung's Disease (congenital megacolon), and Crohn's Disease may require a temporary or permanent colostomy. Diverticulitis is a common affliction of middle-aged persons in Western society and may require a diverting colostomy. Finally, among mature and elderly adults, colorectal cancer is a frequent indication for a temporary colostomy proximal to a resection or for a permanent colostomy when proctocolectomy is necessary. The overall incidence of colorectal cancer in the United States is estimated to be more than 100,000 cases.[3] Obstruction, trauma, and fistulae are other antecedents of colostomy that may occur at any age.

The portion of the colon from which the stoma is raised dictates the type of care the colostomy will need (see Figure 16-1). An ascending colostomy, on the patient's right side, will discharge continuous semi-liquid to semi-solid stools, depending on a person's diet. The effluent will contain digestive enzymes that will quickly denude peristomal skin if the stool comes in contact with it. Patients with an ascending colostomy must use an odor-proof, drainable pouch with a skin barrier. (It should be noted that "appliance" and "pouch" are preferred terms, "bag" suggest a large, conspicuous receptacle.)

A transverse colostomy may be located anywhere in the transverse colon. The amount of large bowel proximal to the stoma will be a key determinant of the consistency of the feces and the frequency of movements. Stool from a transverse colostomy is highly caustic to the skin. A skin barrier and drainable, odor-proof pouch are required. Malodorous stool may be a problem, and patients may feel more secure if they are given deodorants to take orally or drops or powder to place in the pouch after each emptying.

The most common types of transverse colostomies are the loop and double-barrel (see

Figure 16-1 Classification of Colostomies

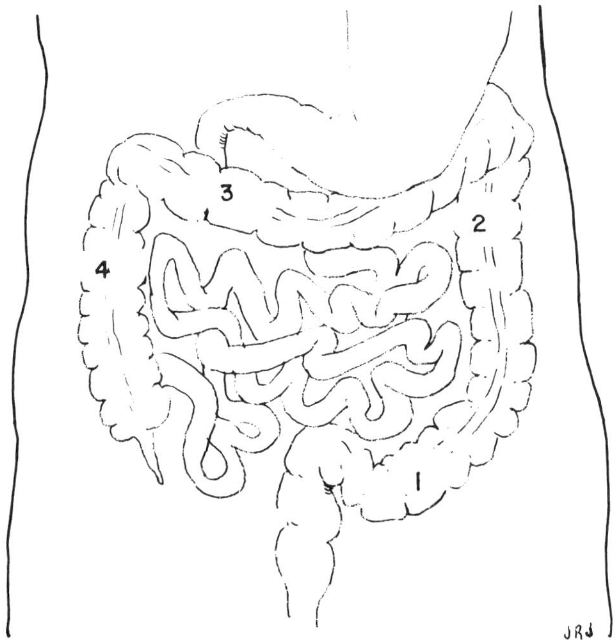

	STOMA	COLON REMOVED OR BYPASSED	TYPE OF EFFLUENT
1.	Sigmoid colostomy	Part of sigmoid colon and whole of rectum	Firm, solid stool
2.	Descending colostomy	Descending colon below splenic flexture and whole of rectum	Formed stool
3.	Transverse colostomy (double-barrel or transverse)	Colon distal to the stoma(s) and rectum	Varying from semi-liquid to toothpaste consistency
4.	Ascending colostomy	All remaining colon and rectum	Semi-liquid

Figure 16-2). Depending upon the nature of the patient's disease, the colostomy will be left in place from six weeks to six months. Loop and double-barrel colostomies are closed when the purpose for which they were created has been accomplished. This closure requires another operation, general anesthesia, and a hospitalization of approximately seven to nine days. It is helpful to call a transverse colostomy a "resting colostomy" rather than a "temporary colostomy." What is temporary to a health professional may be "long-term" to a patient. It is not unusual for patients who are told they have a temporary colostomy to resist learning to care for it and to simply stay at home until it is time to return to the hospital for closure. This is particularly disastrous when it is found that the colostomy cannot be reversed. The goal in all ostomy care is for the patient or family member to become proficient in ostomy management and for the patient to incorporate this body modification into his/her psyche.

Descending and sigmoid colostomies are brought to the abdomen in the lower left quadrant. Stool is generally formed and motions will occur once or twice daily, less often if the patient has a history of constipation. Many patients regulate bowel movements by irrigating daily or several times a week. Between irrigations they wear a small security pouch in case of spillage or to filter flatus and collect mucus that is passed from the exposed intestine. Some patients take pride in not wearing a pouch, covering their stoma with tape and a gauze square between irrigations.

In the immediate post-operative period, the colostomy effluent will be liquid. The stool will not thicken until the patient resumes a normal diet and increased activity. For this reason, it is important that a drainable pouch be used to avoid repeated removal and application of adhesives. Drainable pouch also permit easy measurement of its contents. It is important, too, that the pouch film be transparent to allow frequent assessment of the stoma and effluent.

Several companies manufacture a two-piece appliance, with a flange embedded in a skin barrier and a pouch that snaps on and off the flange like a plastic container lid (see Figure 16-3). In the early postoperative period, it is important to use a model with an accordion flange or free-floating flange which permits a caregiver to attach the flange to the pouch between the fingers, without exerting pressure against a patient's tender abdomen. If this type of two-piece system is not available, then it is important that a two-piece system be snapped together before putting it on the abdomen to minimize the patient's discomfort.

The frequent passage of flatus in the early post-operative period is distressing to patients who are already anxious about their altered anatomy. A hole should never be made in the top of the colostomy pouch to allow the gas to escape. This practice negates the benefits of the odor-barrier films used in most appliances. Pouches should be opened from the bottom to release gas and then immediately resealed. If the patient is able, the best place to perform this procedure is in the bathroom. Otherwise a deodorant should be used in the room. Some pouches have a flatus filter as an integral component. Patients should be assured that flatulence that is present in the early postoperative period will decrease with time. Most manufacturers of ostomy products sell deodorizers. Oral charcoal and chlorophyll tablets are frequently prescribed. Some veteran ostomates recommend bismuth subgallate or bismuth subcarbonate. Patients should be alerted that these medications may make their stool very dark and may also be constipating. Numerous drops and powders are available to be placed into the pouch after emptying. (The deodorizer should not have a

Figure 16-2 Loop and Double Barrel Colostomies

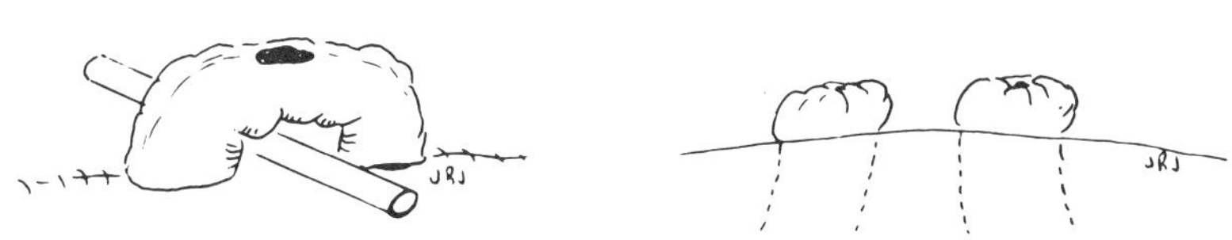

Loop Colostomy **Double-barrel Colostomy**

Figure 16-3 Applying Ostomy Appliances

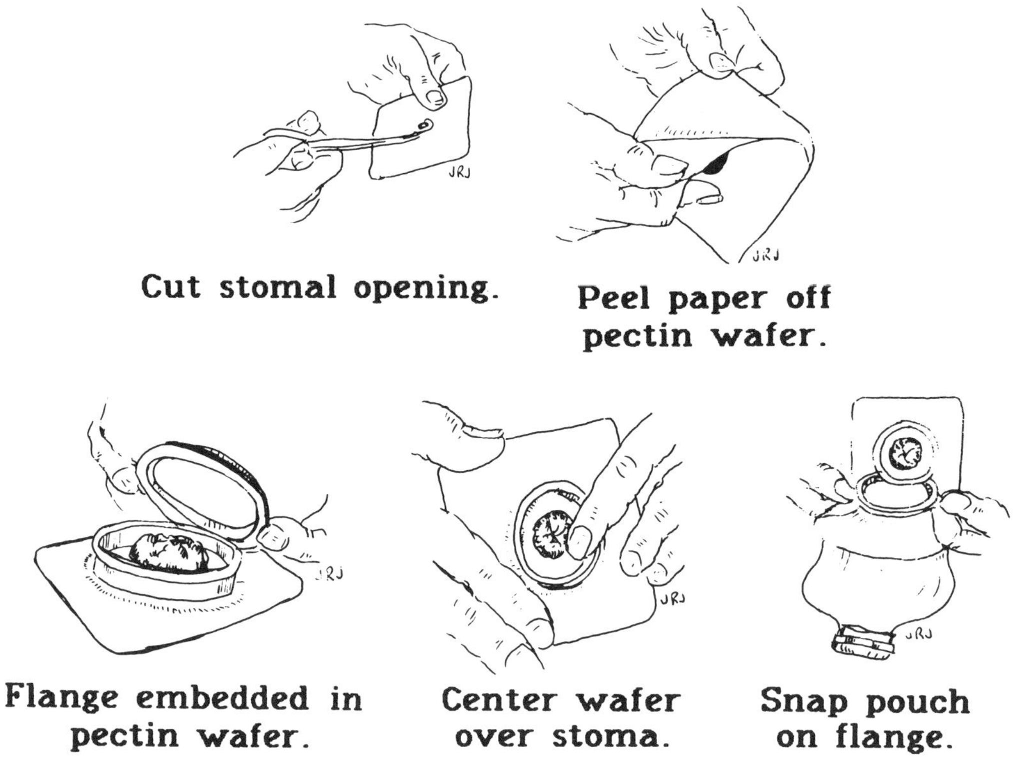

pungent odor of its own.) The old remedy of putting an aspirin tablet in the pouch is ill-advised and should not be recommended. The aspirin may irritate the stomal mucosa and does not affect odor unless it is in contact with feces.

People with colostomies require lifelong follow-up by a surgeon. When colostomates move, they should be encouraged to find a surgeon in their new locale. Whether the colostomy was performed for malignant or benign disease, it is important that patients have annual stomal examinations. If a patient is reluctant to see a new surgeon, an esterostomal therapist (ET) referral would assure knowledgeable follow-up and a link to surgical advice. During the extended postoperative period, common complications associated with colostomy are prolapse, retraction, stenosis and hernia. The occurrence of hernia is reported as high as 33% by the sixth postoperative year; the final incidence may be as high as 50%.[4] If patients complain of bulging around the stoma, they should be referred to their surgeon. Several companies make wide elastic belts with a Velcro closure that provide support. Surgical correction is a last resort. The patient should be advised that post-surgical shrinkage of the stoma will occur and to avoid overstocking with a size that will soon be too large for the stoma.

Skin Care

Peristomal skin damage is a constant threat. The most common cause of peristomal irritation is ill-fitting appliances which leave the area around the stomas exposed to intestinal exudates. Other sources of inflammation and abrasion are mechanical or chemical irritation, allergic reaction, and fungal and bacterial infections. Mechanical irritation is often caused by repeated removal of the epidermis when an adhesive appliance is carelessly stripped off. Chemical irritation may result from using harsh solvents or improper techniques when applying cement or skin protectives. Allergic reactions are not as common as may be imagined, but patients may be allergic to any component of the appliance system - skin barrier, adhesive, or the pouch film itself.

Fungal and bacterial infections are fairly common around stomas. Some patients will suffer in silence with painful, inflamed peristomal skin and accept it as an inevitable burden associated with the "curse of the colostomy." These infections may be treated effectively with topical antifungal and antibacterial agents, respectively. Inflammation secondary to abrasion or contact dermatitis may be relieved by the application of anti-inflammatory products such as Stomacort®. When rubbed in thoroughly, these products allow the application of the pouch without interfering with adherence. In some patients pectin-based barriers will relieve discomfort and restore the integrity of the skin within five to seven days.

Shaving the hair in the peristomal area may contribute to folliculitis, which is exacerbated by appliance removal. It is always recommended that hair be cut with scissors, rather than shaved.

When patients require radiotherapy after colostomy, the surgeon, radiologist and ET should collaborate on a plan to minimize skin problems and gastrointestinal dysfunction and to maximize patient comfort. When the stoma and appliance are within the radiation field, it is important that the collecting device be as thin as possible and that a non-metallic adhesive be used.[5] Sometimes patients must change the type of appliance they are wearing. When this is required, the patient must be given sufficient instruction and time to perfect the new procedure. In some instances, patients are required to remove their pouch during the radiation treatment. It is important that provisions be made in case the colostomy functions during treatment.

Normal age-related changes may cause skin problems in patients who have managed their ostomy successfully for years. Dryness, thinning and wrinkling in their peristomal area may be indications for a new type of skin barrier or adhesive.

Protection of peristomal skin has been enhanced by the development of two types of skin barriers: co-polymer films and solid-form barriers of inert synthetics or karaya amalgams. Synthetic skin barriers have greatly reduced the incidence of painful and costly ostomy-related skin damage. Criteria in the selection of the most appropriate barrier are the type and quantity of effluent; the condition and topography of the skin to be covered; the pouching system that will be used; and the patient's activity, environment, and financial resources.[6] For example, karaya-based and pectin-based wafers melt more rapidly in hot climates. Both are water soluble and require more frequent changing when wearers are engaged in strenuous physical activity that causes heavy perspiration or when they are avid swimmers. Ostomates with the financial resources to change their pouch daily may not use ostomy pastes, but may use skin sealants to protect their skin from damage due to frequent removal and reapplication of adhesives. On the other hand, patients who wear a flange and pouch for five to seven days will probably need products that are more resistant to heat and drainage than a karaya wafer.

Colostomy Irrigation

A colostomy may be irrigated to cleanse the bowel before or after certain diagnostic and surgical procedures. Irrigation, as a means of regulating bowel movements after a colostomy, is a common practice in the United States because the unpredictable elimination of feces from an abdominal stoma is among the most disturbing sequelae of a colostomy. An enema every other day or every third day assures most persons with descending and sigmoid colostomies that they will not have stools between irrigations.

The irrigation procedure requires the slow installation of about one quart of warm tap water to distend the large bowel sufficiently to trigger a massive peristaltic reflex. This ensures that the entire colon forward of the ileocecal valve will empty. Too little fluid, instilled under too high a pressure, will generate activity in the lower half or third of the remaining colon, and the patient will be frustrated by bowel movements between irrigations. Until recently, patients were taught how to irrigate prior to discharge from the hospital. The process of introducing the water and evacuating the colon requires 45 minutes to an hour. This is an exhausting procedure for newly operated patients. In most centers, irrigation now is taught on an outpatient basis in the sixth to eighth postoperative week.

Irrigation is explained as one management alternative for colostomates. It is stressed that this is not a medical necessity but a means of regulating bowel action and eliminating the need for an abdominal appliance. It is important, too, that colostomates understand that they may elect to irrigate for a brief or extended period of time and return to spontaneous evacuations when the practice becomes tiresome or too time-consuming. Older colostomates may find that they are troubled with constipation as colonic peristalsis slows and mucus secretions diminish. They may require stool softeners, bulking agents, or laxatives to stimulate bowel movement, with or without irrigation. People who were laxative-dependent before a descending or sigmoid colostomy will be laxative-dependent after surgery.

Colostomy irrigation is not suitable for many patients. Care should be taken to identify physical conditions that are contraindications to irrigation. (See Table 16-1). It is interesting to note that colostomy irrigation, which was rarely practiced in many foreign countries, has become much more popular outside the United States in the past decade. Conversely, American attitudes have relaxed and irrigation is considered an alternative rather than a mandate. A prospective study of 30 patients compared postoperative management techniques.[7] Of the 22 who agreed to irrigate, 70% chose to continue the practice, but 30% elected to return to spontaneous bowel movements, reserving irrigation for times when they wanted assurance they would be free of stool.

Diet And The Colostomy

Dietary modifications merit only brief mention. There is no diet specific to colostomies. Some people find hard-to-digest food such as corn, nuts and popcorn difficult to pass. Pre-surgical food intolerances will, of course, remain and may be cause for increased attention in the absence of an anal sphincter. Foods that cause gas may be avoided by colostomates or reserved for times when interaction with other people will be minimal. An example of a general food reference list is shown in Table 16-2.

ILEOSTOMY

An ileostomy may be performed anytime - in infancy, early adulthood, and frequently in the fifth and sixth decade of life. In infancy, neonatal necrotizing enterocolitis, meconium ileus, and cloacal exstrophy are relatively rare conditions but ones that may require exteriorization of the small bowel.

Ileostomy is often necessary during the most vital and productive years of life, when patients suffer intractable inflammatory bowel disease (IBD). IBD afflicts an estimated million Americans and the incidence is increasing.[8] The term "inflammatory bowel disease" is used to designate two diseases: ulcerative colitis and Crohn's disease. In the acute stage and in chronic, unremitting cases, symptoms are physically and psychologically debilitating. Surgery is recommended for inflammatory bowel disease when patients become disabled by their symptoms. Other indications for surgery are stunted growth, complications associated with long-term corticosteroid therapy, and the risk of neoplasm.

Ileostomy may be necessary for a patient who is asymptomatic, which complicates rehabilitation. A very ill patient may rationalize that an ileostomy is a small price to pay for restoration of good health; but it is difficult for well and active teenagers and young adults with inherited familial polyposis to be anything but resentful, and disbelieving that they are suffering from a lethal disease. Gardner's syndrome, a variant of familial polyposis manifested as multiple adenomatous polyps in the colon, would be another indication for ileostomy surgery.[9]

When ileostomies were first performed, two factors interfered with the success of the operation. Morbidity and mortality were high as a result of ileostomy dysfunction. This problem was solved by Brooke in the development of the everted Brooke ileostomy stoma.[10] The other impediment to acceptance and rehabilitation was the lack of adherent collecting devices for the continuous semi-solid small bowel effluent. Some of the dressing techniques described by early patients were ingenious, albeit miserable. Appliance components included food cans, coconut shells, balloons, and surgical gloves.

Since the water-absorptive surface of the

Table 16-1 Contraindications to Colostomy Irrigation

Active inflammatory disease	Impaired eyesight, palsy, painful arthritis, and other disabling problems
Postradiation colitis	Mental limitations
History of irritable bowel syndrome	Inadequate bathroom facilities
Residual or recurrent neoplasm	Lack of interest in a time-consuming ritual
Cardiac or renal disease that could be complicated by fluid overload	

TABLE 16-2 Effect of Food on the Colostomy

Gas Producing Foods	Cabbage, Beans, Turnips, Onions, Cucumbers, Radishes, Milk, Carbonated Beverages, Chewing gum, Nuts, Beer/alcoholic beverages
Odor Producing Foods	Fish, Onions, Peanut butter, Strong cheese, Cabbage, Eggs, Garlic, Baked beans, Asparagus, Cod liver oil, Some multi-vit Preparations
Colon Irritant Foods (Increased stools)	Raw vegetables, Green leafy veg, Spices, Beer/alcoholic beverages, Milk, Prunes, Fresh fruit, Raisins, Whole grain wheat, Bran cereals
Foods That Could Obstruct the Stoma (eat with caution)	Nuts, Seeds, Popcorn, Corn, Coconuts, Fibrous foods, Lobster, Shrimp, Crab
Foods Causing Change in Color	Strawberries, Beets, Red Jello, Iron pills, Licorice, Red coloring in baking,
Foods That Control Diarrhea	Bananas, Boiled rice, Peanut butter, Boiled milk, Applesauce, Tapioca,
Foods That Help Eliminate Constipation	Increase fluid intake, Fresh fruit, Cooked fruit, Cooked vegetables, Coffee,
Bulk Forming Foods	Bran, Corn, Lettuce, Noodles, Raw vegetables, Raw fruit, Whole wheat bread,
Foods That Control Odor	Tomato juice, Orange juice, Cranberry juice, Parsley, Yogurt, Buttermilk

large bowel has been removed or bypassed, a drainable appliance must be worn at all times. Excretion from an ileostomy cannot be regulated as can that from a descending or sigmoid colostomy. Generally, the stoma is most active 20 to 30 minutes after a meal and least active an hour or two before eating. Ileostomy output is related to body weight. A 70 kg man will excrete 500 ml to 600 ml per day, and a greater output than that should be regarded as abnormal. Ileostomates generally empty their appliance in the morning when they get up an hour or so after eating, and just before going to bed at night. The essential requirements of a postoperative collection device are a bottom drain that can be opened and resealed, a protective skin barrier, and an odor-barrier film. With current skin barriers, it is possible to protect peristomal skin from the very first post-operative day. The most widely used skin barriers are combinations of gelatin, pectin, and sodium carboxymethylcellulose (e.g., Stomahesive®, HolliHesive®). Karaya-based wafers and other synthetic amalgams are also use. Solid-form barriers have generally replaced the zinc-oxide and latex adhesives, thus eliminating the need for harsh solvents to remove these glues from the skin.

Diet For Ileostomates

It is important to teach patients which food will come through the ileostomy in nearly the same form as when they were eaten, and they should not be alarmed when hard-to-digest foods such as corn and tomato skins appear in the pouch. Patients are instructed to chew food well, but there is no specific diet for people with an ileostomy. Food such as peanuts, popcorn, mushrooms and vegetables may become impacted in the ileostomy, just below skin level. This obstruction may be relieved spontaneously or may require gentle lavage. Lavage should only be done by someone experienced in this procedure. Ileostomies are never irrigated.

People with an ileostomy easily develop electrolyte imbalance when they have diarrhea and during hot weather and strenuous athletic activities that cause profuse sweating. Sodium, potassium, and magnesium supplements may be required, and beverages containing such supplements are available and are helpful to ileostomates. The incidence of gall stones may be higher in patients with ileostomies and is related to the amount of ileum lost.[11] People with an ileostomy also have an increased risk of forming calcium and uric acid stones. Copious fluid intake is considered a key in the prophylaxis of nephrolithiasis. Excess water will be excreted as urine and will not increase ileostomy output. Conversely, ileostomy drainage cannot be manipulated by diet alone, other than by a salt-free diet.[12] Diphenoxylate hydrochloride, loperamide hydrochloride, and codeine phosphate reduce the output; psyllium seed thickens the effluent but increases volume.[13]

Ileostomy Appliances

An appliance to be worn home and whose use is to be continued into the extended postoperative period usually is selected for the patient on the fifth to seventh day after surgery. By this time, the patient is beginning to eat and is recovered enough to attend to instruction and participate in the procedure. It is important to include a family member or other caregiver in the teaching because patients may not be well enough to care for themselves during the first week or two after discharge.

Appliances are available in a variety of styles. Completely disposable styles are worn for three to seven days, then removed and discarded. Other appliances have components that are disposable and parts that are reusable. One or two piece vinyl or rubber appliances may be used for up to six months. When reusable equipment is selected, it is important that the patient have two sets so that one can be cleaned and dried thoroughly while the other is in place. The step-by-step application of a typical appliance is illustrated in Figure 16-3. Many patients wear a cover over the pouch. This helps prevent perspiration and helps some people feel better about the presence of a pouch on their abdomen.

In the early post operative period, patients will not know the type of equipment that is best for them, nor will they have a grasp of the vocabulary and jargon of ostomy care. Members of the United Ostomy Association report that they have received more information from ostomy products suppliers than from anyone else. For this reason, it is crucial that pharmacists who provide ostomy supplies be knowledgeable about the products they sell, their advantages and their limitations. Most manufacturers have training courses to educate their ostomy product suppliers. The International Association for Enterostomal Therapy (IAET) has an annual educational meeting and each region also offers educational meetings, all of which are open to those interested in ostomy care. The IAET has an associate member category which enables pharmacists to join the association and benefit from regional and national activities and publications including the Journal of Enterostomal Therapy.

Unless suppliers are "full-service dealers," they will not have every accessary and product line available to suite the needs of each patient. They should be prepared to refer patients back to an ET, physician, or even to another supplier when product and ostomy management problems persist. Some management problems are the tip off to ileostomy complications that require surgical intervention. The most common complications after ileostomy are prolapse, retraction, stomal stenosis, parastomal hernia, and skin damage.

There are newer operations being performed in the United States and abroad that eliminate the need for an abdominal pouch. These procedures include continentileostomy, popularized by Nils Kock of Sweden, and various ileoanal reservoirs that enable patients to defecate from the rectum (see Figure 16-4). The continent ileostomy is created out of the patient's small bowel that is made into an internal reservoir with a nipple valve that enables the patient to be continent of flatus and stool. It requires periodic intubation of the abdominal stoma to evacuate the pouch. Ileoanal reservoirs result in stooling from six to 12 times per day. Only patients themselves can judge how many stools are "too many" but few would prefer 12 to 15 urgent, loose bowel movements to a well-constructed and well-

FIGURE 16-4 Alternatives to Conventional Ileostomies

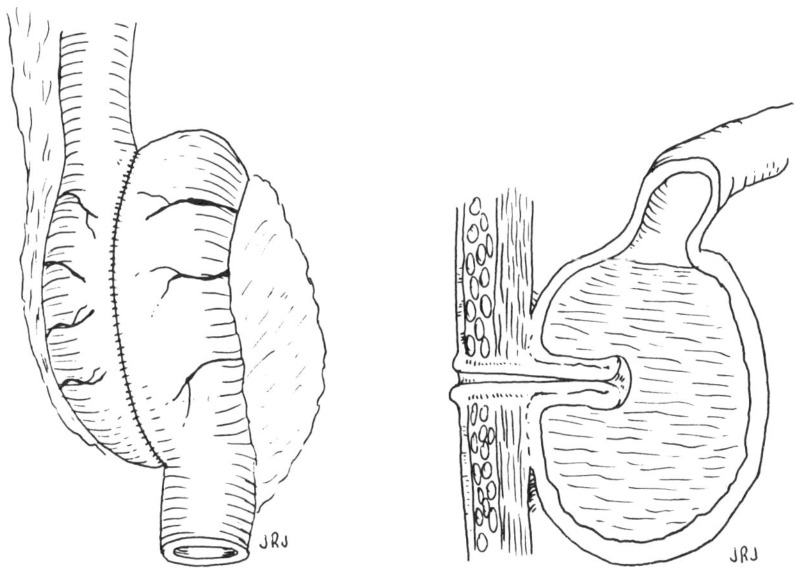

Ileoanal reservoir | Continent ileostomy

managed conventional ileostomy.

The search continues for the cause and cure of inflammatory bowel disease and for the most normal means of diverting feces when the colon must be removed or bypassed. In the meantime, optimal recovery is achieved in the majority of patients and can be attributed to the continuing development of excellent pouching systems and the care and teaching by knowledgeable health care providers and other caregivers.

UROSTOMY

Urostomies are performed in every age group.[1] Congenital and acquired conditions may necessitate temporary or permanent urinary diversion in infancy and early childhood. Bladder exstrophy, neurogenic bladder secondary to myelodysplasia, prune belly, and cloacal exstrophy are all conditions that may necessitate an abdominal urinary stoma for a short or extended period of time. Pelvic and gynecological cancer are the primary reasons for urinary diversion among adults. Trauma to the pelvis or upper urinary tracts, spinal cord injury, neurological disease such as multiple sclerosis, and intolerable urinary incontinence may necessitate a urostomy of one type or another as a temporary or permanent measure. The various types of supravesical diversions are illustrated in Figure 16-5. Urinary diversion with ileal and colon conduits once held great promise. The long-term results however, have been disappointing.[13] The high incidence of reflux, pyelonephritis, and renal deterioration have caused urologists to virtually abandon this operation for young patients with benign disease. It is unlikely that either ileal or colon conduits will provide a satisfactory drainage system for a normal lifetime. However, for adults the ileal conduit is an accepted means of managing urine when a cancerous bladder must be removed. And there is growing interest in a continent urostomy described by Kock and Skinner.[14,15]

Once a satisfactory stoma has been constructed, the appliance becomes the most important determinant of quality of life. Since urinary tract infection is a potential problem, it is preferable to choose a single-use pouch, that is, one that is worn for five to seven days, removed and discarded. The alternative is a reusable pouch that can be removed easily for daily washing, with a clean pouch to replace it. Patients should change their urostomy pouches on a set schedule to reduce the risk of leakage and embarrassing accidents. Patients should be seen four to five times in the first year after their urostomy operation. After that it is important that annual or semi-annual urine cultures be obtained. In addition, many urologists recommend an annual intravenous pyelogram. Urine specimens must never be collected from the urinary appliance. Sterile

FIGURE 16-5 Types of Urostomies

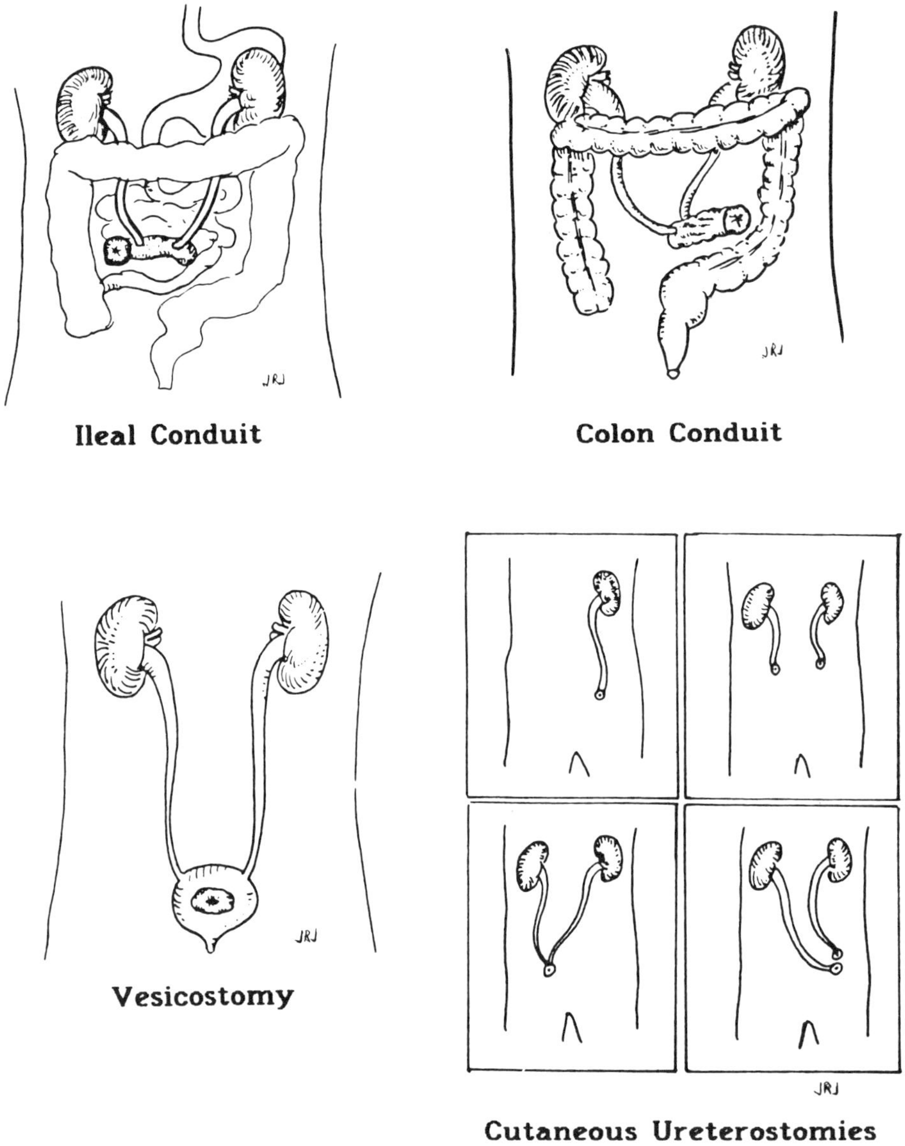

technique should be used after the stoma and peristomal area have been prepared in the usual manner for a urine culture. Many people do not realize that sterile urine can be maintained in patients without a history of pyelonephritis.[16]

Urinary stomas, like colostomy and ileostomy stomas, become smaller during the first weeks after surgery. The appliance opening should be reduced as necessary to protect the peristomal skin from constant contact with urine. Acid urine will burn the skin; alkaline urine will cause warty eruptions that are painful and that actually encroach upon the stoma and contribute to stenosis.

Concerns Of The Urostomate

Since hospital stays are shorter, many patients are returning home with very little understanding or expertise in the care of their urostomy. Follow-up by the ET or home health nurse knowledgeable in urostomy care is important to prevent postoperative complications.

There are many concerns shared by new urostomates, such as risking a swim in the ocean, going on the first business trip, spending the night with children and grandchildren, or sleep-away camp. Attaching the night drainage extension to the bedside receptacle, necessary to carry urine away from the stomal area and to prevent leakage from an overfilled pouch, is one of the most unpleasant aspects of urostomy care. Such accommodations require the assistance and encouragement of a nurse specialist, an experienced surgical supplier, and the empathy of another urostomate. The collaboration of lay people and professionals may be the key to patient compliance with the requisites of ostomy care.[17] The sexual implications associated with urostomies cannot be ignored. The physical effects of cystectomy on female sexual function are not as clearly understood as the effects on male erectile function. Men and women of all ages will be sexually inhibited until they get over the fear of leakage, odor, bulky equipment, and the self-consciousness of a urinary pouch on their abdomen.[18] Many women remain orgasmic. Women have delivered babies vaginally though most women urostomates are beyond the childbearing years. Young boys may have retrograde ejaculation and be infertile, but they should not experience erectile dysfunction after supravesical diversion for non-malignant conditions. Adult men generally are told that they will be impotent. A few men who have undergone cystectomy prior to the age of 50 have retained potency. Men should always be told about the various penile prostheses prior to surgery. They may not be interested then, but it is helpful for them to understand that they may resume sexual activity with the help of a surgically implanted prosthetic device in the future.

There are more complications associated with urostomies than with ileostomies and colostomies. Stomal stenosis is a common occurrence that leads to recurring infection and renal deterioration, ultimately shortening life. The etiology of most problems is fairly straight forward. Poor hygiene, ill-fitting appliances and inappropriate use of equipment and accessories are the usual antecedents, thus the best treatment is simply the elimination of the irritant.[17,19] Urinary tract infection, stomal stenosis, peristomal dermatitis and inflammation are the most common urostomy complications.

Teaching The Urostomate

All urostomy patients should be given these instructions:

1. Single use appliances should be worn for a maximum of five days.
2. Reusable appliances should be disinfected between wearings with an acetic acid solution or with a commercial ostomy disinfectant.
3. Appliances should be emptied frequently and gravity drainage must be used at night.
4. It is important to drink plenty of clear liquids to maintain a dilute, acid urine. The intake of citrus fruits and juices should be kept at a minimum - no more than four ounces daily.

Because any urostomy stomal problem potentiates damage to the upper urinary tracts, patients who complain of stomal bleeding, peristomal irritation or inflammation should be referred immediately to an experienced ET or a urologist.

Many ostomates want to separate themselves from the health care delivery system in order to feel well and cured. This probably explains why veteran ostomates commonly medicate themselves and attempt to solve their own problems without assistance. Some ostomates buy hundreds of dollars worth of remedies and medicaments in an attempt to solve a problem that could be simply treated by an experienced ET. Thus, it is important when urostomates are purchasing creams, lotions, sprays, and antiseptics that the pharmacist inquire about their condition and urge them to seek professional assistance. The relationship between stomal problems and kidney damage cannot be stressed too often to the urostomate.

Urostomy management requires diligent hygiene and knowledgeable follow-up. Meanwhile, the search continues for better forms of urinary diversion that will protect the upper tracts and be socially acceptable, perhaps even eliminating the need for anabdominal appliance.[20,21] Some children who were diverted in the 1960's and 1970's have been undiverted in the past decade and are now using intermittent catheterization successfully.

RESOURCES FOR PATIENTS WITH OSTOMIES

The United Ostomy Association (UOA) is a national self-help organization that had its inception in Philadelphia in the late 1940's. Several ostomates gathered together to discuss their common problems. In those days patients were using zinc oxide around their stoma and primitive rubber appliances with harsh adhesives and solvents, or they were strapping various containers on their abdomen without a leak-proof seal. Understandably, odor, skin irritation, and fear of leakage were nearly crippling after-effects of ostomy surgery. From this beginning, the UOA has grown into a nationwide network of support groups. There are chapters in most major cities and many small towns. The UOA has many publications, including a fine magazine called The Ostomy Quarterly. One of the most important programs of UOA is its volunteer visitor service. Visitors are trained initially and take refresher courses regularly. They are then called in to see prospective and new ostomates. There is no substitute for the encouragement offered by someone "who has been there". To learn more about the United Ostomy Association, write UOA, 2001 West Beverly Blvd., Los Angeles, California, 90057.

PHARMACY SERVICES FOR THE OSTOMATE

Pharmacy services for the ostomy patient include providing products and advice on their proper use, helping to solve problems associated with the ostomy, teaching and supporting the patient, and referring the patient to other health care providers when warranted. An important first step when offering assistance to the ostomy patient is to compile a data base and maintain separate ostomy patient records. The pharmacist should maintain patient records that record the type of ostomy, its output and frequency. In the case of the colostomy patient, it is important to note if it is currently regulated by irrigation. A description of the stoma should also be recorded, including dimensions in inches, centimeters, or with a stoma measuring guide; whether it is round or oval, and flush to the skin or protruding.

Concomitant health problems and a medication profile should also be maintained by the pharmacist for his ostomy patients. The patient's surgeon, ET or nurse specialist, and other caregivers should also be noted.

Ostomy Product Inventory

The foundation of pharmacy services for the ostomate is a complete line of appliances and supplies offered by a pharmacist who is trained in their proper use. A list of the minimal ostomy product inventory with specifications for these appliances and supplies is included in Table 16-3.

Use Of Drugs

Because part or all of the colon is removed and intestinal transit time may be altered, the ostomate may have difficulty in taking prescription, or nonprescription medication (Table 16-4).

Coated or sustained release preparations may pass through the intestinal tract without being absorbed, and the patient may receive a subtherapeutic dose. The ostomate should look for any undissolved drug particles in the pouch. Liquid preparations or preparations crushed or chewed before swallowing are best. Patients should be cautioned about drugs that will discolor the urine or feces because ostomates may be more conscious of these discharges.

The ostomate also must be careful in taking antibiotics, diuretics, and laxatives. Antibiotics may alter the normal flora of the intestinal tract, causing diarrhea or fungal infection of the skin surrounding the stoma. If diarrhea occurs, fluid and electrolyte intake should be increased. Antidiarrheal and antimotility drugs may affect ileal excreta. The physician may prescribe nystatin powder to treat fungal overgrowth.

Sulfa drugs should be used with caution. Crystallization in the kidney may occur more often in patients having difficulty with fluid balance. To minimize this problem, fluid intake should be increased, and the urine should not be acidified. In ileostomy patients, whose fluid and electrolyte balance is more difficult to maintain, diuretics should be given with care because additional loss of fluid may cause dehydration and electrolyte imbalance. The ileostomate should be monitored for signs of hyponatremia if salt substitutes are prescribed.

Laxatives may be used in colostomy patients, but only under close supervision. Ostomates tend to become obstructed, and the laxative's particular action may cause perforation. If the colostomate is constipated, a stool softener may be recommended. Antacids may also cause problems and should be taken with caution. Calcium-containing products may cause calcium stones in the urostomate; magnesium products may cause diarrhea in the ileostomate; and aluminum products may cause constipation in the colostomate. To alleviate any anxiety, the patient should be counseled on drugs that may discolor the feces (Table 16-5).

SOLVING PROBLEMS FOR THE OSTOMY PATIENT

In certain instances the pharmacist can help resolve ostomy related problems. However, some complaints from ostomy patients require consultation and in many cases referral to the patient's surgeon and/or ET. Appendix 16 - B lists common problems associated with ostomies. Also included are clarifications (i.e., additional information) that should be

Table 16-3 Ostomy Product Inventory

One-piece drainable pouch (disposable)
Pre-cut with a full range of openings from 3/4" to 3".
Custom cut (starter hold and patient cuts opening to fit stoma).
One-piece urostomy pouch (disposable)
Full-range of stoma openings from 3/4" to 2".
Custom cut (starter hole and patient cuts opening to fit the stoma).
Solid form skin barriers
Karaya rings, Coll-Seel®, Stomahesive®, HolliHesive®, Curagard®.
Karaya powder and paste
Stomahesive® powder
Stomahesive® HolliHesive® paste
Double-faced adhesive discs
Skin cement remover
Tape
Paper, plastic and waterproof pink tape.
Colostomy irrigation sets
Replacement irrigation sleeves
Belts
Night drainage systems
Attachments for the various urostomy pouches must be in stock, e.g., United, Sur-Fit, Coloplast and Hollister.
Skin creams/lotions
Only creams that permit the application of adhesives and pectin barriers are acceptable, e.g., Sween® Cream, Aloe vera gel and Stomacort®
Skin sealants
Aerosol and packaged wipes, e.g., Bard Barrier Film®, Skin-Prep® and Sween-Prep®
Pouch deodorants
Tablets or drops for the pouch.
Oral deodorants
Bismuth subgallate, bismuth subcarbonate, charcoal, or chlorophyll.
Two-piece pouch systems (disposable)
It is important that each flange size have a corresponding pouch size, and that flanges and pouches are from the same manufacturer, e.g., Coloplast, ConvaTec or Hollister.
Pouch covers
Educational booklets
Booklets from the United Ostomy Association, manufacturers or nearby hospitals.

obtained by the pharmacist from the patient. Lastly, alternative interventions are suggested. It is important to stress that these "textbook" interventions should not replace sound professional judgement based upon an assessment of the patient and accepted standards of care.

CONCLUSION

With proper instructions and equipment, ostomates can lead normal, healthy lives. Pharmacists can help by giving patients the necessary information concerning treatment, ostomy supply services, and appropriate referrals to an ET nurse.

Table 16-4 Drug Effects on the Ostomate

		Colostomate	Ileostomate	Urostomate
DOSAGE FORMS	Chewable tablets	1	1	1
	Enteric-coated tablets	1	3	1
	Sustained release medication	1	3	1
	Liquid medication	1	1	1
	Gelatin capsules	1	1	1
COMPOUND	Alcohol	1	1	1
	Antibiotics (poorly absorbed)	1	2,3	1,2
	Antidiarrheal agents	1,2	1	1
	Calcium-containing antacids	2	2	2
	Corticosteroids	1	2	1
	Diuretics	1	2	2
	Magnesium-containing antacids	2	2	1
	Opiates	1,2	1	1
	Salicylates	1	1	1
	Salt substitutes	1	2	1
	Stool softeners	1	2	1
	Sulfa drugs	1	1	2
	Vitamins	1	2	1

1, Probably no adverse effects; 2, may cause an increase in adverse effects, patient should be monitored; 3, may be ineffective, patient should be monitored.

Table 16-5 Drugs That May Discolor Feces

Drug (brand name)	Effect
Aluminum antacids	Whitish color or speckling
Antibiotics (oral)	Greenish gray
Anticoagulants (excess)	Pink to red to black (bleeding)
Bismuth salts	Black
Charcoal	Black
Ferrous salts	Black
Heparin	Pink to red to black (bleeding)
Indomethacin (Indocin)	Green
Oxyphenbutazone (Tandearil)	Pink to red to black (bleeding)
Phenazopyridine (Pyridium)	Orange red
Phenolphthalein	Red
Phenylbutazone (Butazolidin)	Pink to red to black (bleeding)
Pyrvinium Pamoate (Povan)	Red
Salicylates	Pink to red to black (bleeding)
Senna (and other anthraquinone derivative)	Yellow-green to brown

Reprinted from S. Strauss. Your Prescription and You - A Pharmacy Handbook for Consumers," 3rd ed., Medical Business Services, Ambler, PA, 1978.

Appendix 16-A Discharge Instructions for the Ostomy Patient

Squibb Sur-Fit® System

Supplies Needed: Sur-Fit Flange 1 3/4" ___Flexible___Regular

Sur-Fit drainable pouch___opaque ___transparent
___10" ___12"

Stomahesive paste

Optional Supplies:

Change pouch every 5th day or if leakage occurs. Change pouch on a schedule to prevent unexpected accidents. Remeasure the stoma frequently during the first 3 months. Decrease the size opening as the stoma shrinks.

1. Using the pattern provided, or the pattern that you make as the stoma shrinks, cut opening in the flange to correspond with the size of the stoma.
2. Attach pouch to the flange.
3. Peel circular paper to expose Stomahesive® wafer.
4. Squeeze Stomahesive® Paste around the inner circle that you have just cut. This will form a caulking to prevent leakage and melt out.
5. Peel off square paper to expose adhesive. Set prepared pouch aside.
6. Remove entire pouch system from your body. Do not throw away clamp.
7. Wash skin around the stoma and up to it with mild soap. Rinse will. Blot very dry.
8. Carefully center flange over stoma. Check in mirror to see that you have centered it. Remove two narrow paper strips.
9. Attach clamp.

Please make an appointment in my office on the day you are going to see your surgeon. If you should feel too tired, don't hesitate to cancel the appointment and reschedule. I just want to follow-up. If you have any questions in the meantime, please do not hesitate to call.

The Ostomy Association meets on the second Monday evening of every month at 7:30 pm at the Health Department, which is just down the street from the hospital. We hope you will join us as soon as you feel able.

Appendix 16 - B Common Problems of the Ostomate

Pouch leaks and requires changing more frequently than every 3 to 7 days.

If it's a fecal ostomy . . .

1. Is the stool very liquid, causing the skin barrier to melt away or the adhesive surface of the pouch to loosen?
   A. An ostomy paste (Stomahesive,® Hollihesive®) might be used as a "caulking" around the stoma to prevent stool from undermining the skin barrier or adhesive.
   B. The patient might take Metamucil® or Fiberall® to thicken the stool. This often makes the effluent more manageable. (Reassure the patient that you know this product says it is for constipation and you are recommending it for loose stools. Explain the thickening effect.)
2. Is the stool too thick and bulky, actually "unseating" the flange or faceplate as it comes out of the stoma?
   A. The patient might take a stool softener, drink prune juice, or eat foods with a laxative effect (see Table 16-2).
   B. The pouch opening may be enlarged to permit evacuation of bulky stool. The exposed skin should be covered with a skin sealant to protect it from irritation.
3. Are there scars or wrinkles around to the stoma or is the stoma situated in a crease? The patient may benefit from additional convexity in the flange or faceplate. This person probably should be evaluated by an ET.

If it is a urostomy . . .

4. Is a skin barrier being used?
   Some skin barriers, such as United's XL-14®, are more resistant to urine and do not melt as fast as others.
5. Is the patient drinking enough fluids?
   Some patients report that dilute urine does not melt away skin barriers and undermine adhesive as badly as highly concentrated, alkaline urine does. Encourage hydration.
6. Are there scars or wrinkles adjacent to the stoma or is the stoma situated in the crease?
   The patient may benefit from additional convexity in the flange/faceplate. Ostomy paste may be used as a caulking. The patient should be evaluated by an ET.

Odor

If it is a fecal ostomy . . .

1. Is the odor associated with food?
   Certain foods cause malodorous stool (see Table 16-2). The patient may either avoid the food or take charcoal, chlorophyll, or bismuth subgallate tablet by mouth.
2. Is the odor offensive when the pouch is sealed?
   If there is odor when the pouch is sealed, either the pouch is leaking; the patient is wearing old equip ment that retains odor (and the patient should be encouraged to replace it); or the patient is wearing cheap, disposable pouches that are not odor proof. Brands such as Coloplast®, Hollister®, and Sur-Fit® insure that odors do not permeate their film pouches.
3. If recommended brands are being used and odor persists...
   The application procedure is probably not correct; the patient has stool seeping under the flange; or the patient is overly self-conscious and needs reassurance. Review the application procedure with the patient. Inquire about leakage. Reassure the patient as indicated.
4. Offensive odor lingers in the bathroom.
   Room deodorants such as CBC's Medi-Air®, Sween's Hex-On®, or D-Odor's® drops are excellent deodorants that do not mask offensive odors with a more offensive smell.
5. The odor is just offensive when the pouch is emptied.
   Patients should be reassured that everyone's bowel movement has a smell. Charcoal tablets and deodor-

Appendix 16 - B Common Problems of the Ostomate (cont.)

izing drops can be placed directly in the pouch. A solution of mouthwash and water may be helpful in rinsing the pouch if the patient has a need to be fastidious. Oral deodorizers such as charcoal, chlorophyll or bismuth subgallate can also be used.

If it is a urostomy . . .

1. The odor is in the pouch.
   Probably the patient is wearing reusable pouches and should be encouraged to clean it more vigorously with a deodorizing soap or discard it and buy new one.
2. The odor is in the night drainage unit.
   The night drainage unit should be washed more vigorously with a disinfectant soap or discarded and replaced. Sometimes, two aspirin in the night drainage unit everyday, after it has been cleaned, will discourage odor. Besides commercial antiseptics, a solution of equal parts of white vinegar and water is an excellent disinfectant/deodorizer.
3. The urine smells terrible when the pouch is emptied.
   This may be caused by the interaction of a pectin skin barrier with urine. The only solution is to discontinue the use of the pectin barrier or try several deodorizers for the pouch until the most effective one is found. Foul-smelling urine is the first sign of infection. It is important to determine whether the urine is malodorous as it leaves the stoma or as it accumulates in the pouch. The patient should remove the pouch and collect urine directly from the stoma to assess its color, smell and clarity. A urine specimen for analysis and culture should only be obtained by a physician or ET and should be done with a sterile catheter, using aseptic technique.

Flatus

1. Is it associated with gas-producing foods?
   Review the food list (Table 16-2) of gas-producing foods with the patient.
2. Is it causing the pouch to bulge excessively?
   There are pouches that come with gas filters and there are gas filters such as Filtrodor® that can be used with standard pouches
3. Is gas a frequent, unexpected annoyance, unrelated to meals?
   Newly operated patients often complain of gas. They should be reassured that this will diminish over time, in 6 to 8 weeks. People who eat 5 to 6 small meals, rather than 1 or 2 large meals, report they have less problems with gas. Suggest mechanisms, such as the quick placement of a hand over the stoma to muffle the noise. Foods such as yogurt and buttermilk are recommended by some people. Commercial products are safe and may be recommended.

Denuded skin/peristomal discomfort

1. Is this a new problem? Does the pouch opening fit properly?
   The pouch opening should not exceed the size of the stoma by more than 1/8". With some of the new pectin barriers, it is safe to use an opening that is the exact size of the stomal base. The placement of a pectin skin barrier, such as Stomahesive® or HolliHesive®, will permit the application of a pouch over the denuded skin; and healing will take place underneath. The pouch should not be removed for 5 days unless leakage occurs. The patient should be referred to an ET to determine the cause.

2. Is this a chronic problem?
   Patients often self-medicate with ointments or creams that prevent their pouch from adhering and actually contribute to leakage. Some physicians prescribe creams or ointments and should be informed that they are not compatible with pouching systems. Patients with chronic skin problems should be referred immediately to an ET. When this is not possible, the peristomal area may be treated with an ulcer dressing, such as J&J Ulcer Dressing®, Comfeel Ulcus®, or DuoDerm®. These products will absorb

Appendix 16 - B Common Problems of the Ostomate (cont.)

more moisture than other solid-dorm skin barriers. Their use may be discontinued when skin integrity has been restored.

Depression, anger, frustration, or hopelessness expressed by or apparent in patient's behavior.

1. Is this a new affect? Is it related to the disease that required the ostomy or the ostomy itself? Psychological adjustment to ostomy is enhanced by association with others who have had similar operations. Patients should be referred to the local volunteer who has had similar surgery and is of the same sex, socioeconomic status and of similar age. Ask patients if they would mind an ostomy volunteer calling. Alert the physician to the patient's behavior. There is no harm in telling patients that you noticed a reaction and asking if there is anything that you can do to help.

REFERENCES

1. Strategic Planning Report. International Association for Enterostomal Therapy, Newport Beach, CA June 1982.
2. Druss RG, et al. Changes in body image following ileostomy. Psychoanal. 1972; Q41:196-206.
3. Fazio V. Cancer of the colon and rectum. Principles of Ostomy Care. D Broadwell and B Jackson, Eds. St. Louis, CV Mosby. 1981.
4. Thompson JPS. Cecostomy and Colostomy. Part 1: Surgical Complications. In Brooke DN, et al. Eds. Clinics in Gastroenterology. 1982; 11:2.
5. Breckman B. Stoma Care. Beaconsfield, England: Beaconsfield Press, 1981.
6. King NHL. Utilization of solid-form skin barriers. J Enterost Ther. 1983; 10:224-226.
7. Williams NS and Johnston D. Prospective controlled trial comparing colostomy irrigation with "spontaneous-action" method, Brit Med J. 1980; 12:107.
8. McGarity WC. Ulcerative colitis and Crohn's disease. Principles of Ostomy Care, D Broadwell and B Jackson Eds. St. Louis, CV Mosby. 1982; p114-131.
9. Goode PS. Nursing management of disorders of the gastrointestinal system. Principles of Ostomy Care, D Broadwell and B Jackson, Eds. St. Louis, CV Mosby. 1982; p257-289.
10. Brooke BN. The management of an ileostomy including its complications. Lancet. 1952; 2:102-104.
11. Brooke BN and Jeter KF. Stomal function and care. Bockus Gastroenterology, Vol. 4, EJ Berke, et al. Eds. New York, WB Saunders. 1985.
12. Fawaz KA, et al. Ulcerative colitis and Crohn's disease of the colon - a comparison of the long-term postoperative courses. Gastroenterology. 1976; 71:372-378.
13. Jeter KF. Ostomy: Part 4, Urostomy. Family Practice Recertification. 6(6):99-121, 1984.
14. Kock NG, et al. Urinary diversion via a continent ileum reservoir: Clinical experience. Scand J. Urol Nephrol (Suppl), 49:23-31, 1978.
15. Skinner DG, et al. Technique of creation of a continent internal ileal reservoir (Kock Pouch) for urinary diversion. Urologic Clinics of North America, 11(4):741-749,1984.
16. Watt RC and Thomas EL. Relating urinary diversion and appliance bacteriology. J Enterost Ther. 1978; 5(4):5-11.
17. Jeter KF. Managing the patient with the urinary stoma. Weekly Urology Update. 1980; 30(2).
18. von Eschenback AC and Rodriguez DB. Sexual Rehabilitation of the Urologic Cancer Patient. Boston: GK Hall. 1981.
19. Jeter KF. Hyperplasia or what? J Enterst Ther. 1983; 10:181-184.
20. Kock NG, et al. Urinary diversion via a continent ileal reservoir: Clinical results in twelve patients. J Urol. 1982; 128:469-475.
21. Gerber A. The Kock continent ileal reservoir for suprevesical urinary diversion: An early experience. Am J Surg. 1983; 146:15-21.

17 The Treatment of Pressure Sores

Thomas M. Chamberlain, Pharm.D., FASCP, Thomas J. Cali, Pharm.D., FASCP, Jan Cuzzell, R.N., M.A. and Steven F. Bauwens, Pharm.D., FASCP

When pressure sores develop they do so for many complex reasons. However, many individuals incorrectly view pressure sores as a chronic problem associated with poor quality of care. Yet pressure sores are wounds of an acute nature, and should be managed accordingly. Pressure sore management should always focus first on preventive strategies, thereby reducing the need for specific wound care treatment.

By applying the principles of pharmaceutical care and adopting an outcomes management approach to their practice, home health care (HHC) pharmacists can play an important role in enhancing the quality of care, and minimizing the financial and personnel resources required to manage this prevalent condition.

In long term care (LTC) settings, pressure sores are a widespread problem involving significant morbidity and mortality. Fifty percent or more of all pressure sores occur in the elderly. The risk of mortality among elderly with pressure sores has been reported to increase fourfold compared with other populations. The failure of a pressure sore to heal has been associated with a six fold increase in morality.[1] Pressure sore prevalence varies from 15% to 20% in the LTC setting,[2] and the risk of developing pressure sores in this environment may be five times as great as noninstitutionalized elderly.[3] Osteomyelitis is present in 26% of nonhealing pressure sores, and bacteremia in 50% of those patients whose sores are debrided.[3]

The economic impact of pressure sores on the health care system is substantial. The average cost of treating a pressure sore has been estimated to be between $500 and $30,000,[4] and the total cost to the health care system is estimated at over $3.5 billion per year.

PATHOPHYSIOLOGY

Pressure sores are localized areas of necrosis that develop when skin and soft tissue are compressed between a bone and an external surface for a prolonged period of time.[5] Although pressure sores can occur anywhere, they typically develop directly over bony prominences. Therefore, the most common locations of pressure sores are the sacrum, greater trochanter, ischial tuberosities, heels, malleoli of the ankles, scapulae, and elbows.[6]

Pressure sores range in severity from simple erythema to deep wounds with extensive muscle and bone involvement.[5,7] Ischemia leading to tissue necrosis has been identified as the primary factor in producing pressure sores. The process begins when prolonged pressure, shearing, or friction distorts affected tissue and increases interstitial fluid pressure. As a result, capillary blood flow to skin and underlying tissue is impaired, oxygen and nutrient supply is reduced, and ischemia is produced.

Although the mechanism causing the formation of pressure sores is not completely understood, a precise sequence of physiologic changes leading from ischemia to tissue necrosis has been proposed.[5] When tissue pressure remains above capillary closing pressure (32 mm Hg) for prolonged periods of time, local circulation is compromised, and the tissue is deprived of oxygen and nutrients resulting in the accumulation of waste products. An inflammatory response is triggered resulting in localized edema, blood clot formation, impaired circulation, and eventual cell death. The result is necrosis of muscle and subcutaneous tissue, and ultimately of the dermis and epidermis. The hypothesis suggests that destruction of muscle and subcutaneous tissue occurs before necrosis of the dermis and epidermis. The suggestion that deeper tissue is already damaged by the time necrosis is observable at the skin surface[8] is consistent with the widespread undermining often observed in severe pressure sores.[5]

Wound Healing Physiology

Following tissue ischemia and cellular necrosis, a predictable cascade of events occur to heal the skin defect and re-establish the skin's normal protective barrier. The three phases of biochemical and cellular responses that occur during wound healing are the: (1) reaction (inflammatory) phase, (2) regeneration (proliferative) phase, and (3) remodeling (maturation) phase.[9] Although the process of healing is a continuous one and these phases overlap, understanding the characteristic features of each phase can help health care professionals identify problems resulting from impairment or prolongation of the healing process. Assessment of wound progress through each phase of healing provides a basis for selecting rational treatment modalities. See Table 17-1.

Reaction Phase

The reaction phase of healing, also called the inflammatory phase, begins at the time of ischemia and presents as a transient or blanchable (i.e., removes color from skin with pressure) erythema. An immediate response of vasoconstriction and clot formation at the site of injury is followed within 5-10 minutes by active vasodilation of the same vessels. With vasodilation, capillary permeability increases, allowing plasma to leak into the surrounding tissue. Simultaneous blockage of the local lymphatic channels with fibrin prevents reabsorption of tissue fluid. Continued accumulation of fluid within the wound tissue results in compression of the sensory nerves. These events result in the classic signs of inflammation: localized edema, erythema, heat, and pain.

The cellular changes that occur during the reaction phase are responsible for removal of wound debris and prevention of infection. White blood cells

Table 17-1 The Three 'R's of Wound Healing

	Response	**What Happens**	**How It Looks**
Reaction (injury to 72 hrs)	Vascular	Vessels constrict	Clot formation
		Vessels dilate	Erythema
		Vessel permeability increases	Warmth
		Lymph channels block	Edema
		Pressure on sensory nerves increases	Pain
	Cellular	Leukocyte migration	erosanguinous wound exudate
		Epithelial cell migration	pink wound margins
			"Budding" of hair
Regeneration (up to 3 weeks)	Vascular (growth factors)	Capillaries bud to form new blood vessels	Granulation tissues fills the wound cavity
		Fibroblasts lay down new collagen	
	Wound Contraction	Myofibroblasts migrate into wound space	Wound becomes smaller and changes shape as edges pull together
Remolding (3 weeks to 2 yrs)	Reorganization of Collagen	Collagen interacts with collagenase	Scar becomes flat and brittle with collagenase. Color of scar changes from pink to white
		Increase in wound strength	Wound edges stay together and resist being pulled apart

migrate to the site of injury, entering the wound through the blood vessels. Polymorphonuclear leukocytes (PMNs) predominate during the first two to three days after injury. Lysis of PMNs leads to liberation of proteolytic enzymes which initiate the tissue necrosis process. PMNs soon are replaced by macrophages. In addition to removing bacteria and cellular debris by phagocytosis, the macrophage is thought to release growth factors that stimulate the remainder of the repair process. The macrophage, therefore, may be thought of as the coordinator of tissue repair.

Epidermal cell migration also occurs during this phase. In pressure sores where minimal tissue loss occurs, epithelial cells migrate from the wound edges and hair follicles until skin integrity is restored. When more extensive tissue involvement occurs, epithelial cell migration plays a limited role in wound closure.

A nonblanchable erythema of intact skin will resolve promptly if the cause of pressure is removed. In acute injuries with minimal tissue destruction, the inflammatory response usually subsides in three to five days as capillary permeability returns to normal and tissue fluid drains. In cases of untreated pressure sores, inflammation often is sustained. A prolonged inflammatory phase delays the healing process, and recurrence of inflammatory signs and symptoms usually is associated with continued tissue trauma or wound infection.

Regeneration Phase

The regeneration phase, also referred to as the proliferation phase of healing, begins approximately four days after injury and continues for about three weeks. Granulation or scar tissue is formed during this phase of healing. Stimulated by macrophages, uninjured capillaries begin to bud (i.e., develop new branches), forming new blood vessels. In addition, fibroblasts are stimulated by macrophages to produce collagen. Budding capillaries, combined with collagen synthesis, create the red, thick, pebble-like appearance of granulation tissue.

Granulation plays a major role in pressure sore healing when extensive tissue loss is present. Granulation tissue serves to fill the crater-like defect that occurs when necrotic tissue is removed, and gives structural stability to the wound. Adequate protein stores are required for collagen synthesis. Protein and calorie malnutrition, and certain vitamin and mineral deficiencies, cause a wound to remain in the regeneration phase of tissue repair indefinitely, resulting in diminished tissue resistance to infection.

Contraction of a deep, open pressure sore occurs during the regeneration phase. Specialized fibroblasts in the wound bed called myofibroblasts exert a mechanical force on the wound edges. The result is a pulling together of the wound while the surrounding skin is stretched and thinned. Clinically, wound contraction is observed as a gradual decrease in wound surface dimensions. The shape of the wound also may change during contraction due to differences in the elasticity and mobility of surrounding skin.

Remodeling Phase

The remodeling or maturation phase of tissue repair begins as early as three weeks after injury and continues for a year or more after wound closure. During this phase, the strength of the scar tissue increases and prevents the wound edges from pulling apart through reorganization of the collagen. The result is firm, elastic tissue that provides minimal padding for the underlying bone.

There are many factors that can slow or even halt the progression of healing through the various phases. Infection, unrelieved pressure, and inadequate nutrition are primary concerns. Adequate tissue oxygenation is needed for optimal leukocyte and fibroblast function, as well as epidermal cell proliferation. Therefore, patients with a chronic reduction in blood oxygen saturation (e.g., chronic obstruction pulmonary disease and cardiopulmonary disease) or those with reduced blood flow to the wound (e.g., arteriosclerosis, vasoconstriction, peripheral vascular disease, etc.) generally heal more slowly. Table 17-2 outlines factors that impair healing such as age-related physiologic decline, stress, corticosteroid therapy, and local tissue trauma.

PATIENT ASSESSMENT

Assessment procedures in the prevention and management of pressure sores should include a comprehensive evaluation of each patient. When pressure sores develop, a physical evaluation of the wounds should be performed.

Although the recommended interval for assessment is every two weeks, the specific frequency should be determined by patient acuity. When patients at risk are identified, the staff must take appropriate steps for prevention of pressure sores in these individuals.

Table 17-2 Factors That Impair Healing of Pressure Sores

INTRINSIC FACTORS	EXTRINSIC FACTORS
Malnutrition • Protein depletion (serum albumin < 3.0 g/dL) • Calorie depletion • Vitamin deficiency • Trace element deficiency (zinc, copper, ferrous iron, manganese)	**Necrotic Tissue** Physical obstacle to epidermal cell migration and wound contraction; pablum for bacterial proliferation
Prolonged reaction phase; impaired revascularization, fibroblast function, and collagen synthesis; impaired wound remodeling; decreased resistance to infection	
Prolonged reaction phase; impaired remodeling phase	
Altered fibroblast function (Vitamin C): poor quality of healing (Vitamin A and C); impaired healing of bone (Vitamin D)	
Altered enzymatic reactions	
Tissue Hypoxia (from atherosclerosis, small vessels disease, hypovolemia, cardiopulmonary disease, etc.) Impaired capillary budding; impaired fibroblast function; decreased epithelia cell regeneration; impaired leukocyte function and increased wound infection	**Tissue Trauma** (from unrelieved pressure, too aggressive cleansing or inappropriate use of dressing materials) Cellular injury and reinitiation of inflammation
Infection (>10^5 organisms/gm of tissue) Prolonged or recurrent reaction phase	**Topical Antiseptics/Antimicrobials** Potentially cytotoxic to cells when used inappropriately
Advanced Age Decreased epidermal turnover; increased skin fragility; prolonged rate of repair (all phases); increased incidence of malnutrition; impaired respiratory and immune systems; increased risk of ischemic injury due to decreased number of dermal blood vessels	**Tissue Desiccation** Impairs epithelial migration and fibroblast proliferation
Steroids Suppressed reaction phase	**Dead Space** (wound space left unfilled with dressing material) Pooling of wound exudate encourages bacterial proliferation and abscess formation
Diabetes Impaired circulation leading to tissue hypoxia; impaired leukocyte function; increased incidence of wound infection	

Nursing home patients are twice as likely as hospitalized patients to develop pressure sores, primarily because of the presence of multiple risk factors.[10] These risk factors fall under two broad categories: physical immobility and age-related medical conditions.

Patients who are immobile, bedridden, or unable to ambulate are at increased risk. Immobility is present whenever a patient is totally dependent on assistance with his activities of daily living. This restriction of spontaneous movement causes pressure to be exerted over an area for a prolonged period of time.[11] A less dependent condition, impaired activity, is present when a patient is confined to a bed or chair. Impaired activity may result from a decline in neurologic functioning secondary to Alzheimer's disease, multi-infarct dementia, cerebrovascular accident, sedation from medication, or any form of paralysis.

Age-related medical conditions associated with the formation of pressure sores or the prevention of healing include malnutrition, dehydration, incontinence, alteration in mental status, and other underlying medical conditions that may impair skin integrity.

Malnutrition, especially protein-calorie malnutrition,[12] increases a patient's risk of pressure sore development. This risk increases when serum albumin concentrations fall below 3.5 gm/dL. Malnutrition can result from reduced food intake, loss of appetite, gastrointestinal fluid losses secondary to prolonged vomiting or diarrhea, or increased metabolic demand. Pinchofsky-Devin and Kaminiski have documented the relationship between protein malnutrition and pressure sores.[13] Evaluation of protein parameters, including serum albumin, total leukocyte count, and serum transferrin may help predict the patient's relative risk. Assessment of lean body weight and recent weight loss history may indicate problems with calorie malnutrition. Pressure sores most commonly are seen in individuals with a moderate (78-87%) or severe (<78%) reduction in lean body mass in conjunction with protein malnutrition. Pinchofsky-Devin and Kaminiski report that serious sores occur in individuals with a substantial reduction in protein status as evidenced by a decreased serum albumin concentration.[13] Revising these factors is essential for the effective management of pressure sores.

Assessment of dehydration in the elderly is complicated by inconsistent symptomatology and absent or minimal physical findings. Laboratory evaluation of blood urea nitrogen (BUN) concentration, BUN to serum creatinine ratio, and other parameters indicative of dehydration is recommended.

Fecal and urinary incontinence, if not promptly and effectively evaluated and managed, increase the risk of skin breakdown and the development of pressure sores.[5] Incontinence promotes maceration, decreasing tissue tolerance to pressure, friction, and shearing forces. Fecal enzymes are caustic and cause rapid tissue breakdown with prolonged exposure.

Alteration in mental status is a frequent complication in LTC patients. A decline in mental status contributes to the development of pressure sores by decreasing awareness of pressure or painful stimuli.[11, 14] This is especially true with drug-induced sedation or in patients who are comatose.

Other underlying medical conditions, such as decreased circulation secondary to peripheral vascular disease or diabetes mellitus, impaired host immune competence (e.g., diabetes mellitus or chronic infection), and localized infection in pressure-supporting areas contribute to the development of pressure sores and impair the healing process.[11]

Several practical instruments have been developed to evaluate patient risk for pressure sore development. These instruments assess various aspects of a patient's condition, including mental status, continence, mobility, activity, nutrition, general health, fluid intake, concurrent disease, circulation, infection, mechanical factors, musculoskeletal status, and skin condition. Although laboratory tests are an important source of objective information,[12] perhaps the single most important assessment is direct examination of skin integrity.[15]

PRESSURE SORE ASSESSMENT

Because accurate pressure sore assessment is a prerequisite for successful treatment, a thorough evaluation of each pressure sore must be performed. Unfortunately, adequate assessment of procedures are infrequently performed in community settings. Typically, pressure sores are classified according to severity and extent of tissue involvement. Various wound-staging systems are used for this purpose, notably Shea's four-state system,[16] and the International Association for Enterostomal Therapy's (IAET) systems.[8] Although the Shea and the IAET systems focus only on depth as the major criterion for staging, they remain in use because documentation of pressure sores in terms of stages is useful in evaluating the severity of the wound. The value of staging systems is debatable, however, because the stages are not definitive and often are difficult to determine. For example a necrotic wound cannot be assessed accurately until the eschar (i.e., the crusty surface layer of dead tissue and exudate) is removed. In addition, there is a low degree of interrater reliability in staging.

The National Pressure Ulcer Advisory Panel (NPUAP) has attempted to develop a universally accepted system by combining elements of the most commonly used staging systems.[17] The NPUAP categorizes pressure sores according to the following stages:

- Stage I - Nonblanchable erythema of intact skin; the heralding lesion of skin ulceration.
- Stage II - Partial thickness skin loss involving epidermis and/or dermis. The sore is superficial and presents clinically as an abrasion, blister, or shallow crater.
- Stage III - Full thickness skin loss involving damage or necrosis of subcutaneous tissue that may extend down to, but not through, underlying fascia. The sore presents clinically as a deep crater with or without undermining of adjacent tissue.
- Stage IV - Full thickness skin loss with extensive destruction, tissue necrosis or damage to muscle, bone, or supporting structures (e.g., tendon, joint capsule, etc.).

Although staging systems are useful for classifying wounds according to severity and extent of tissue involvement, they are limited in their ability to guide product selection. An evaluation that characterizes wounds as healing, infected, or necrotic, more accurately describes the status of a pressure sore and, therefore, can better guide product selection. Thorough pressure sore assessment should include the following procedures:

- Document the location of the wound;
- Measure and record wound size in centimeters at greatest length, width, and depth;
- Draw a picture of any irregularly shaped wound in the progress notes;
- Determine the stage of the wound;
- Describe the appearance of the wound, check for pus, exudate, necrotic debris, eschar, granulation tissue, drainage, color, type and odor;
- Assess for pockets, tracts, and undermining;
- Assess appearance of wound margins for induration, tenderness, rash, tape burns, maceration, or any other condition;
- Determine wound status, healing, infected, or necrotic; and
- Document findings in the medical record.

GOALS OF MANAGEMENT

Effective management of pressure sores requires an interdisciplinary approach and should focus on both preventive care and the development of individualized wound treatment regimens. Although pressure sores develop for many complex reasons, they continue to be synonymous with poor quality of care, adding to the perception that pressure sores are a chronic problem. However, pressure sores are wounds of an acute nature and should be managed accordingly. Since specific wound care treatment is unnecessary when a pressure sore is prevented from developing, pressure sore management should focus on preventive strategies.

Prevention Strategies

Reduction of pressure, especially over bony prominences, and maintenance of skin integrity and nutritional competence are essential to pressure sore prevention. Frequent turning of patients is a well-established preventive intervention. Patients who cannot move themselves must be repositioned at regular intervals. Although a two-hour interval generally is accepted as the optimum, individual tolerances for different times and pressures vary considerably.[5] The frequency of repositioning depends on the patient's risk factors and the supporting surface. Patients at high risk of developing pressures sores must be carefully monitored on a daily basis for signs of erythema over pressure points. Turning patients is labor intensive and must be continually monitored if this intervention is to be successful.

Relief of Pressure

A variety of pressure relieving devices are used to counteract point pressures on bony prominences. Although foam or static air mattresses are used widely, their effectiveness is questionable. Localized devices, such as donuts and Una boots, which are used to reduce pressure, should be avoided because they increase pressure of the wound periphery and can promote ischemia on the sacrum and heels. Alternating air mattresses also have proved effective but are costly and complex to operate and maintain.

Other mechanical causes must be prevented as well. When the head of the bed is elevated to more than 30° (e.g., nasogastric tube fed residents) the sacral area is exposed to shearing forces.[5] When a patient slouches in the sitting position, shearing forces are produced in the ischial tuberosities and the sacrum.[18] These shearing forces can be reduced or prevented with foam-padded chairs and stretchers, wheelchair cushions, and soft pillows for positioning.

Caregivers can minimize the patient's risk of developing pressure sores by implementing the following general care procedures:

- Turn patient every two hours if patient does not turn self;
- Shift patient's weight every two hours while in chair;
- Relieve pressure sore area with appropriate pressure-relieving devices;
- When patient is in bed, keep heels propped off mattress surface;
- Encourage patient to be out of bed and to walk when possible;
- Use pressure pad or foam in chair;
- Perform range of motion every shift;
- Perform back rub at least daily to stimulate circulation, except in Stage I area (massage of these areas may cause tissue damage); and
- Avoid sedating medications.

Skin Protection

Although urinary incontinence usually can be managed or reduced with behavioral or habit retraining, medication, surgery, or various supportive emissaries, the following guidelines for skin protection are recommended:

- Clean patient thoroughly with soap and water after urination and defecation;
- Apply moisture barrier cream as needed to protect skin from contact with urine and feces;
- Keep all skin areas clean and dry and perform perineal care;
- Identify the cause of skin breakdown in high-risk patients - reverse or improve when possible; and
- Identify and treat the cause of diarrhea.

Nutrition

Nutritional interventions are important preventive and therapeutic measures. Since well-nourished patients usually do not develop pressure sores,[19] and patients with pressure sores require adequate protein stores for normal wound healing, HHC providers should continually monitor their patients' nutritional status. In patients with impaired protein status, as evidenced by decreased serum albumin concentrations, nutritional support is indicated. Both calorie and protein competence is critical to wound healing. Optimal protein intake to assist wound healing varies from 1.2-1.8 g/kg of lean body mass for patients with normal renal function.[13] Adequate caloric intake is necessary to prevent protein breakdown.

Guidelines that should be implemented to maintain adequate nutritional status in a patient with a pressure sore include:

- Encourage oral intake of protein and calorie-containing fluids unless contraindicated;
- Observe and record food intake at meals;
- Weigh patient weekly; and
- Obtain dietary consult for increased nutritional requirements and supplements, and evaluate need for alternative delivery methods (i.e., tube feeding, parenteral nutrition).

TREATMENT STRATEGIES

The ultimate goal of pressure sore treatment is complete closure of the wound. As a wound progresses through the various phases of healing, predictable changes occur in wound status, appearance, and size. Therefore the clinician must continually monitor wound status and modify therapy accordingly.

A multitude of products are available for the topical treatment of pressure sores. HHC pharmacists should assess the advantages, disadvantages, and unique qualities of these products and provide recommendations for patient-specific treatment regimens. Although a comprehensive discussion of each treatment option is beyond the scope of this article, a brief description of the various product categories is provided in Tables 17-3 through 17-5. HHC pharmacists and other health care professionals must be cognizant of the relationship between wound status and product selection. Effective pressure sore management relies on the clinician's ability to select specific products based on wound assessment.

Pressure sores may be characterized as necrotic, infective/exudative, or healing. The development of general treatment guidelines for each type of wound should assist the interdisciplinary team in establishing a patient specific plan of care.

Necrotic Wounds

Necrotic wounds are full thickness pressure sores covered with thick black, gray, or brown necrotic tissue or eschar. The eschar of necrotic wounds serves as a physical obstacle to wound healing and readily supports bacterial growth, especially once it becomes moist or contaminated. In Stage IV wounds, eschar can mask an infection that, if untreated, can penetrate more deeply causing osteomyelitis or systemic infections. Therefore, the goal of therapy for necrotic wounds is debridement.

Treatment options for necrotic wounds are listed in Table 17-3. In general, infected necrotic wounds require surgical intervention to quickly remove the source of sepsis. Enzymatic, mechanical, and autolytic methods of debridement, which take more time to achieve results, are appropriate for non-infected necrotic wounds, and in patients in whom surgical treatment is inappropriate. When enzymatic debriders are prescribed, they are applied topically to

Table 17-3 Treatment Options for Necrotic Wounds

TREATMENT GOAL: REMOVE ESCHAR

Specific Treatment Options by Category	Description by Category	Advantages by Category	Disadvantages by Category
Surgical Debridement:	Surgical excision of eschar by physician. May require concomitant treatment with systemic antimicrobials.	Rapid removal of necrotic tissue. Large wounds may be partially debrided reducing risk to patient.	May require hospitalization for procedure. Caution must be used with those who are immunosuppressed, debilitated, or have bleeding disorders. May leave some necrotic debris in place.
Enzymatic Debridement: Fibrinolysin deoxyribonuclease (Elase®), Papain (Panafil®), Collagenase (Santyl®), Sutilains (Travase®)	Enzyme topically applied to necrotic surface. Usually covered with wet gauze and/or transparent dressing. Applying a protectant (i.e., moisture barrier cream) to surrounding tissue may be indicated. Often requires concomitant treatment with topical or systemic antimicrobials. Discontinue when wound is red and granulating or if it bleeds easily when cleansed.	Less traumatic than surgical deriding. Ease of application. Cost-effective debridement therapy.	Cross-hatching recommended if thick eschar is present. Some detergents and antiseptics may inactivate certain products. Effect on viable tissue varies by product. May require longer treatment period.
Mechanical Debridement: Wet-to-dry dressings Hydrotherapy	Removal of eschar using mechanical forces that pull off necrotic tissue. Discontinue when wound is red and granulating or if it bleeds easily when cleansed.	Promotes softening and loosening of eschar. Potentially less traumatic than surgical debridement.	Generally not as effective in severely necrotic wounds. Must monitor for signs of injury to healthy tissue.
Autolytic Debridement:	Use of occlusive dressings or dressings which impart moisture to soften and liquefy necrotic tissue.	Selective form of debridement (does not harm healing tissue). Effective alternative for debridement of small wounds. Readily available.	May lead to infection in large necrotic wounds. Not indicated for clinically infected wounds due to increased bacterial growth beneath dressing.

the eschar surface and usually are covered with a moist gauze or transparent dressing. If thick eschar covers the wound, cross-hatching of the eschar should be performed before applying the enzymatic debrider to enhance penetration of the drug and hasten the debridement process. Enzymatic debriders also may be used in infected necrotic wounds. When used in this manner, they may require concomitant treatment with a topical or systemic antimicrobial. Enzymatic debriders should be discontinued when granulation tissue begins to form or if bleeding occurs easily during cleansing. Debridement of a necrotic wound usually results in an infected/exudative wound.

Infected/Exudative Wounds

These pressure sores generally have some necrotic tissue or "slough" ranging in color from creamy ivory to yellow-green. Tenacious exudate, pus, fibrous material, and other cellular components also may be present. Necrotic tissue in the presence of moisture readily supports bacterial proliferation.

Table 17-4 Treatment Options for Infected or Exudative Wounds

TREATMENT GOALS: REMOVE PUS, EXUDATE, AND NECROTIC DEBRIS; REDUCE BACTERIAL GROWTH

Specific Treatment Optons by Catagory	Description by Category	Advantages by Category	Disadvantages by Category
Absorption Dressings: Dextranomer (Debrisan®) Flexible hydroactive granules and paste (DuoDerm®, Bard®) absorption Calcium sodium alginate fibers (Kaltostat®)	Includes granules, flakes, paste, and pads. Placed directly into wound bed to absorb exudate. Provides minor debriding action by retaining wound debris.	Absorbs wound exudate while maintaining wound moisture. Cleanses wound bed.	Some dressings require irrigation to remove from wound. May increase time for dressing changes. May impair granulation and epithelialization by drying wound bed, if exudate is minimal.
Topical Antibiotics: Silver sulfadiazine cream (Silvadene®), Povidone iodine ointment (Betadine® ointment), Triple antibiotic ointment (Neosporin®)	Antimicrobial solutions, ointments and creams. Indicated for prophylaxis or for treatment of an infected wound.	Easy to a apply. Water miscible creams easy to remove. Helps control bacterial growth until necrotic tissue can be debrided.	May have (cytotoxic effects which may delay wound healing. Ointments are difficult to remove. Allergic reactions may occur. Bacteria may become resistant with prolonged use.
Enzymatic Debridement: Fibrinolysin desoxyribonuclease (Elase®), Papain (Panafil®), Collagenase (Santyl®), Sutilains (Travase®)	See Table 17-3. May be adjunctive therapy. Applying a protectant (i.e. moisture barrier cream) to surrounding tissue may be indicated. Apply selectively to necrotic area.	See Table 17-3.	See Table 17-3. May be difficult keep on a highly exudative wound.
Non-adherent Dressings: Telfa®, Exu-Dry®, Vaseline® gauze, Adaptic®	Nonocclusive, absorbent dressing. May be used with topical medications.	Easy to use. Inexpensive.	Nonocclusive. Does not physically protect wound site from injury. May be difficult to remove.
Gauze Dressings: Wet-to-dry dressings	Coarse mesh gauze dressing (i.e., 4x4). Mechanical removal of infected material and necrotic tissue.	Economical. Readily available. Good mechanical debridement.	May adhere to wound bed. May cause bleeding, pain and removal of healthy granulation tissue and epithelium. Requires increased nursing time because more frequent dressing changes are needed to remain effective

Table 17-5 Treatment Options for Clean or Healing Wounds
TREATMENT GOAL: PROTECT, KEEP MOIST, AND PROMOTE HEALING

Specific Treatment Options by Category	Description by Category	Advantages by Category	Disadvantages by Category
Solutions: Normal saline Shur-Clens ® Lactated Ringers	Cleansing solution that is not harsh to healing tissue.	Cleanses wound. Maintains moist environment.	None
Gels: Carrington Wound Dressing (TM) Vigilon ® Intrasite ®	Topicals with absorptive and moisturizing properties.	Non-adherent. May cool and/or soothe wound. Easy to apply.	Usually requires protective outer dressing. May require multiple daily dressing changes. May macerate surrounding tissue.
Transparent Dressings: Op-Site ® Tegaderm ® Bioclusive® Acu-Derm® Blisterfilm®	Adhesive transparent thin film type semipermeable dressing. Semipermeable membrane allows moisture and oxygen exchange.	A barrier to contamination that also keeps wound moist. Allows for easy visual inspection. Good adhesive properties. Waterproof dressing allows patient to shower. Reduces pain. Time saving.	May lead to tissue maceration in extremely moist wounds. Some products are difficult to apply. May promote infection if necrotic tissue is present. Potential for adhesive injury. Expensive.
Hydrocolloid Dressings: DuoDerm ® Restore ® Comfeel ®	Dressing that reacts with exudate to form a gel. Creates a physical barrier and maintains a moist/acidic environment.	Totally occlusive; protects wound from physical injury and contamination. Maintains moist environment. Easy removal without adhesion to wound surface. May remain on wound for up to five days. Waterproof dressing allows patient to shower.	Difficult to observe wound. May promote development of infection in deep wounds. May accumulate excess fluid and macerate tissue. Dressing may soften and wrinkle with prolonged wear, wrinkles may increase pressure on wound base.
Non-Adherent Dressing Telfa ® Exu-Dry ® Adaptic ® Vaseline ® gauze	Nonocclusive absorbent dressing. May be used with topical products.	Inexpensive. Easy to use.	Does not physically protect wound site from injury. Some products may be difficult to remove. Nonocclusive.
Gauze Dressings	Fine mesh gauze dressing used as vehicle for soaks, lubricants, or antimicrobials.	Economical. Readily available. Effective delivery of solution if kept moist. Cost-effective filler for large wounds.	May cause bleeding, pain, and remove healthy granulation tissue if allowed to dry. Requires increased nursing time to keep dressing moist.
Lubricating Sprays Granulex ®	Aerosolized oil to encourage healing.	Easy to apply. Cools and moisturizes. Prevents premature drying/cornication of epithelial tissue.	Usually flammable. Inhalation of aerosol spray should be avoided. Difficult to apply to a small contained area. May stain skin, clothing and linens.

For this reason, the goal of therapy for this type of wound is to remove slough and exudate and reduce bacteria on the wound surface.

Infected/exudative wounds require aggressive cleaning with daily hydrotherapy or physiologic saline irrigation. Mechanical cleansing helps to remove the soft, loose necrotic tissue and colonized surface debris. In very large or deep sores, local tissue defenses may not be adequate enough to reduce the bacterial load and wound infection results. If signs of local infection are present, topical antimicrobial therapy is indicated to help control bacterial proliferation on the wound surface. If the infection is severe and has progressed to bacteremia, systemic antibiotic therapy should be administered in addition to topical treatment.

Treatment options for non-infected wounds include enzymatic debriding agents or hydrophilic absorption dressings to facilitate separation of soft necrotic tissue and to absorb exudate. Wet-to-dry saline dressings also can be used to mechanically lift loose necrotic tissue from the wound surface. However, wet-to-dry dressings are a non-selective form of debridement and also can remove healthy tissue if used inappropriately. For this reason, they should be discontinued if bleeding is observed during a dressing change. Treatment options for these wounds are summarized in Table 17-4. Effective use of these treatments should result in a clean healing wound.

Clean Healing Wounds

Pressure sores that are completely free of pus, exudate, and necrotic tissue and are actively healing should be considered clean healing wounds. Full thickness pressure sores (Stage II and IV) are covered with clean, granulation tissue. Superficial sores (Stage II) are pink and moist with pearly pink margins indicating reepithelialization. The goal of therapy for this type of wound is to maintain a clean, moist environment and protect the healing tissue from infection and trauma.

Healing wounds should be cleansed gently with an aseptic syringe and physiologic saline or with a non-toxic wound cleanser. High-pressure irrigation or aggressive scrubbing with gauze pads should be avoided as this can traumatize tissue and delay healing. Antiseptic solutions (hydrogen peroxide, iodophors, etc.) and detergents (chlorhexidine, soap, etc.) should not be used for cleansing due to the potential cytotoxicity of these agents. A clean, moist wound environment can be maintained with a variety of dressing materials (Table 17-5). By promoting a slightly moist wound surface, cells important to the healing process function more efficiently and the wound heals faster. For this reason, air-drying wounds and using heat lamps is contraindicated for clean healing wounds. If gauze is used to dress the wound, it should be kept moist with saline at all times to prevent over-drying. Gauze dressing may need to be remoistened before removal to prevent debridement of healthy tissue. Occasionally, healing wounds become infected, especially if it is a deep wound with an underlying osteomyelitis. If systemic signs and symptoms of infection are present, topical and systemic antimicrobials need to be considered. Treatment options for clean healing wounds are summarized in Table 17-5.

ROLE OF THE HOME HEALTH CARE PHARMACIST

Although HHC pharmacists are not the primary health care professionals responsible for the assessment and management of pressure sores, they are in an excellent position to use their administrative, clinical, and educational skills to enhance the quality of care for patients at risk for developing pressures sores.

Administrative Functions

Administratively, HHC pharmacists can have a dramatic impact on patient care by encouraging the development and implementation of policies and procedures for all aspects of pressure sore management. In particular, the HHC pharmacist can take an active role by:

- Encouraging the development of an interdisciplinary specialty team that performs routine periodic assessment of all patients with pressure sores;
- Assisting in the development of policies and procedures for assessing and managing pressure sores;
- Assisting in reducing unnecessary expenditures;
- Promoting research to determine the effectiveness of pharmacologic therapy and other treatment modalities; and
- Assisting the staff in complying with federal and state regulations.

Clinical Role

There are many areas in which HHC pharmacists can apply their clinical skills producing a major impact on the overall management of pressure sores, resulting in a positive patient outcome and enhanced quality of life. By monitoring the patient, the HHC pharmacist can recommend cost-effective and appropriate use of products and devices, and develop individualized treatment regimens, based on the patient's condition and status of each pressure sore. Therapeutic recommendations also should focus the attention of the nursing staff and the attending physician on exacerbating conditions and include recommendations for alternative therapy. For example, concomitant disease states (e.g., urinary incontinence, diabetes mellitus) can contribute to the development of pressure sores, as well as impair the healing process. The physician also should be alerted to medications known to impair the wound healing process, such as tetracycline and corticosteroids.

In all areas, clinical monitoring should focus on desired therapeutic endpoints and the prevention of drug-related problems. To effectively assess these monitoring parameters, the HHC pharmacist must work closely with the nursing staff to ensure proper selection of wound care products and devices. Documentation of all clinical findings and procedures in the nursing notes is an essential step in facilitating continuity of care.

Educational Activities

The educational role of the HHC pharmacist may focus on programs for the various caregivers in the home setting. Suggested topics may include prevention of pressure sores, patient assessment and wound status evaluation, accurate nursing documentation of wound assessment and response to treatment, development of pressure sore care plans, and a review of product categories and specific treatment options available for achieving treatment goals.

CONCLUSION

Prevention, assessment, and management of pressure sores present many challenges to health care professionals practicing in the HHC setting. HHC pharmacists can play an important role in improving the quality of care and enhancing the quality of life of patients suffering from pressure sores.

The morbidity, mortality, economic, and emotional impact of pressure sores mandates that HHC professionals undertake a clearly defined and comprehensive approach to outcomes management. By utilizing an interdisciplinary team to develop and implement such a management strategy, they can effectively improve the quality of care of their patients. HHC pharmacists should participate in and facilitate the work of this team. With an expanded knowledge of the pressure sore disease process, assessment procedures, and management practices, HHC pharmacists can provide significant assistance in achieving positive outcomes from this persistent, widespread, and costly problem.

Adapted with permission from The Consultant Pharmacist, 1992; 7:1328-1340.

REFERENCES

1. Emanuele JA, Katz T, Levien DH. Pressure sores: how to prevent and treat them. Postgrad Med. 1992; 91:113-20.
2. Cowart V. Pressure ulcers preventable, say some clinicians. JAMA. 1987; 257:589-93.
3. Moss RJ, LaPuma J. The ethics of pressure sore prevention and treatment in the elderly: a practical approach. J Am Geriatr Soc. 1991; 39:906-8.
4. Steward T. Pressure points. Decubitus. 1988; 1:12-6.
5. Goode PS, Allman RM. The prevention and management of pressure ulcers. Med Clin N Am 1989; 73:1511-24.
6. Iverson-Carpenter MS. impaired skin integrity. J Gerontol Nurs. 1988; 14:25-9.
7. Woolsey RM, McGarry JD. The cause, prevention, and treatment of pressure sores. Neurol Clin 1991; 9:797-808.
8. Lyder CH. Conceptualization of the stage 1 ulcer. J ET Nurs 1991; 18:162-5.
9. Peacock EE. Wound healing and wound care. In: Schwartz Sl. Shires GT, Spenser FC, Stover EH, Eds. Principles of surgery. 4th ed. New York: McGraw-Hill, 1984.
10. Scheckler WE, Peterson PJ. Infections and infection control among residents in eight rural Wisconsin nursing homes. Arch Intern Med. 1986; 146:1981-4.
11. Sparks S. Nurse validation of pressure ulcer risk factors for a nursing diagnosis. Decubitus. 1992; 5:26-35.
12. Holmes R, Macchiano K, Jhanigiani SS, et al. Combating pressure sores nutritionally. Am J Nurs. 1987; 10:1301-3.
13. Pinchofsky-Devin GD, Kaminiski MV. Correlation of pressure sores and nutritional status. J Am Geriatr Soc. 1986; 34:435-40.
14. Gosnell DJ, Pressure sore risk assessment: a critique. Part I: the Gosnell Scale. Decubitus. 1989; 2:32-8.
15. Pajk M, Craven GA, Cameron-Barry J, et al. Investigating the problem of pressure sores. J Gerontol Nurs. 1986; 12:11-6.
16. Shea JD. Pressure sores: classification and manage-

ment. Clin Orthop. 1975; 112:89-100.
17. The National Pressure Ulcer Advisory Panel. Pressure ulcers: prevalence, cost, and risk assessment. Decubitus. 1989; 2:24.
18. Allman RM, Laprade CA, Noel LB, et al. Pressure sores among hospitalized patients. Ann Intern Med. 1986; 105:337-42.
19. Aronovitch SA. A retrospective study of the use of specialty beds in the medical and surgical intensive care units of a tertiary care facility. Decubitus. 1992; 5:36-42.

18 Establishing a Home Infusion Pharmacy Service

David M. Melikian, Pharm.D.

Over the past ten years the general home health care (HHC) market, which represents approximately fifteen billion dollars annually, has seen significant growth, averaging 15 - 30% for most market segments.[1] This rapid and sustained growth has attracted the interest of many pharmacists and independent investors, who would like to become a part of this growing industry. The home infusion therapy market, which represents approximately 19% of total home care dollars, is currently projected to be approximately three billion dollars.

The therapies classically provided by home infusion companies include total parenteral nutrition (TPN), anti-infective (antibiotic, antiviral, antifungal), pain management, chemotherapy, enteral nutrition and hydration (see Table 18-1). Other therapies include alpha-1-antiprotease, dobutamine, deferoxamine, growth hormone, intravenous immunoglobulins (IVIGG), colony stimulating factors (filgrastim, sargramostim), epoetin, inhalation pentamidine and catheter care. These market segments are projected to grow approximately 15% per year for the next three to five years.[1,2]

Table 18-1 Number of Patients, by Type of Therapy[1]

		NUMBER	PERCENT
THERAPY	Antibiotcs	9,537	23.3
	Pain Management	1,611	3.8
	Chemotherapy	2,050	4.8
	TPN	4,551	10.7
	Enteral Nutrition	7,259	17.0
Total of 5 Major Therapies		**25,007**	**58.6**
OTHER Therapies*		17,649	41.4
ALL		**42,656**	**100**

* Includes human growth hormone, catheter care, hydration, intravenous blood transfusions, aerosolized pentamidine, blood products, durable medical equipment and others

Over the past ten years a significant awareness has developed within the network of payer sources which emphasizes the potential cost savings of home infusion. Therapies such as inhalation pentamidine, which were not reimbursed five years ago, are now commonly approved for home use. Implementation of more rigid cost containment measures, managed care, per diem charges and drug use review have prompted physicians and discharge planners to release patients as soon as possible to the HHC setting. Also adding to the growth of the HHC industry is the belief that HHC services are less expensive than the same service provided in the hospital.

THE PHARMACIST'S ROLE IN HOME INFUSION THERAPY

All successful home infusion therapy programs have the support of competent pharmacy services. The pharmacist plays a pivotal role in the formulation and delivery of infusion therapy. At this time approximately 65% of the home infusion market (based on revenues) is serviced by the fifteen largest national home infusion therapy companies.[3] Thirty-five percent of the home care market is provided by franchised infusion companies, regional infusion companies (2 or more infusion locations in a limited geographic area), and independent pharmacies.[3]

Many independent pharmacy practitioners are beginning to provide infusion therapy as a part of their current services. However, providing home infusion services requires a significant amount of clinical and operational expertise, which is uniquely different than the traditional forms of community and hospital practice. In addition to the traditional knowledge of sterile compounding techniques and handling of chemotherapy and biohazardous waste, pharmacists must also be knowledgeable about medical and surgical supplies which are necessary to support catheter patency, catheter site care and equipment required to deliver the medication, i.e., parenteral and/or enteral pumps, elastomeric or spring-loaded infusion devices.

Over the last five years there has been increasing pressure on home infusion companies to show measurable competence and commitment to quality care. As a result, many infusion companies seek accreditation from nonprofit organizations which provide recognition for qualified organizations. This voluntary accreditation process has become the "standard" to which all infusion companies are compared. Two accrediting bodies are the Joint Commission on Accreditation of Healthcare Organizations[4] (JCAHO) and the Community Health Accreditation Program[5] (CHAP). (See also Chapter 4.)

The following are common activities and responsibilities of pharmacists who provide home infusion services: (see also Chapter 1.)

- compounding parenteral solutions and medications using accepted standards of practice;
- dispensing/documentation and monitoring use of medications, catheter care and medical/surgical supplies;
- monitoring/documentation of side effects, adverse drug reactions, drug-drug and drug food interactions, and evidence of positive response to therapy (positive patient outcomes);
- coordinating the provision of appropriate medical/surgical supplies and distribution/delivery of the products to the patient's home;
- managing the purchasing function, and establishing appropriate guidelines and procedures for stock levels and inventory control;
- providing direct or indirect training/educational information in written or verbal form to patients, caregivers and nursing staff regarding enteral and parenteral pump programming, and routine operational function; aseptic technique and reconstitution/administration instructions; general medication information including; generic/trade name, intended use, dose, administration instructions, storage common side effects, unusual adverse reactions and practical/potential drug-drug or drug-food interactions;
- ongoing communications with nursing staff, referring and attending physicians, discharge planners, social workers, and other referral sources;
- providing initial and ongoing support for sales and marketing efforts, emphasizing the uniqueness and quality/level of services provided by the pharmacy; and,
- participating in quality assurance and quality improvement. (See also Chapter 4.)

MARKET ASSESSMENT AND SALES PLAN

In order to establish and maintain a successful home infusion pharmacy, several areas of business analysis must be performed prior to providing patient care.[6-9] An important first step is to plan and establish a data base to analyze the potential market for infusion services. Assessing the market may be the most difficult aspect of establishing a data base for the pharmacist. A market analysis of the intended geographic location of services must be conducted. Markets and referral sources should be analyzed, in order to select markets with the fewest competitors and with the greatest potential.

Components of Market Analysis

1. Market Size
   a. Investigate the number of hospitals, health maintenance organizations (HMO) and nursing homes that have the potential for patient referrals.
   b. Categorize the type of specialties offered in the hospital (e.g., pediatric, rehabilitation, hospice), and by physician groups. Certain physician groups are more likely to refer patients to the HHC pharmacy. These include infectious disease, gastroenterology, orthopedics, oncology, internists, general practitioners, neurologists, podiatrists, pulmonologists, and endocrinologists.
   c. Determine the patient population demographics, age, gender, economic status/payer mix (number of patients who are private pay vs. medicaid and medicare, discounted capitation, etc.), and urban or rural population.
   d. Evaluate the number of support services available to compliment the home infusion pharmacy, i.e., home health agencies

(HHA), visiting nurse association.
   e. Assess the competition. Know the services they provide, strengths and weaknesses, and marketing strategies.

2. Market Trends

These trends must be continually evaluated to determine their influence:
   a. patient population; growth or decline
   b. reimbursement demographic changes
   c. changes in the number of diagnoses of diseases treated with infusion therapy
   d. local changes in the economy of the region
   e. changes in the number and type of competitors in the area
   f. labor shortages or gluts, and wage/salary trends

3. Sales Planning

Developing a detailed sales plan is vital to the successful growth of any home infusion program. HHC patients are most commonly referred by case managers, physicians or discharge planners. Promoting the infusion pharmacy service is best accomplished by face-to-face meetings, but may also be accomplished through hand-carried or mailed literature. Many pharmacists are inadequately trained in formal sales skills and would probably benefit from working with a sales professional. These sales skills may be learned "on-the-job", or may be obtained through partnership or contracting with a sales consultant.

Tips for Making Sales Calls

1. Face-to-face sales call to referral sources
   a. Once an appointment has been scheduled, the total time allotted for the presentation will be short. Plan and organize any information or materials needed for the presentation ahead of time.
   b. When speaking with the referral source, thank them for the opportunity and time. Ask questions to determine the referral source's objectives or needs, and listen carefully to learn their "prime objective". Avoid prolonged casual conversation and stick to the sales point.
   c. By no means monopolize the conversation with the referral source. A 50/50 or 60/40 conversation with the referral source doing more of the talking should be the goal.
   d. The referral source will only retain approximately 10% of what is discussed, so keep the presentation simple and focused. Discuss the key services provided by the pharmacy service that distinguishes it from the competition.
2. Presentation or sales call to HHA
   a. These are usually related to current patients on service, or results from a request for information regarding infusion/enteral pumps, and/or equipment used by the pharmacy service.
   b. Educational seminars on new therapies, or in-services on parenteral/enteral pump equipment are common. The pharmacist should prepare an agenda for the presentation, with an outline or handout material of the subject matter to be discussed.
   c. Meetings to discuss clinical monitoring and updates of current patient information are also common. These may be accomplished via telephone conversations or face-to-face meetings.
3. Direct mailing of literature to referral sources
   a. The advantage of direct mailing is that specific information may be sent to the greatest number of referral sources in the shortest period of time.
   b. The direct mailing should consist of two mailings: First mailing is a formal announcement to all possible referral sources announcing the intent to provide services and what those services entail. Second mailing is a business letter introducing the program and discussing the services, include brochures and business cards.
4. Establish a referral source list which contains key information regarding each referral source, i.e., personal notes, likes/dislikes, professional information, and other items which may help in future sales calls.

A good sales plan involves return calls to referral sources to inform them of new services and therapies provided by the pharmacy, and to reacquaint them with the company. Informing the medical community and promoting the home infusion program should be a rewarding challenge, the results of which will produce increased revenues, if performed efficiently and effectively. The most important component in the promotion of the infusion is the provision of high quality service to patients and all referral sources.

Capital Investment and Pharmacy Design

The most costly portion of the initial capital investment and building process is the pharmacy case work (cabinetwork and shelving) and sterile compounding equipment. If adequate space already exists within a current licensed pharmacy, the initial expense can be considerably less than building a new licensed area. When an adequately sized refrigerator/freezer and suitable computer/printer already exists, the costs may be further minimized. Table 18-2 lists the typical expenses associated with equipping a home infusion pharmacy.

Physical Facilities

A sterile area for compounding of solutions and medications is essential. The sterile compounding area may exist within the pharmacy as a separate work area; however, it must be functionally separate from other activities. Traffic flow must be restricted to only sterile compounding activities. Separating the compounding activities from other areas of the pharmacy by building a separate clean room is the ideal approach. New proposed standards for sterile compounding may affect this aspect of the infusion pharmacy operations.[10,11] These proposed guidelines may require the construction of a filtered clean room, with attached anteroom. This filtration system increases the sterility of the compounding area, however, it will also increase the building cost. A separate work area for checking compounded items, labeling, paperwork/files and gathering of medical/surgical supplies is needed. When the infusion pharmacy has dedicated personnel to the operation and clinical services, specific work areas or offices should be planned for these individuals.

A work area for customer service representatives, pharmacists, nurses, accounts receivable, accounts payable and sales/marketing should be provided. When the infusion pharmacy employs a nurse(s) to support the administration and function of the operations, they should be located in proximity to the pharmacy operations. Communication between nursing and pharmacy staff is vital for smooth operations.

A warehouse for storage of large and small volume parenterals, legend drugs, legend and nonlegend medical/surgical supplies, OTC products, parenteral and enteral pumps, and IV poles is necessary. Purchasing and inventory control is an important component in ensuring the survival of an infusion pharmacy operation. Obtaining the best possible prices from wholesalers, pharmaceutical manufacturers and other vendors is crucial for maximizing the pharmacy's profit margin. Use of direct contracts with manufacturers will minimize the expenses of the wholesaler's handling fees. Group purchasing programs may provide substantial savings for small pharmacy operations. By estimating current and projected usage numbers, a goal to turn over inventory 9-12 times per year may be

Table 18-2 Initial Capital Costs

Case work	$10,000 — 20,000
Laminar Air Flow Hoods (Vertical and/or Chemotherapy)	3,500 — 8,000
Refrigerator/Freezer	1,000 — 2,000
Computer System & Printer	1,500 — 2,500
Balance with Weights	1,000
IV Cart	500
Incubator	400
Miscellaneous (Computer Labeling Package, References Anti-Fatigue Mats, Stools, etc.)	2,000
Estimated Total Expenses	$ 16,000 — 36,400

(Inventory, personnel, and related expenses are not included in capital costs.)

achieved using weekly or semimonthly ordering. The cost of goods sold should be kept as low as possible. Ideally with strict purchasing guidelines and excellent contracts, this number should be approximately 20-25% of total sales, but frequently is 30-45%.

PERSONNEL

Hiring and retaining qualified personnel to oversee the financial, operational and clinical activities is the key to the success of the infusion pharmacy program. Recruitment of qualified individuals who know the home infusion business well may prove to be a challenge because individuals with extensive HHC expertise are difficult to find. Reimbursement, pharmacy, and nursing functions are very different in the HHC arena compared to ambulatory and/or the acute care setting. Many skills are similar to those required for acute care/hospital operations and clinical care.

The costs involved in hiring and retaining professional personnel represents a major component of the infusion program's budget. Typical HHC staff include the following:

1. Customer Service Representative (CSR), Billing/Reimbursement: The CSR is extremely important in the HHC operation. These individuals generally gather initial admission information from the referral source and verify the patient's coverage with the payer source to determine acceptance of the case. Because reimbursement for home infusion therapies varies greatly, it is important to hire individuals with previous HHC medical billing experience. In a small operation, the billing function may be provided through an outside contracted service. However, the preferred operational structure is to include this function as part of the full-time staff.
2. Pharmacy Staff: The pharmacist must have current knowledge and skills regarding sterile compounding technique and equipment, parenteral and enteral delivery systems, and medical/surgical supplies used to support intravenous and central catheters. In a small start-up operation, one may elect to contract with a pharmacist who already possesses these skills. This function may also be accomplished through additional education at schools of pharmacy or continuing education programs, working with local hospitals, or hiring a consultant pharmacist to provide individual training. Several pharmaceutical manufacturers have produced video tapes which effectively train pharmacy personnel in sterile compounding technique, and are available upon request.

   Pharmacy technicians are an important asset to the home infusion pharmacy, and play a significant role in cutting costs and improving operational efficiency. When allowed by pharmacy state law, pharmacy technicians may be used for the common clerical and compounding functions. Important skills and knowledge necessary to perform the pharmacy technician function are related mainly to sterile technique and compounding of parenteral solutions.
3. Nursing Staff: The home infusion therapy nurse plays a vital role in the development of the overall home infusion program. Referral sources and patients frequently identify the quality of the product/program (pharmacy service) with the nurse providing care. In a small start-up operation the nursing component may be contracted out to a HHA, or independent certified IV nurse. Establishing a relationship with a Medicare-certified HHA within the geographic service area is very important, because they can supply the nursing component for patients in outlying locations, or for difficult patients that the pharmacy's nursing staff cannot service.
4. Sales Staff: As mentioned in a previous section of this chapter, the sales/marketing component is a very important function within the home infusion pharmacy program. Without the continual support of assertive sales staff to seek out new business and potential clientele for therapy, the infusion program may not prosper. In the initial weeks of the program the pharmacist and nurse can effectively be used as sales staff. As the business volume increases, it will become more difficult for the pharmacist or nurse to devote enough time to promote the program effectively. One should consider employing a person whose primary responsibility is focused on promoting the program to key referral sources and support organizations.

PATIENT SELECTION CRITERIA

Patients referred to the home infusion therapy program usually have no previous exposure to this form of health care delivery. A significant amount of information must be evaluated prior to accepting or rejecting a patient to the infusion program. An evaluation of the following criteria and questions is important in making the final determination:

Screening Referrals

1. Confirmation of reimbursement for services provided is the most important first step in making the decision to accept or reject patients. Understanding the process for verification of coverage from payer sources (managed care/ indemnified insurance programs, HMO, Medicare, Medicaid, etc.) is vital to the continued success of the infusion program.
2. The pharmacist should evaluate of the proposed therapy and services necessary to provide care including
   a. Can the therapy be administered safely in the home environment? What literature is currently available?
   b. What type of venous access will be used, and can the drug be administered safely using this device?
   c. What is the stability of the drug and mode of administration of the therapy?
   d. Is the drug readily available to the pharmacy? Is it approved for the intended use?
   e. Is staff adequately trained to compound and administer the therapy?
   f. Has the patient received the therapy previously in a controlled environment (hospital, clinic, home), and is the patient medically stable?
   g. Is the patient located within the normal geographic range, and can the therapy be delivered in a reasonable (safe) period of time that does not compromise patient care?
3. Evaluation of the home environment:
   a. Patient has a permanent/fixed address for delivery and administration of therapy;
   b. Home has adequate refrigerator/freezer storage space;
   c. Telephone is available for emergency calls;
   d. Environment is safe for administration of therapy; no electrical hazards, clean home environment, etc.
   e. Home has running water and electricity;
4. Evaluation of the patient/caregiver:
   a. Patient comprehends the extent of self-care, can read, and is willing to actively participate (or with help of caregiver) in the plan of treatment;
   b. Patient has appropriate intelligence, manual dexterity and eyesight which allows them to administer and monitor therapy when appropriate;
   c. Substance abuse potential is minimized.

PATIENT TRAINING AND EDUCATION

In order to successfully complete home infusion therapy, the patient and/or caregiver must be adequately taught the basics of drug administration, catheter care, and supplies/equipment management. Approximately 55-65% of medication administration and personal hygiene care is done by the patient's family and/or caregiver.[12]

A comprehensive education/training plan, which includes return demonstration of drug administration skills, is necessary to ensure that all components of the treatment plan are understood. It must be a simple process for the patient/caregiver to understand, yet be individualized for the specific and unique needs of each patient. Training time is dependent on the degree of difficulty of the therapy and the learning ability of the patient. Both written and verbal instruction should be presented, including information on storage and disposal.

Preprinted patient teaching instructions are available through several consulting firms, or may be developed internally by the nursing and pharmacy staff. The instruction process should include the following steps:

1. Introduction and initial patient assessment: This is the first meeting for the clinician and patient/caregiver. It usually takes place in the hospital or clinic setting, but may occur in the home at the first nursing visit. At this time the clinician explains the process of the treatment program and begins the paperwork to admit the patient on service. Assignment of benefits, rights and responsibilities, acknowledgment of financial responsibilities and other forms may be completed at this time (Appendix 18-A). The clinician should also try to set the patient's mind at ease by assuring the patient that the instruction process and follow-up visits will continue until the patient is independent, and can provide self-care.
2. Patient training materials: Verbal and written

instructions should be provided to the patient/caregiver during the subsequent teaching visits. All training should be documented in the patient's record. An in depth description of the infusion program, including the reason for a specific therapy, type of catheter care, administration schedule, right to medication counseling by the pharmacist, and overall goals and plan of treatment should be covered. If the small start-up operation does not have the resources to develop the teaching/training materials, they may be purchased. There are several commercially available programs that contain patient teaching materials, visual illustrations/aids and medication information sheets. In addition, pharmaceutical manufacturers have video tapes which are effective for patient teaching.

3. Observation of care through return demonstration: In this phase of training/education, the clinician observes the patient/caregiver perform the routine administration of medications, techniques of catheter care, and equipment management. The patient should be able to demonstrate to the clinician the ability to perform each necessary procedure correctly. The time required for this step varies, depending on the patient's/caregiver's ability and treatment modality.
4. Documentation of patient teaching: It is very important that clinicians document the patient's proficiency to correctly perform each task required to successfully administer the therapy prescribed. A patient teaching/training checklist may be developed for this documentation. A patient teaching checklist is included in Appendix 18-B.

Documentation By the Home Infusion Pharmacist

Documentation plays a significant role in the day-to-day functioning of a home infusion pharmacy. Clear and concise documentation of daily activities is necessary in order to perform normal operations. Correct documentation is also necessary to meet the requirements of federal and state laws/regulations, accreditation standards of practice, and to minimize the potential for litigation. Specific policies and procedures which address standards of practice, correct documentation and communications, incident/occurrence reporting and proper monitoring guidelines also reduce the chances for litigation.

It is the direct responsibility of the provider to ensure that the patient is able to assume the burden of self-care. When complications occur, accusations of failure to inform and properly train the patient/caregiver can complicate the issue, and may bring about litigation. Providers can reduce the risk to themselves by making certain that all aspects of patient care are properly documented, and that errors in communication are avoided.

ESTABLISHING POLICIES AND PROCEDURES

Policies and procedures should be established for all aspects of the home infusion program, include nursing services, pharmacy services, and operations. Within each service area the policies and procedures should outline the company's policy regarding specific aspects of operations or clinical practice and the procedures necessary to carry out the outlined policy. If the small start-up infusion program does not have resources necessary to develop the policies and procedures, they may be purchased from several commercially available sources. Consultants may also be hired to develop policies and procedures specific for the company's needs.

Quality Assurance/Improvement Program and Outcome Indicators

Over the last few years there has been a greater emphasis on improving the quality of care provided by home infusion therapy companies. In order to be competitive in the home infusion pharmacy market it is imperative to develop a quality assurance/improvement program. (See also Chapter 4.)

Currently most major referral/payer sources and JCAHO are requesting trending data on the home infusion therapy provider's quality assurance/improvement program. These referral sources are looking for data that indicates that the home infusion services are linked to improved patient outcomes, and have a positive influence on the disease process. The JCAHO has developed guidelines for "Indicators" of quality of care/service that meet these requirements.[13] These indicators should represent all disciplines of care provided by the infusion company, including nursing, pharmacy, equipment management and patient satisfaction. Examples of indicators include number/percentage of thrombophlebitis and catheter infections per year for the company; number of readmissions to the hospital per therapy; number of medication errors/occurrences recorded by pharmacy and/or nursing per year; and satisfaction of patients related to the providers services.

Development of pharmacy and nursing care plans are very important tools which can be used to emphasize to referral sources that positive patient outcomes can be directly linked to appropriate goal setting and patient monitoring.[14,15] The monitoring that is required by plans of care should be realistic because of the many operational duties of the clinicians. Follow-up documentation in the patient record that indicates that the care plans are being used, and are effective in accomplishing the intended goals, is crucial to the quality improvement program. If the infusion therapy company does not possess the expertise to develop this type of program, consultants may be hired to develop and implement the quality assurance/improvement program.

Another area of emphasis is patient/client satisfaction. Many referral/payer sources request data that show that patients serviced by the infusion therapy pharmacy are satisfied with all aspects of services provided. Positive results may show that patients are satisfied with the quality of care and services provided.

CONCLUSION

The home infusion pharmacy market is continuing to change. With the advent of managed care on the horizon, profit margins for many therapies will begin to erode, and the once lucrative home infusion market may begin to decrease. Many opportunities still exist in niche markets, and will continue to grow in these niche areas for the next few years. The successful pharmacy provider who will survive in the future will be very competitive, possess excellent clinical staff, and be operationally and financially efficient.

REFERENCES

1. Parver AK, Dozier JL. Itemizing Infusion: National Alliance for Infusion Therapy. Homecare 1992; 10:54-58.
2. Winters RW, et al. Home Infusion Therapy. Nat'l Alliance For Infusion Therapy, Washington DC 1993.
3. Anon. Managed Care Digest. Marion Merrell Dow, Kansas City, 1993.
4. Joint Commission on Accreditation of Health Care Organizations; One Renaissance Boulevard, Oakbrook Terrace, IL. 60181, (708) 916-5600.
5. Community Health Accreditation Program, Inc., A subsidiary of the National League of Nursing; 350 Hudson Street, New York, NY. 10014, (212) 989-9393.
6. Cherney A. Market Assessment. Homecare. 1993; 1(Supp.)12-14:21.
7. Kraemer P, Kraemer P. Components of a Strategic Plan. Homecare. 1992; 10:96-102.
8. Boesch D. Taking the First Steps to a Successful Intravenous Therapy Business. Consult. Pharm. 1993; 8(2):119-124.
9. Tanner DJ. Marketing Considerations in Home Health Care. Am Jour Hosp Pharm. 1985; 42:2695-99.
10. Draft Technical Assistance Bulletin on Quality Assurance for Pharmacy-prepared Sterile Products and Draft Guidelines on Compounding of Nonsterile Products in Pharmacies. Am Jour Hosp Pharm. 1993; 50(Jul):1440-52,1452-61.
11. Sterile Drug Products for Home Use. U.S.P. Forum [1206] 1993; 19(3):May-June, 5380-5409.
12. Conaway F. Marketing to Caregivers; A New Generation of Customer. Homecare. 1993; 8:134-135.
13. Joint Commission on Accreditation of Healthcare Organizations. Transitions: From QA to CQI; Using CQI Approaches to Monitor, Evaluate, and Improve Quality. 1991; 1-51.
14. Gold ML, Feduer DO. Developing a Pharmaceutical Care Plan. U.S. Pharmacist 1992; 10:53-60.
15. Brushwood DB, et al. OBRA 90; What It Means to Your Practice. U.S. Pharmacist 1992; 10:64-74.

Appendix 18-A Consent Form for Home Parenteral/Enteral Therapy

1. I ___________________________, have agreed to participate in the home infusion pharmacy program.

2. I am aware of and understand the risks and benefits involved in the therapy, and agree to abide by the rules and guidelines as outlined in the treatment protocol.

3. I understand either myself or my caregiver will be trained to self-administer this therapy.

4. I understand I have the right to ask any questions and receive answers during my participation in this program.

5. I may withdraw from the infusion program at any time.

6. I assign to the provider any and all insurance benefits otherwise payable to me for services provided. I request payment of authorized Medicare, Medicaid or other carrier benefits to, or on my behalf, for any services furnished to me by the provider.

7. I authorize the provider to disclose all or any part of my medical record to any third party payer who might be responsible for the bill, including but not limited to, Medicare and Medicaid, indemnified insurance companies, workers' compensation carriers, or the employer of the person responsible for the bill. Release of information will be limited to that which is necessary to obtain payment for services rendered by the provider.

8. I acknowledge that the provider has informed me of my right to declare any advanced directives and living wills as allowed by the state.

9. I have been informed by the provider of their policies and procedures regarding the return of goods, and understand that now medications or legend items may be returned to the pharmacy.

Patient Signature: ______________________________ Date: _______

Witness: ________________________________

Appendix 18-B Patient Teaching Checklist

Patient's Name:____________________ Evaluating Nurse:____________________
Physician:________________ Hospital:__________________ Date:______________
Additional Person Trained:________________________ Relationship:____________

Procedure	Initial	Minimal Help	Independent	Comments and/or Recommendations
1. Introduction to Home Therapy A. Understands Theory, Purpose				
B. Understands Policies Including: • Returned Goods Including Defective Equipment • Forms to be Signed • Delivery of Supplies • Inventories • Nurses Role and On-Call System				
2. Basis Aseptic Technique A. Environmental Preparation				
B. Hand washing				
C. Use of Sterile Equipment				
3. Catheter Dressing Changes A. Type of Catheter				
B. Method and Frequency				
C. Showering, Bathing, Swimming				
D. Site Observation				
4. Handling of Solution A. Storage				
B. Preparation for Infusion				
5. Admixture A. Prescription Interpretation				
B. Labels				
C. Inspection				
D. Units of Measure				
E. Method of Admixing (Adding Vitamins)				
6. Solution Administration A. Pump - Type				
B. Infusion Sets, Filters				
C. Lipids				
D. Ancillary Medications				
E. Sets Up Infusion				
F. Begin Infusion, Set Rate				
G. Terminate Infusion				

Appendix 18-B Patient Teaching Checklist (cont.)

Procedure	Initial	Minimal Help	Independent	Comments and/or Recommendations
7. Heparinization A. Method				
B. Frequency				
8. Self Monitoring A. Weight				
B. Urine Testing				
C. Intake and Output				
D. Temperature				
9. Complications & Trouble Shooting A. Mechanical				
B. Metabolic				
C. Discontinuing IV (Support Person)				
10. Understanding Emergency Procedures, knows who to call if having problems				
11. Proper Disposal of Contaminated Equipment				
12. Supply and /or Usage Changes				
A.				
B.				
C.				

13. Remarks:

______________________________ ______________________________

Patient Signature Date Instructor Signature Date

______________________________ ____________________

Additional Person Trained Date Relationship

19 Pumps, Controllers, and Catheters

Robert A. Louie, Pharm.D. and
Barbara C. Bolinger, Pharm.D.

Inpatients who have been stabilized on sophisticated parenteral drug therapy may require a high degree of medical monitoring but not hospitalization. These increasingly complex therapies may be administered in home health care (HHC) settings. Types of intravenous medications that HHC patients may receive include antibiotics, cancer chemotherapies, antithrombolytics, fluid and electrolyte replacement regimens (i.e., hydration), inotropic therapy, iron overload therapy, analgesics, nutrition and tocolytic therapy. Due to the nature of these therapies, infusions may be administered by a variety of electronic infusion devices. This chapter will describe the different types of home infusion pumps and controllers, and the criteria that should be considered when selecting a pump for patient use. In addition, the various catheters that may be used in ambulatory patients receiving infusion therapy will be discussed.

CLASSIFICATION OF ELECTRONIC INFUSION DEVICES

Home electronic infusion devices may be designed as either pumps or controllers. Pumps generate pressure to deliver intravenous (IV) fluids while controllers rely on gravity to create the driving force for the delivery of the solution. Controllers are used for the administration of noncritical and nonviscous fluids. The flow rate of controllers is usually regulated by the counting of drops in a reservoir chamber. Since controllers do not generate a positive infusion force, minor occlusions can impede fluid flow. In some instances, raising the height of the infusion container may overcome the impedance and resume the proper infusion rate.

Pumps may generate a positive infusion pressure by one of several methods. The first method is described as a linear peristaltic mechanism, whereby fingerlike projections move the fluid through the IV tubing to the patient. In some pumps, a section of the IV tubing is wrapped around a rotary cam and the rate of fluid administration is regulated by the speed of the cam rotation. This type of propulsion is called rotary peristaltic. In both types of peristaltic systems, fluid flow is unidirectional since the projections or cam compress the tubing from the IV container to the patient in a successive fashion. (See Table 19-1.)

Another mechanism by which pumps infuse fluids is through the use of a cassette or syringe that is incorporated into the administration set. In this method, the cassette/syringe sequentially fills and then delivers the fluid in a pulsating manner. The rate of infusion is controlled either by the filling volume or the frequency of compressions.

In general, pumps provide a more accurate and consistent infusion of therapies and therefore are most commonly used in those therapies where an irregular delivery could be potentially harmful to the patient. Therapies that may cause harm include pain management, cancer chemotherapies and some antibiotics. While pumps may be more precise in drug delivery, they also tend to be more expensive than controller devices. In addition, some types of therapies do not require a high degree of fluid control. In the study conducted by Winters, et al., 30% of patients receiving antibiotics used the gravity method for drug administration.[1] Since antibiotics are usually administered on a scheduled basis for a period of weeks, patients can incorporate infusions into their daily routine.

Parenteral nutrition therapies should always be infused by a pump. This type of therapy is commonly administered over twelve to fourteen hours each day especially at night. More advanced pumps are capable of special programming which allows tapering or ramping of infusion rates. In ramping of rates the fluids are initially administered

Table 19-1 Representative Pumps

	Pump Mechanism	Flow Rates KVO (a) Infusion Volume	Alarms	Power Requirements (Battery Operation)	Dimensions: H x W x D (Weight)
LifeCare 4 Abbott Laboratories, Abbott Park, IL	Piston-actuated diaphragm cassette	1-999 ml/hr KVO 1-4 ml/hr 1-9999 ml	Upstream & downstream occlusions, infusion complete, air in line, flow error, low battery, depleted battery	105-129 VAC, 60 Hz, (6 hours at 50 ml/hr)	8 x 9 x 11 (12 pounds)
Flo-Gard 6200 Baxter Healthcare Deerfield, IL	Linear peristaltic	1-999 ml/hr KVO 1-5 ml/hr 1-9999 ml	Upstream & downstream occlusions, infusion complete, air in line, flow error, door open, low battery, depleted battery	115 VAC, 60 Hz (6 hours at 125 ml/hr)	9.5 x 6 x 11 (14 pounds)
Gemini PC-1 IMED Corporation San Diego, CA	Linear peristaltic	0.1-999 ml/hr KVO < 1ml/hr 0.1-9999 ml Note: Device can function as pump or controller	Upstream & downstream occlusions, infusion complete, air in line, flow error, door open, low battery, depleted battery	90-130 VAC, 50/60 Hz (5 hours at 125 ml/hr)	8 x 6.5 x 10.75 (9.5 pounds)
560 IVAC Corporation San Diego, CA	Linear peristaltic	0.1-999 ml/hr KVO 5 ml/hr 1-9999 ml	Upstream & downstream occlusions, infusion complete, air in line, flow error, door open, low battery, depleted battery	95-135 VAC, 50/60 Hz (5 hours at 125 ml/hr)	11 x 5 x 7 (14 pounds)

(a) Flow rate to keep vein open (KVO)

slowly, then gradually increased and maintained at that rate for a prolonged period. As the infusion nears completion, the infusion rate is again slowed. The purpose of this type of administration is to minimize the possibility of rebound hypoglycemia which may result from a sudden increase in carbohydrates followed by a sudden decrease as the parenteral nutrition is completed.[2]

Alarms

Most pumps and controllers alert the user when one of the following situations occur: air in IV line detected; occlusion or high pressure which may prevent IV fluid flow; door/latch open; cartridge improperly inserted; low volume of IV fluid remaining; end of the infusion program; and, off mode status. The alerting formats are usually audible and/or visual alarms which require the operator to correct the situation before the infusion can continue.

The need to prevent the "free flow" of the IV fluids has recently become an important issue. During 1991, there were five documented incidents in hospital settings in which an IV infusion set was removed from the infusion device without clamping the tubing. This resulted in free-flow of the IV fluid into the patient. Two instances resulted in patient deaths.[3] Consequently, most institutions have now initiated policies and procedures which mandate that IV pumps and controllers utilize IV tubing sets which prevent free-flow. These sets have clamps which automatically close before removal from the infusion device. Free flow cannot occur unless the clamp is manually (purposely) opened by the operator. Unfortunately, anti-free-flow IV sets also have an increased cost over unprotected sets.

AMBULATORY INFUSION PUMPS

In the past five years there has been an

increase in the number of ambulatory infusion pumps which have application in HHC practice. These pumps have the advantage of being small enough that patients can receive infusion therapies without significantly disrupting their activities of daily living. Older patients prefer these ambulatory pumps because they weigh less and are less intrusive. However, these same patients may be intimidated by the electronic gadgetry and the array of audible pump alarms.

The ambulatory pumps utilize drive mechanisms which are similar to the full size bedside pumps with the exception of their smaller size. The ambulatory pumps range in weight up to 31 ounces, compared to twelve pounds or more for a standard hospital IV pump. (See Table 19-2.) In addition, the standard pump requires an IV pole while the ambulatory pump can usually be carried in a small pouch or fanny pack.

While the ambulatory pumps have the ability to infuse fluids from a standard IV bag, most of these pumps use a minibag, syringe or cassette to contain the drug. The choice of the container may be determined by the volume of fluid to be administered which is a function of the drug concentration. The minibag has the advantage of being interchangeable with other pumps and thus could decrease the cost of disposables. The cassette system is essentially a minibag within a plastic housing. This arrangement makes the cassette unique to a specific brand of pump and cannot be used by other pump manufacturers. Each cassette requires individualized preparation. In addition, the cost for the empty cassettes is significantly higher than minibags or syringes of similar volume. While these factors may make the cassette system seem undesirable, some patients are more comfortable using this type of drug container since the drug is more protected within the plastic housing. This preference is especially true with patients receiving cancer chemotherapy. Because the cassette is attached to the pump, there is no separate IV bag and thus the pump is more compact. If large volumes of fluids must be administered, a "pass through" cassette is available to allow use of the pumping mechanism, but necessitates the use of a separate IV bag.

Pumps are available which are capable of using prefilled syringes that can minimize preparation costs and manufacturing time by the pharmacist or technician. However, it should be noted that some patients have an aversion to syringes and may be opposed to using this type of infusion pump.

The ambulatory infusion pumps have many of the alarm features as the larger bedside pumps. The battery condition is a significant feature for the ambulatory pumps since this is the primary source of power. Most pumps alert the operator when the battery power is low but still capable of driving the pump. An additional alarm occurs when the battery is "dead" and the pump cannot be powered. This type of alarm allows the patient to replace the battery with minimal disruption of the infusion. Due to the ambulatory pump's smaller size, alarms may not be as noticeable by the patient. Visual alarms usually require the patient to read an LED message and audible alarms are at a lower volume than bedside pumps. Elderly patients have an especially difficult time being alerted to an ambulatory pump's alarms. All patients should be instructed to check the pump display periodically during the day to insure proper operation.

One reason for the increased use of ambulatory infusion pumps in the HHC setting is the range of infusion capabilities. Despite their relatively small size, these pumps have many of the same capabilities as the larger bedside pumps. These pumps can be programmed to deliver medication either by continuous infusion, intermittent infusion with or without a baseline infusion, continuous infusion with patient controlled bolus, large volume infusion over a prolonged period of time, very low infusion rates to maintain the patency of the vein, referred to as KVO, or keep vein open.

Continuous Infusion

This type of infusion is commonly used for therapies where there is no need to adjust the infusion rate. Patients receive infusions at a constant rate (e.g., ml/hr, ml/day). If the medication can be administered at a higher concentration, the patient may be able to receive a longer course of medication with fewer cassette or IV bag changes. Examples of continuous infusions are cancer chemotherapy, antithrombolytics, tocolytics and stable pain control.

Intermittent Infusions

Intermittent infusions are utilized primarily with antibiotic regimens. Patients can receive a 24 hour supply of medication without having to use separate IV bags or change the pump fluid container. Some pumps require a small basal flow (e.g., 0.2 ml/hr) between the primary infusions while others are

Table 19-2 Representative Ambulatory Infusion Devices

	Infusion Delivery	Flow Rates (a)	Pump Mechanism (Power source)	Reservoir	Dimensions H x W x D Weight (w/batteries)
CADD-1 (Model 5100 HFX), Pharmacia-Deltec, St. Paul, MN	Continuous only	1-299 ml/day	Linear peristaltic (9V Alkaline)	Cassette, Bag adaptor	6.3 x 3.5 x 1.1 (15 ounces)
CADD-Plus (Model 5400), Pharmacia-Deltec, St. Paul, MN	Continuous, Intermittent	0.1-75 ml/hr KVO 0.2-10 ml/hr	Linear peristaltic (9V Alkaline)	Cassette, Bag adaptor	6.3 x 3.5 x 1.1 (15 ounces)
CADD-PCA (Model 5800), Pharmacia-Deltec, St. Paul, MN	Continuous, PCA bolus	0-20 ml/hr (0-99.5 mg/hr)	Linear peristaltic (9V Alkaline)	Cassette, Bag adaptor	6.3 x 3.5 x 1.1 (15 ounces)
CADD-TPN (Model 5700), Pharmacia-Deltec, St.Paul, MN	Continuous w/wo taper	10-400 ml/hr	Linear peristaltic (9V Alkaline)	Bag adaptor	5.3 x 3.5 x 1.1 (13 ounces)
Provider One Plus, Abbott Laboratories, Abbott Park, Il	Continuous w/wo taper	1-250 ml/hr KVO 1 ml/hr	Rotary peristaltic (Two 9V Alkaline)	No captive reservoir	5.2 x 3.4 x 1.3 (14 ounces)
Provider 5500, Abbott Laboratories, Abbott Park, IL	Continuous, Intermittent, PCA bolus	0.1-250 ml/hr (0.1-9999.9 mg/hr) KVO 0.1 ml/hr	Rotary peristaltic (Two 9V Alkaline)	No captive reservoir	5.2 x 3.4 x 1.3 (14 ounces)
Bard Ambulatory PCA, Bard MedSystems, North Reading, MA	Continuous, PCA bolus	0-20 ml/hr	Linear peristaltic (9V Lithium)	Bag (Up to 250 ml)	3.4 x 4.7 x 1.2 (11 ounces)
Bard Cormed III, Bard MedSystems, North Reading, MA	Continuous only	0.1- 9.99 ml/hr	Linear peristaltic (9V Alkaline)	Bag (100 ml & 250 ml)	3.4 x 4.7 x 1.2 (11 ounces)
Infu-Med 300, MedFusion Inc., Duluth, GA	Continuous only	0.1-9.9 ml/hr	Linear peristaltic (9V Alkaline)	No captive reservoir	4.1 x 4.4 x 1.8 (12 ounces)
Infu-Med 420 I/C, MedFusion Inc., Duluth, GA	Continuous, Intermittent	0.1-30 ml/hr KVO 0-9.9 ml/hr	Linear peristaltic (9V Alkaline)	No captive reservoir	4.1 x 4.4 x 1.8 (12 ounces)
Infu-Med 430 PCA, MedFusion Inc., Duluth, GA	Continuous, PCA bolus	0.1-30 ml/hr (0-199.9 mg/hr)	Linear peristaltic (9V Alkaline)	No captive reservoir	4.1 x 4.4 x 1.8 (12 ounces)
WalkMed 440 PIC, MedFusion, Inc., Duluth, CA	Continuous, intermittent, bolus PCA	0.01-19.99 ml/hr	Linear peristaltic (9V Alkaline)	No captive reservoir	4.1 x 4.4 x 1.8 (12 ounces)

(a) KVO is the flow rate necessary to keep the vein open.

capable of no infusion at all. The effect of basal fluid flow on the patency of the IV line has not been determined.

Continuous Infusion With Controlled Bolus

Patients receiving pain management therapies utilize infusions which allow them to control bolus injections while also receiving a baseline infusion of analgesic. This type of therapy is referred to as patient controlled analgesia (PCA). (See also Chapter 22.) These bolus injections are intended to provide relief for any uncontrolled pain which can vary depending on the time of day and physical activity of the patient. This type of pain is referred to as breakthrough pain and is characteristically seen in oncology patients who become refractory to conventional types of oral or intermittent injections of narcotics.[4] Pumps for PCA have the additional feature of regulating the time period between bolus injections and/or limiting the number of bolus injections per hour. The number of bolus injections given as well as the total amount of medication administered (i.e., baseline plus bolus doses) can be retrieved from the pump memory. This feature can be of value to the clinician in determining whether to adjust the baseline infusion rate. More sophisticated pumps can also record the number of attempted bolus injections. If there is a significantly larger number of attempted vs. administered bolus injections, the patient may need a more immediate adjustment to the baseline infusion rate. These attempts could also indicate that the patient is dependent upon the narcotic, or does not believe that the pump is actually administering any medication. In both instances, evaluation of the patient's regimen and their understanding of pump operation is important. Representative PCA pumps are listed in Table 19-2.

Large Volume Infusions

Therapies which require a tapering infusion rate will utilize pumps which are capable of sophisticated programming with minimal impact on the patient. Parenteral nutrition regimens commonly use this type of infusion. Since this therapy is usually given at night, patients simply start the infusion and go to sleep. There is no need to awaken during the night to adjust the infusion rate. A special backpack carrier is necessary to hold the infusion pump and IV bag due to the large volume of IV fluid to be administered. While this type of therapy can be termed ambulatory, many patients tend to limit their physical activities because of the weight of the pump and IV bag. In addition, parenteral nutrition infusions produce a constant drain on the power source and batteries may be depleted after a short period (e.g., four hours). Thus, most patients utilize AC adapters which can be plugged into an electrical outlet. Battery power is reserved for short outings where electrical current is not readily available.

DISPOSABLE PUMPS

Disposable infusion pumps are sometimes referred to as elastomeric pumps. The IV fluid is contained in an elastomeric membrane and produces a positive pressure which supplies the medication at a preset infusion rate for short periods of time (i.e., 24 hours). Patients may prefer the disposable pumps since these weigh less than electronic infusion devices and may not interfere with their daily activities. IV poles and batteries are not necessary, and patients seem to be less intimidated with these pumps since there is no electronic gadgetry. In addition, the pumps produce no noise when operating.

Preparation of the earlier versions of these pumps was laborious and in some instances hazardous if cytotoxic drugs were used. A tremendous amount of manual pressure was required to fill the elastomeric membrane. Consequently, "back spray" and leakage could occur. Despite these problems, disposable infusion pumps may cost less than electronic infusion devices.

In recent years, tremendous improvements have also been made with disposable infusion pumps. Newer versions of disposable pumps have been made safer by incorporating a valve which allows IV fluids to flow in one direction only. This design eliminates the possibility of backspray. In some instances, pump manufacturers have developed special devices to expedite the filling of pumps so that pumps can be filled faster and in larger quantities. In recognition of the great potential for disposable devices, manufacturers have developed pumps with a wide range of preset flow rates (0.5 ml/hr to 250 ml/hr). This feature allows them to be used for both continuous and intermittent infusions of medications. The lower infusion rates allow patients to receive a longer courses of therapy (i.e., 5 day course) with a single pump.

Disposable pumps are available in different volume capacities. This feature increases the number of medications that can be administered by disposable pumps, because stability is often a function of drug concentration. Refrigerating or freezing pumps might allow providers to supply patients with an entire course of therapy and thus minimize deliveries. Training of patients and caregivers is still necessary with disposable infusion pumps. They must be instructed on aseptic connecting and disconnecting of the pump from the IV catheter. However, the lack of programming steps, battery changes, and alarms makes this training less rigorous and intimidating to the patient.

More recently, a reusable pump with disposable inserts has been marketed. The pump produces positive pressure using a spring system. This new system utilizes the advantages of the disposable pumps (i.e., light weight and size) with the added benefit of decreased cost of disposables (i.e., insert). The only constraint is the volume capacity which limits application to certain medications.

Disposable infusion devices provide another alternative to administering medications to patients at home. They are especially attractive when short courses of therapy are desired and when patients or caregivers have limited abilities. Representative disposable pumps are detailed in Table 19-3.

NEW TECHNOLOGY

New advancements continue to be made in pump technology. Most of these high technology pumps have been designed for the hospital setting but some are being marketed directly for the HHC environment. There are a growing number of devices that have multiple channel abilities. These multi-channel pumps may be programmed to infuse

Table 19-3 Representative Disposable Pumps

	Flow Rate	Capacity	Wear Time	Special Features
Infusors Baxter Healthcare Deerfield, Il	2.0 ml/hr 0.5 ml/hr 2.0 ml/hr 0.5 ml/hr	65 ml 65 ml 100 ml 95 ml	24 hours 5 days 2 days 7 days	Elastomeric pressure driven
Intermates Baxter Healthcare Deerfield, IL	50 ml/hr 100 ml/hr 200 ml/hr 250 ml/hr 50 ml/hr 100 ml/hr	105 ml 105 ml 105 ml 275 ml 275 ml 275 ml	2 hours 1 hour 0.5 hour 1 hour 5 hours 2.5 hours	Elastomeric pressure driven
Homepump Block Medical, Inc. Carlsbad, CA	50 ml/hr 100 ml/hr 200 ml/hr 2 ml/hr 5 ml/hr 175 ml/hr	60 ml 110 ml 110 ml 110 ml 110 ml 205 ml	1 hour 1 hour 0.5 hour 2 days 1 day 1 hour	Elastomeric pressure driven, In line filter to remove and particulate matter
Paragon Ambulatory Pump I-Flow Corporation Irvine, CA	0.5 ml/hr 1.0 ml/hr 2.0 ml/hr 4.0 ml/hr	110 ml 110 ml 110 ml 110 ml	8 days 4 days 2 days 1 day	Spring driven, Reusable pump, Disposable bag insert, In line air-eliminating filter
Sidekick I-Flow Corporation Irvine, CA	50 ml/hr 100 ml/hr 200 ml/hr	50 ml 50 ml 50 ml	1 hour 0.5 hour 0.25 hour	Spring driven, Reusable pump, Disposable bag insert, In line air-eliminating filter

more than one medication from either an IV bag or syringe. In its simplest form, the multi-channel pump is merely two pumps in one that operate independently of each other. This arrangement allows patients to have only one pump device and provides them with greater physical stability when walking.

Other pumps have up to four channel capabilities. These pumps deliver four separate medications as continuous or intermittent infusions, and in some instances, the operator can program a flush between incompatible drugs. Obviously these types of pumps are reserved for more complex therapies and are more commonly seen in intensive care and bone marrow transplant units. Examples of multiple channel pumps are listed in Table 19 - 4.

New technology has also been applied to the programming of pumps. Some pumps are now capable of bar code reading to simplify the programming process. In the HHC setting, bar codes could be attached to the IV bag and the patient would scan the pump directions prior to each dose. Theoretically, this feature should decrease the likelihood of programming errors especially when the patient receives multiple therapies.

The Intelliject® pump by Ivion is controlled by a special computer chip which has been programmed using an external computer. Complex infusions by circadian administration (i.e., variable drug doses during a specific time period) can be

Table 19-4 Representative Pumps with Multiple Channel Capabilities

	Pump Mechanism Number of Channels	Flow Rates KVO (a)	Dimensions H x W x D (Weight)	Features
LifeCare Omni-Flow 4000 Abbott Laboratories Abbott Park, IL	Piston diaphragm Four channels	1.4-800 ml/hr KVO 1-99.9 ml/hr	11.3 x 9.1 x 7 (13.25 pounds)	Can deliver up to four fluids at independent rates, automatic flush between medication infusions, automatic air elimination. Infusion delivery: continuous and intermittent
LifeCare Plum 5000 Abbott Laboratories Abbott Park, IL	Piston diaphragm Two channels	0.1-999 ml/hr KVO 1 ml/hr	7 x 9 x 9 (13 pounds)	Can deliver two fluids at independent rates, can function as pump or controller. Infusion delivery: continuous and intermittent
Provider 6000 Abbott Laboratories Abbott Park, IL	Rotary peristaltic Two channels	0.1-250 ml/hr KVO 0-1 ml/hr	6.8 x 4.7 x 2.2 (31 ounces)	Can deliver two fluids at independent rates, channels can be programmed to start at different times. Infusion delivery: continuous, intermittent, bolus PCA
Gemini PC-2 IMED Corporation San Diego, CA	Linear peristaltic Two channels	0.1-500 ml/hr (C) 0.1-999 ml/hr (P) KVO 1 ml/hr	11.9 x 10.6 x 7.2 (18.5 pounds)	Can deliver two fluids at independent rates, can function as pump or controller. Infusion delivery: continuous
Intelliject Ivion Corporation Broomfield, CO	Rack and pinion drive Four channels	0.3-40.54 ml/hr	9.9 x 6.5 x 2.8 (3.4 pounds)	Can deliver four fluids at independent rates, channels can be programmed to start at different times, flush between medication infusions. Infusion delivery: continuous, intermittent, bolus PCA, circadian administration, Requires computer chip programming

(a) KVO is the flow rate necessary to keep the vein open.

delivered to a patient with minimal pump manipulation.

Some pumps allow communication between the clinician and patient by way of a telephone modem. Patient requirements can be monitored by the clinician and infusion adjustments can be made from a great distance. This remote control ability might be especially attractive with pain management patients who have less stable therapies. These new methods of programming have only been incorporated into devices with multiple channel deliveries. However, it is possible that the same technology might be applied to single and dual pumps in the future. With the pending changes in health care in the United States, it is possible that more complex therapies will be administered in the home using these technologically advanced devices. See also Table 19-5.

JCAHO REQUIREMENTS

The Joint Commission on Accreditation of Health Care Organizations (JCAHO) has specific guidelines regarding equipment utilized in the HHC setting. Since all types of infusion devices are included as equipment, clinicians should be familiar with these guidelines. It is beyond the scope of this chapter to cover all aspects of the requirements and the reader should refer to "Equipment Management" in the JCAHO manual.[5,6] (See also Chapter 4.)

In general, these guidelines address the selection, delivery, setup and maintenance of pumps so that the needs of the patient are met. Training and education of the provider and patient are also discussed. Topics include equipment safety checks and troubleshooting; routine and emergency response procedures; communication and teaching skills of the provider; access to 24 hour emergency services for

Table 19-5 Representative New Technology Pumps

	Pump Mechanism	Flow Rates KVO (a)	Dimensions H x W x D (Weight)	Features
Verifuse Block Medical, Inc Carlsbad, CA	Linear peristaltic	0.1-300 ml/hr KVO 0.1 ml/hr	6.4 x 3.1 x 1.1 (16 ounces)	Can be programmed, monitored and verified at a remote site, can be programmed using bar codes. Infusion delivery: continuous. intermittent, PCA bolus. Requires: pump programmer and modem
Vivus-4000 I-Flow Corporation Irvine, CA	Linear peristaltic	0.1-200 ml/hr KVO 0.1-5 ml/hr	7.8 x 4.5 x 1.9 (37 ounces)	Can be programmed, monitored and verified at a remote site, can deliver up to four fluids at independent rates, also available as a two channel pump (Vivus-4000/2), optional printer provides record of therapy. Infusion delivery: continuous, intermittent, PCA bolus. Requires: pump programmer and modem
Ally Ambulatory Drug Infusion System Q-Life Systems, Inc. Kingston, Ontario, Canada	Spring driven NOTE: This pump is scheduled for 1994 release in the United States	0.1-30 ml/hr KVO 0.1-10 ml/hr	3.2 x 2.2 x 0.8 (3 ounces)	Programmed vial optical link, very small and lightweight, uses manufacturer cassette system (50 & 100 ml), optional printer provides record of therapy. Infusion delivery: continuous, intermittent, PCA bolus. Requires: pump programmer

(a) KVO is the flow rate necessary to keep the vein open.

equipment maintenance or replacement; procedures to receive, clean, and sterilize (if appropriate) reusable items; documentation of the manufacturer, model, serial number, and maintenance instructions; process for obtaining timely and accurate information about equipment hazards, defects, and recalls; monitoring of the safety and working condition of pumps; and patient education provided by a qualified individual.

PUMP SELECTION

Several aspects must be considered in the selection of infusion devices. The first consideration is the type of therapy to be delivered. For example, whether the patient is to receive hydration or chemotherapy by continuous infusion, antibiotics by intermittent infusion, or pain management by continuous and bolus infusion will dictate the required pump capabilities. The length of therapy will also impact the selection of pumps. If therapy is of short duration, disposable pumps may be the most cost effective. An electronic pump may be a better choice with longer courses since multiple daily doses require fewer line manipulations.

Operational aspects of the pump should also be considered. How user friendly a pump is may affect the patient's therapy. Programming should be simple and logical for the patient, caregiver, pharmacist and nurse. Many after hour calls are due to programming problems and clinicians need to be able to relay instructions by phone to patients.

Selecting a pump will also depend on the needs of the clinician, such as in pain management therapies where bolus doses given and attempted may determine the need to adjust baseline infusions. A desirable feature of some pumps is the ability to produce a hard copy printout of patient pump parameters. This printout will provide a summary of the patient's therapy, and may serve as quick documentation for the patient's chart.

Obviously, the cost of a pump is a primary consideration. It is important to include the cost of IV administration sets and any additional equipment (e.g., manifolds, syringes, caps) when calculating total expenses for pump usage. Pumps which can use universal type IV administration sets will have lower operating costs.

Manufacturer support is another factor when selecting an IV pump. Support can be provided in many ways. Most pump manufacturers have a variety of training materials ranging from printed manuals to instructional videotapes intended for patients and clinicians. These types of teaching aids are of great help when training the patient and caregiver. Technical assistance should be available 24 hours a day to help resolve problems that the clinician might encounter. The manufacturer should be able to provide maintenance and repair service. If pumps need to be returned to the manufacturer, loaner pumps should be available at minimal cost. Finally, the manufacturer should keep the clinician informed of pump improvements with the possibility of upgrading existing inventories.

The purchase of IV pumps represent a capital expenditure that can have a significant impact on the provision of services to HHC patients. Selection of an appropriate pump can minimize complications and unnecessary deliveries to the patient's home. While no single pump can be used for all patients, clinicians should select pumps which have the greatest application for their patient population.

VENOUS ACCESS DEVICES

Innovations in the design of venous access devices for home IV patients have facilitated the expansion of home IV therapy. Peripheral catheters, central catheters, and implantable ports have become relatively routine components in HHC practice. A special consideration for infusion therapy patients at home is the need for maximum patient self-sufficiency in light of sporadic nursing support. Caring for HHC patients with venous catheters requires special knowledge about appropriate catheter maintenance. See Table 19-6.

Peripheral Catheters

Peripheral venous access catheters are the most commonly used means to establish IV access and may have a variety of uses in the hospitalized patient. For home use, however, these lines are converted to a heparin lock by the addition of a resealable injection cap and are most often used for short-term (less than two weeks) administration of intermittent fluids or blood sampling.[7] Traditional peripheral catheters, due to their rigidity, may subject the patient to an increase in associated problems such as phlebitis (both mechanical and chemical) and infiltrating IV sites which are common and may result in unscheduled nursing visits.[8]

Types of Peripheral Catheters

Table 19-6 Peripheral and Central Catheter Care[14]

TYPE OF CATHETER	INDICATION	FLUSHING	CAP CHANGE/ SITE CARE
Peripheral Catheters (Abbocath, Jelco, Quick-Cath, Surflo)	Short-term therapy, Quick venous access	Heparin: 1 ml (100U/ml) Q12 hrs and after each use. Saline: 1ml before and after each use or Q12 hrs if not used.	Cap : Q72 hrs Site: Every 3 days.
Peripherally Inserted Central Catheter (PICC)	Access beyond 7 days	Heparin: 2.5-3 ml (100 U/ml) Q12-24 hrs, and after each use. Saline: 3 ml before and after each use or Q12-24 hrs if not used.	Cap: Q72 hrs (clamp before removal of cap). Site: Every 3 days.
Central Venous Catheters (Hickman, Broviac, Leonard)	Long-term central access	Heparin: 2.5 ml (100U/ml) after each use or Q12-24 hrs. Saline: 2.5 ml before and after each use or Q12-24 hrs if not used	Cap: Every 7 days. Site: Every 7 days.
Groshong Central Venous Catheter	Long-term access, Patients allergic to heparin	Heparin: DO NOT USE Saline: 5 ml after each use or Q7days if not being used.	Cap: Every 7 days. Site: Every 7 days.
Implanted Port (Port-a-Cath, Infus-a-Port)	Long-term access	Heparin: 5 ml (100U/ml) after each use and Q4weeks if not used. Saline: 5 ml before and after each use or Q4weeks if not in use.	Cap: NOT REQUIRED, Site: Every 3 days when in use. Not needed when not in use.

Abbocath®, Jelco®, Quick-Cath®, and Surflo® are examples of peripheral catheters. These catheters are inserted directly in a vein in the hand or arm and are made of teflon or other synthetic materials. They are fairly inexpensive and relatively easy for a registered nurse to insert in the patient's home, provided the patient does not have compromised venous access. These catheters are normally primed with 1 ml of fluid, depending on the type of extension set being used. When using this type of catheter in the home, it is advisable to utilize an extension set in order to lessen the stress on the insertion site of the catheter and ultimately allow for decreased vein irritation and longer indwelling time. Therapies often administered include isotonic fluids, medications, blood transfusions, and as a means of obtaining venous blood specimens.[7-9]

Care of Peripheral Catheters

Removal of the catheter and insertion of a new one to a different site every 48-72 hours with injection caps being changed at that time as well are standard procedures. Dressings should be changed every 48-72 hours, and routine flushing with 1 ml heparin (100 U/ml every 8-12 hours and after each use (after saline) to maintain patency. Flushing with 1 ml saline should be done before and after each use, or every 12 hours if the catheter is not being used. In general, the IV site should be maintained with a cleansing routine of povidone-iodine or alcohol. Povidone-iodine ointment at the site of insertion may be applied, but this is gradually losing favor. A transparent occlusive dressing should be applied and maintained for as long as the catheter remains in place. The Centers for Disease Control recommends changing the dressing every 48-72 hours.[8-11]

The advantage of these types of peripheral catheters is the ease of insertion and the availability of immediate access. Disadvantages include frequent site changes (every 48-72 hours), a higher incidence of phlebitis, and the fact that irritant drugs or parenteral nutrition cannot be infused through this line.

Complications

Although peripheral catheters are convenient, they are not without problems. One minor complication that can occur is a ruptured vein which requires removal of the catheter and application of a pressure dressing to minimize the development of hematomas. Also, if infiltration occurs the catheter must be removed and the site treated appropriately. Another complication is an IV that becomes occluded by a blood clot, especially if the rate of infusion is slow or heparin flushes are not routinely being administered. In most cases the IV line must be restarted. Major complications include local site infections, disseminated infections, and IV associated phlebitis. Treatment generally involves IV antibiotics with a change of the IV site.[9,11]

Other Types of Peripheral Catheters

One specialized type of peripheral catheter is the hydrating catheter, such as the Streamline® and the Intima®. Once these catheters are exposed to the bloodstream they become hydrated and pliable, thus reducing the risk of phlebitis. The care of these catheters is the same as those mentioned above. While nursing standards dictate that the insertion site be changed every 48-72 hours, in practice the indwelling time of these catheters may be much longer. In fact, hydrating catheters may remain functional and without complications for up to three weeks using the same site.[8-10]

Another type of peripheral catheter is the Landmark Midline® which may be used in cases requiring longer indwelling time or for irritant medication (such as erythromycin). These catheters are inserted above or below the bend of the arm and may be single or double lumen. Again, there is controversy over how frequently the site must be rotated, but the injection cap must be changed after 40 punctures or seven days.[7]

Peripherally Inserted Central Catheter

A peripherally inserted central catheter (PICC) is a radiopaque central catheter composed of polyurethane and silastic that is inserted peripherally, usually into a vein in the antecubita fossa through an introducer. The tip of the catheter is placed into the superior vena cava and is suitable for virtually any type of therapy lasting beyond seven days. This catheter is commonly used for parenteral nutrition administration, chemotherapy, long-term antibiotics, pain management, and any other therapy that requires large vein access and may be used for up to three months. Because the catheter terminates in the antecubital space, an extension tube with a self-sealing injection cap is often added to the line in order to make it easier for the patient to use.[7]

Care of the PICC Line

In order to maintain patency of this line, 2.5-3 ml (100 U/ml) of heparin should be used as a flush after each infusion (after saline flush) of fluid for a patient on intermittent therapy. If the catheter is not being used, it should be flushed every 12-24 hours. If the patient is receiving medication that is incompatible with heparin, the line must be flushed with saline before and after medication is administered, or every 12-24 hours if not being used. The injection cap should be changed at least every 72 hours and as needed if rubber coring occurs. The subclavian catheter must be clamped before removal of the injection cap.[7-11]

Care of the PICC line also requires care at the insertion site. This care consists of removal of the old dressing, inspection of the site, cleansing with povidone-iodine solution and allowing the skin to air dry at least two minutes to maximize action. Some protocols call for applying a povidone-iodine ointment to the sutures and insertion site before applying a transparent dressing. These dressing changes should be done every three to five days or when the dressing becomes moist or loose.[7]

The advantages of the PICC line are that it may be inserted by a qualified registered nurse, it may remain in place indefinitely, it is easily inserted, and has increased comfort and less arm restriction than other types of catheters. Disadvantages include the need for x-ray verification of superior vena cava placement and the potential for complications associated with central line placement. These complications include site infection, sepsis, catheter migration, clot formation, air embolus, and extravasation.

Patient Teaching

The patient or family caregiver must know, understand, and demonstrate the purpose of the central catheter, the importance of not touching the catheter or tubing with the hands, the need to report any pain in the arm, neck, or ear, difficulty in breathing, or fever. The patient should be told to avoid crowds and persons with infections. It is extremely important that all who care for the patient be educated in aseptic technique, handwashing, catheter care, flushing, dressing changes, and how to obtain supplies and solutions. A list of medications and solutions, their purpose, dosage, side effects, and time and length of administration should be readily available.[11]

Central Venous Lines

Central venous lines are recommended for IV therapy that lasts more than four weeks or for those who require multiple courses of intermittent IV medications. These catheters are available as single or multiple lumen and are commonly used for infusions of TPN, IV fluids, antibiotics, chemotherapy, and blood products as well as blood sampling. If the catheter has at least two lumens and will be used for blood sampling, it is recommended that one lumen, usually the largest, be designated for drawing blood.[10] Other patients who may benefit from this type of catheter are those who require frequent venous access, frequent blood sampling, vesicant therapy, or have venous thrombosis and sclerosis from previous peripheral IV therapy.

Types of Central Catheters

Examples of trade names of central catheters are Broviac®, Hickman®, and Leonard®. These catheters are surgically inserted and tunneled through the subcutaneous fascia and then threaded into the subclavian vein. Tunneling allows for tissue growth around the catheter, thus blocking the introduction of microorganisms up the exterior of the catheter. Once the site has healed and tissue growth occurs, the need for extensive site care is reduced making maintenance easier. A Dacron cuff is placed on the subcutaneous portion of the catheter and allows for fibrous tissue growth and thus a means of anchoring the catheter into place.[7,10]

Care of Central Catheters

Because any break in the integrity of the skin provides a potential place for bacteria to enter the patient's system, it is important that proper site care be followed. This care includes removing the old dressing, cleansing the site with alcohol and povidone-iodine, and covering the site with an occlusive dressing. Initially site care must be done every 72 hours, and after the site heals, every seven days thereafter. In home use, the patient and family members are taught to change the dressings themselves. Injection caps should initially be changed every 72 hours and then after 40 punctures or seven days. In order to maintain patency each lumen of the catheter must be flushed with 2.5 ml (100 U/ml) of heparin after each infusion of fluid. If the catheter is not being used, it should be flushed routinely every 12-24 hours. In a patient who is receiving medication that is not compatible with heparin, the line must be flushed with saline before and after medication is administered.[7,10,11] The advantages of this type of catheter are that they may be used for a wide variety of therapies, they have a lower risk of infection, and they may be used for an extended period of time. Disadvantages include the need for surgical placement and removal.

Other Types of Central Catheters

The Groshong® catheter is very popular for home infusion therapy because it does not require the use of heparin. This catheter is made of silicone and has a closed distal tip with a pressure-sensitive two-way valve that opens inward with aspiration and opens outward with infusion. When the valves are closed they prevent blood from backing up into the catheter, thus eliminating the need for heparin. In addition, the Groshong catheter does not need to be clamped when injection caps are removed. This catheter should be flushed with saline after every medication administration and every seven days when not in use. Injection caps should be changed initially after 18 punctures or seven days and subsequently after 40 punctures, seven days, or after blood aspiration through the cap.[10]

Patient Teaching

The patient or family caregiver must demonstrate all aspects of care associated with the catheters. In addition, if multiple lumens are being used the patient must know which is designated for medication and which for blood testing. If a pump is to be utilized, the patient must be educated as to its use and programming instructions. Complications as listed below must be reported to a physician as soon as possible. Most importantly, the patient must be given instructions regarding resumption of activity as tolerated, to change transparent dressings after a shower if wet, and that one may swim if allowed by the physician.[11]

Complications With Catheter Use

In addition to patients knowing how to safely care for their catheters, they must also know how to prevent, recognize, and treat complications. One complication that may arise is site infection which may be prevented by proper site care. Patients must be informed to be alert for any temperature elevation and to inspect the site for redness, swelling, or any drainage. Improper site care may result in bacteria ascending the catheter and causing sepsis. Thrombosis can develop in the vessel in which the catheter is placed. Signs of thrombosis include tenderness and swelling in the arm, neck, and shoulder on the catheter side of the body as well as sluggishness in the flow of IV solutions. Catheter migration, to either side of the atrium, may be detected and while the catheter is routinely flushed. If routine flushing is not performed a clot can form in the catheter. Patients are told to never force any fluid through a catheter since partial or total blockage may have occurred and must be treated with urokinase. Patients must also be able to recognize a torn or leaking catheter. In order to minimize the risk of this happening, patients should be taught to clamp the catheter when changing injection caps; rotate the site of the clamp; and tape the catheter up in order to prevent tugging of the line. If patients do not clamp the catheter when changing injection caps or if a tear develops, the patient may be at risk of developing an air embolus. If this occurs the catheter must be clamped immediately and emergency assistance obtained.[7,11,12]

Implantable Port

Subcutaneous or implantable ports have many of the same applications as central catheters. Implantable ports may be designed as single or double lumen. Acceptance and use of these devices has grown rapidly, especially in the HHC patient who requires intermittent courses of IV therapy and is ideal for active patients or those who are not capable of extensive site care and flushing procedures. There are no external parts to the port and nothing can be seen when the port is not in use, which is a feature many patients find attractive. These devices may be used for fluid administration and blood sampling. These ports may be contraindicated in patients with inadequate body tissue to support the device, or in obese patients, or on a postradiated chest.[7,10,11,13]

Types of Implantable Ports

Examples of implantable ports include Infus-a-Port®, Port-a-Cath®, and Medtronic®. These ports are composed of a silicone catheter and either a metal or plastic injection port with a self-sealing rubber septum. Implantation of the port usually takes 30 minutes to one hour and is performed in the operating room under local anesthesia. The device is placed in a small subcutaneous pocket and the silicone catheter attached to the injection port is threaded into the subclavian vein. A backstop/base is sutured over the bone for stability and the pocket containing the port is closed creating a completely implanted device.[13] These ports have been made available for venous access and for infusion of fluids into the arterial, peritoneal, and epidural spaces. Huber needle with a 90° bend is inserted for continuous infusion to increase comfort and decrease the chance of accidental needle removal or puncture. Once the port has been located by palpation, the needle and extension tubing are primed with fluid and inserted perpendicularly through the skin, into the reservoir against the needle stop.

Care of the Implantable Port

Because the entire device is in the subcutaneous tissue, the care regimen for these ports is fairly simple. Once the surgical incision has healed, no site care or dressing is required. However, when the port is in use, the skin should be prepped and an occlusive dressing should be applied which secures the needle in place. Injection caps for ports are not required. For maintaining patency, 5 ml (100 unit/ml) heparin flushes are used before and after each use, and at least every four weeks if not in continuous use. If fluids being administered are not compatible with heparin, it is necessary to flush with 5 ml of normal saline before and after each use. As with central venous catheters, double lumen devices require separate flushes based on their use.[7,10,11,13]

A port offers several advantages over an external venous access device such as less risk of infection, less interference with the patient's normal daily activities, no external catheter when the port is not in use, and easier care. Potential disadvantages include some discomfort associated with the needle stick, initial expense for surgical placement and for Huber needles. Other drawbacks include the limited lifetime of the port based on the number of needle sticks (usually 1000-2000 sticks), and the possibility of missing the septum with the Huber needle and injecting the medication subcutaneously.[10,13]

Complications

Because the port system is placed in the right atrium, there is a similarity between complications that may occur in the implantable port and central venous catheters. Patients should be taught to prevent, detect, and treat such complications as site infection or breakdown, sepsis, thrombosis, catheter migration, clot formation, and air embolus that may occur only when the port is in use. One must also watch for port migration and the risk of extravasation if the needle is not properly placed through the septum.[7,11,13]

Patient Teaching

The patient or family caregiver must demonstrate the same procedures as with other types of venous access devices, including handwashing technique, knowledge of the system, and assessment of the system for potential complications. Flushing and administration of medications ordered must be taught, as well as use of an infusion pump. One must also understand instructions pertaining to daily activity, such as showering, and the possibility of swimming, if allowed.[11]

PHARMACIST'S ROLE

The pharmacist's involvement with infusion therapy has traditionally been limited to drug preparation and dispensing. However, statements on the pharmacist's role with respect to IV infusion devices have been published.[15] (See also Chapter 1.) Suggested areas of involvement include:

1. Research and development of innovative drug delivery systems and administration devices.
2. Evaluation and research to determine the direct and comparative efficacy, safety, and cost-effectiveness of specific drug delivery systems and administration devices.
3. In conjunction with pharmacy and therapeutics committees (or other appropriate medical staff committees), decisions to choose or exclude particular drug delivery systems and administration devices for use in specific organizational settings.
4. Development of organization-specific policies and procedures regarding the acquisition, storage, distribution, use, maintenance, and ongoing product quality control of drug delivery systems and administration devices.
5. Choice of a particular drug delivery system or administration device for use in a specific patient's drug therapy.
6. Direct communication with patients to instruct them in the use of such systems and devices and to gather information necessary to monitor the outcome of their therapy.
7. Monitoring of the ongoing clinical effectiveness and suitability of specific drug delivery systems or administration devices with respect to specific patients and the communication of clinically relevant observations and recommendations to prescribers and other health professionals involved in the patients' care.

In the HHC setting, the pharmacist has the opportunity to be actively involved with drug therapy and the selection of infusion devices. The pharmacist should work directly with physicians and nurses in the selection of the pump to deliver the prescribed therapy, because of the multitude of ambulatory infusion devices which have a wide range of pump features. In addition, assessments must be performed on an ongoing basis to determine whether the equipment is appropriate for an individual patient's use.

One area where the pharmacist has important patient involvement is education and training. The pharmacist usually has a thorough understanding of pump operation and programming since they prepare the IV doses. Drug concentration and volume are factors that must be carefully calculated to deliver the medication in the desired manner. The pharmacist serves as a resource person regarding drug compatibility, stability and administration. Thus training is not limited to patients, but may also include the other members of the health care team.

In addition, the pharmacist is often called upon to help solve problems that may occur with a patient's drug therapy or the infusion device. The importance of excellent communication skills cannot be overemphasized. Patients at home need to be assured that they are receiving their therapy as prescribed.

As pump technology advances, the pharmacist will be more involved with the assessment of these new products. New pumps represent capital expenses which may have variable additional benefits to the HHC patient. In light of the current emphasis on limiting the cost of health care expenses, pump selection and evaluation may be an especially important role for the pharmacist.

CONCLUSION

The use of pumps, controllers, and catheters in HHC settings has helped to revolutionize health care in recent years. These devices facilitate the provision of infusion therapy without the need for hospitalization. Rapidly changing technology will result in the development of more complex delivery systems for use in the home in the future.

REFERENCES

1. Winters RW, Parver AK, Sansbury JD. Home Infusion Therapy. National Alliance For Infusion Therapy, Washington DC. 1992.
2. Sax HC. Complications of total parenteral nutrition and their prevention. In: Rombeau JL, Caldwell MD, Eds. Parenteral nutrition. Philadelphia, PA: WB Saunders. 1993; 373.
3. Hospital risk control update. 1991; 12:1-5.
4. Foley KM, Arbit E. Management of Cancer Pain. In: Devita VT, Hellman S, Rosenberg SA, Eds. Cancer principles and practice of oncology. Philadelphia, PA: JB Lippincott. 1989; 2067.
5. Equipment management. In: Accreditation manual for home care, Oakbrook Terrace, IL: JCAHO. 1991; 71-76.
6. Scoring guidelines. In: Accreditation manual for home care, Oakbrook Terrace, IL: JCAHO. 1991; 1-35.
7. Handy C. Vascular Access Devices Hospital to Home Care. JIN. 1989; 12(Supp.1):S10-17.
8. Lyons L. New Technologies Are Expanding Uses Of Peripheral Catheters. Infusion. 1992; 2(1):1-2.
9. Rostad M. Intravenous Access Part 1. Peripheral IV's. Urologic Nurs. 1992; 12(1):18-22.
10. Tillman K. Venous Access Devices: Guidelines for Home Healthcare Nurses. Home Healthcare Nurs. 1991; 9(5):13-17.
11. Tucker S, Canobbio M, Paquette E, Wells M. Patient Care Standards, 5th ed. St. Louis, MO; Mosby-Year Book Inc., 1992; 53-58.
12. Rostad M. Intravenous Access Part 2. Central Venous Lines. Urologic Nurs. 1992; 12(3):108-110.
13. Camp-Sorrell D. Implantable Ports: Everything You Always Wanted To Know. J Intraven Nurs. 1992; 15(5):262-273.
14. Anon. Venous Access in Home Care. 1992; 2(1):3-6.
15. Avon. ASHP Statement on the Pharmacist's Role with respect to Drug Delivery Systems and Administration Devices. Am J. Hosp Pharm. 1989; 46:2342-3.

20 Concepts of Parenteral and Enteral Nutrition

Ronald R. Conte, Pharm.D.

Home total parenteral nutrition (TPN) is a lifesaving intervention for patients with severe gastrointestinal dysfunction. With proper parenteral or enteral nutrition therapy, malnourished patients can dramatically improve their physical status. In this chapter, the pharmacist is provided with information to assist in the successful management of patients at home on parenteral or enteral therapy. Practical points about patient assessment and monitoring as well as basic discussions of parenteral nutrition formulations are included. Information is also presented on nutritional support for the pregnant patient, the pediatric patient, and the AIDS patient.

Since 1984, the Oley Foundation and the American Society for Parenteral and Enteral Nutrition (ASPEN) has provided outcome data on patients receiving parenteral and/or tube enteral nutrition therapy in the home health care (HHC) setting. Longitudinal data on 7917 patients shows an increase of 3% in parenteral nutrition as compared to an increase of 31% in enteral therapy.[1] Cancer is the most frequent diagnosis requiring such therapy. The percentage of new patients infected with the human immunodeficiency virus (HIV) and diagnosed with acquired immune deficiency syndrome who receive parenteral nutrition now equals the number of new Crohn's patients. Outcome data from the ASPEN report indicates that most patients on home TPN had either no hospital readmissions or one. Sepsis is the number one complication for readmission in almost 62% of the cases. Mortality related to home parenteral nutrition is only 3%. No deaths have been related to home enteral nutrition.[1]

Approximately 29,000 patients with intestinal failure require home parenteral nutrition. Statistics show that one half of all Crohn's disease and congenital bowel disease patients (pediatrics) resume oral nutrition. Only 25% with chronic motility disorders and 17% of the patients with ischemic bowel or radiation enteritis will fully recover.[2]

INDICATIONS

No disease process benefits from starvation. However, it is still difficult to determine whether nutritional improvement produces positive outcomes for all cases. The argument rages on about the role of parenteral nutrition in the cachectic cancer patient. Weight gain can be achieved in most cachectic cancer patients, but it can be questioned whether it improves survival. In patients with lymphomas, testicular cancer, sarcoma, and lung cancer, there is no difference in survival between TPN treated and untreated groups.[3,4] However, cancer is still the most frequent diagnosis for home parenteral nutrition. The most common tumors are of the bowel or genitourinary tract.[5]

TPN therapy is clearly indicated for Crohn's disease (regional enteritis), motility disorders, radiation enteritis, short bowel syndrome, severe malabsorption syndrome, high output enterocutaneous fistulae, ulcerative colitis and congenital bowel dysfunction. There are several other groups of patients where TPN shows some limited benefits. In patients undergoing bone marrow transplants (BMT), TPN does provide increased calorie and protein intake during cytotoxic therapy. Survival is improved with TPN, although outcomes have not been uniformly successful. Enteral therapy may still offer advantages in the BMT patient.

Both intradialytic parenteral nutrition (IDPN) and intraperitoneal nutrition (IPN) provide nutrition for patients with end-stage renal disease (ESRD). It is not possible to review the complex physiologic basis for hemodialysis or peritoneal dialysis in this chapter. However, it is important to note that not all ESRD patients will benefit from

IDPN therapy. More studies are needed to determine its efficacy in reversing malnutrition. IDPN is reserved for those patients who have failed conventional measures.[6] Additional studies are needed to determine the full merit of IPN and optimal formulary mixtures must still be assessed.[7]

During pregnancy, certain patients develop hyperemesis gravidarum, intractable vomiting with dehydration, electrolyte imbalance, ketonuria and weight loss of greater than 5% of body weight. Peripheral parenteral nutrition (more so than TPN) is indicated, especially if the patient develops severe protein and calorie malnutrition.

CLINICAL FINDINGS AND ASSESSMENT OF NUTRITIONAL STATUS

The degree of starvation is dependent on to what extent the body is depleted of protein. Protein-calorie malnutrition (PCM) results from increased energy expenditure, anorexia and skeletal muscle breakdown.[8] In dissecting the components responsible for body energy needs, one must understand what occurs with basal metabolic rates. In the resting state, energy is generated for protein synthesis and degradation, as well as for carbohydrate and lipid metabolism. In addition, basal energy is needed to pump ions across cells, to pump the heart, to provide diaphragmatic movement for the lungs, and for brain function. In simple starvation or fasting states, the energy requirement may be reduced up to 20% of the basal metabolic rate.[8]

Cancer Patients

In patients with neoplasms, there are several altered metabolic processes involving carbohydrates, protein and fat. The results are abnormal gluconeogenesis and glucose intolerance. With an increase in glucose production, there is an increase in protein breakdown and an increase in lipolysis. Tumors require glucose for growth. It has been shown that a one kilogram tumor consumes 140 Gm of glucose daily. That amount can be up to 40% of the total carbohydrate consumption in a hospitalized cancer patient.[9] With this usage occurs a futile cycling of carbohydrates: glucose is metabolized from anaerobic glycolysis with lactate production and is then reconverted to glucose in the liver by the Cori cycle. This results in abnormal energy expenditure and negative nitrogen balance. With the increase in mobilization of free fatty acids, there is a corresponding increase in immunosuppression.

In pediatric cancer patients, the goal of nutritional support is to prevent/reverse nutritional deficits; promote normal growth and development; minimize morbidity and mortality; and maximize the patient's quality of life. The pediatric cancer patient presents with caloric deficiencies with a hypermetabolic state, hallmarks of cancer cachexia. Chemotherapy in children is the main contributor to treatment-related nutritional compromise. Antimetabolites can inhibit the utilization of essential vitamins, as well as purines, calcium, magnesium, potassium and phosphorus.[10]

Pediatrics

Assessment criteria for malnutrition in children includes a weight loss greater than 5%, a weight for height of 90% or less, an albumin level less than 3.2, and an energy reserve of the fifth percentile or less. In addition, the weight or height percentile should be two percentiles lower than pre-illness.[10] As with adults, baseline nutritional assessments need to be completed for each patient. Initial laboratory assessment is the same as that for adults. Vital signs, weight, and fluid input and output are to be done initially as well as daily.[11]

Pregnancy

In pregnancy, parenteral nutrition is necessary when indicated to prevent perinatal mortality, congenital CNS malformation, or low birth weight or size. In the first half of pregnancy, there is maternal storage of fat, protein, minerals and fluid. Fluid accumulation during pregnancy may give dilutional values for albumin as well as electrolytes. Anergy and a decrease in total lymphocyte count indicate nutritional deficiency in pregnancy.[5]

AIDS

Unlike uncomplicated starvation where fat stores are depleted to conserve muscle mass, adipose tissue is spared in AIDS patients. Wasting is not intrinsic to the degree of immunodeficiency and is best characterized by loss of body cell mass, mainly muscle protein.[12] It is the degree of wasting rather than the etiology that leads to death.[13] Death occurs when body weight reaches two-thirds, or body cell mass is one-half, of normal values.[14] Wasting in AIDS is associated with four interrelated processes:

1. Inadequate intake. This is due to a number of cytokines including tissue necrosis factor (TNF). TNF increases hepatic synthesis of

fatty acids by stimulating peripheral lipolysis. A futile cycling of fatty acids results.[15] Although a hypertriglyceridemic state is part of this process, there is no relationship with TNF activity. Interferon alfa sometimes induces hypertriglyceridemia. Evidence suggests both interleukin-1 and interferon alfa may induce anorexia or cachexia.[16]

2. Hypermetabolism. Resting energy expenditure (REE) is elevated early in the HIV infection, even in asymptomatic patients with normal CD4 counts. REE increases even more with systemic infection in AIDS. Although REE alone does not equate with weight loss, AIDS patients with secondary infections have a weight loss of 5% in 28 days.[17]
3. Altered Metabolism. In AIDS, there is an increase in fatty acid oxidation and ketogenesis as well as an inhibition of limited carbohydrate stores.
4. Malabsorption. There is a breakdown in mucosal integrity leading to significant malabsorption as the disease of AIDS progresses. With systemic infections, there is actual blunting of intestinal billi. Mycobacterium avium intracellular (MAI) and Cryptosporidium parvum are two of the more common systemic pathogens responsible in part for extensive malabsorption.[18]

From these four processes, a few clear-cut statements can be made about nutritional status in HIV patients: There is an initial loss of storage fat with subsequent decreases in lean body mass. There then follows weight loss paralleling a decrease in food intake and breakdown in intestinal mucosal integrity.[19]

Weight standardization can be accomplished by calculating the body mass index (BMI). The patient's weight in Kg is divided by height, in meters. BMI values up to 21 indicate wasting; up to 19 indicates severe wasting.[20] Iron, zinc and selenium blood tests are important to do initially since decreases commonly seen in HIV patients may be a prognostic marker for inadequate nutritional status. Zinc is necessary for protein and lipid metabolism; deficiencies in lipid metabolism hypothetically contribute to the increased lipid composition of the HIV envelope.[21] This creates a very rigid cellular structure. However, enhancing the membrane is also essential in maintaining immune competency. Triglyceride levels also are elevated in HIV patients with or without a compromised immune system. This is due to profound alterations in lipid metabolism mediated by interferon, TNF or both. Of particular note, Vitamins E, as well as A, B12 and folate are also decreased in HIV disease and should be monitored initially and periodically throughout the course of the disease.

Assessment Guidelines

Assessing a patient for home parenteral or enteral nutrition can be very complex. ASPEN has clearly outlined guidelines in assessing patients for home TPN.[22] Obviously, home TPN is appropriate for those patients unable to tolerate oral food or meet their nutritional needs orally. The severity of the patient's underlying medical condition(s) as well as the degree of malnutrition are two very important factors in determining the appropriateness of TPN delivery at home. Active medical conditions should be stabilized in the hospital before patients are discharged to home infusion services. It is paramount that the home TPN patient have support systems which assist in a stress-free, relaxed atmosphere for delivery of high technology therapy. Emphasis is placed on there being an active, knowledgeable caregiver who can assume responsibility for the care of the patient at home as well as understand the steps involved in TPN therapy. The caregiver and the patient may be one and the same, but usually it is a family member, close friend or neighbor. Sometimes the caregiver is a nurse from a home health agency who is responsible for the total nursing care of the patient.

Although the patient's physician is ultimately responsible for the overall care of the home TPN patient, no home therapy is complete without a team of individuals to assist the physician. The team usually includes HHC pharmacists, nurses, dieticians, social workers and vendors for various medical equipment and supplies. The environment for home TPN delivery should be safe and free from potential infection.

Assessing the patient's psychosocial status is as important as any other factor outlined. Many times infusion therapies at home overwhelm the patient, presenting barriers to the overall improvement of the patient's condition. Both medical fears as well as non-medical fears (lack of money, support, dysfunctional family members or other social problems) contribute to delays in the patient's ability to improve medically at home.

After all of the above are evaluated, the potential benefits of therapy must outweigh the known risks. Patients should not be subjected to home TPN therapy when (1) the active medical condition(s) require in-hospital care; (2) home enteral feeding is the preferred route of nutritional support; (3) the patient or caregiver is unable to learn the techniques and procedures or the patient's psychosocial state or home environment interferes with safety; (4) or the patient or legal guardian does not desire home TPN.[22] In many cases a complete evaluation for a patient being considered for home TPN can be done prior to discharge from a hospital by an experienced HHC nurse.

Assessment Parameters

Physical parameters in initial nutritional assessment include the following:[23]

1. Height in centimeters.
2. Weight in kilograms.
3. Basal energy expenditure (BEE) in kilocalories/ day.
4. Actual weight as a percentage of ideal body weight.
5. Actual triceps skinfold thickness as a percentage of the standard.
6. Actual mid-upper arm muscle circumference as a percentage of the standard.
7. Creatinine / height index.
8. Serum albumin level.
9. Serum transferrin level or total iron-binding capacity.
10. Total lymphocyte count.
11. Measure of cell-mediated immunity (developed hypersensitivity reaction).
12. Nitrogen balance.
13. Apparent net protein utilization.
14. Weight changes as percent of usual weight.
15. Caloric intake.
16. Body surface area.

A summary of how some parameters are calculated can be found in Appendix 20-A.

The percentage of ideal body weight, tricep skinfold thickness, and arm muscle circumference are termed anthropometric measurements. These calculations are usually performed by a dietician and give estimates of body muscle mass and fat stores. Visceral protein status can be approximated from serum transferrin or from total iron binding capacity (TIBC). Lymphocytes are known as infection fighters. They have actually been referred to as "bags of protein". These cells migrate to the site of infection, identify the pathogen(s), phagocytize them and then leave. The severity of the deficit is based on total lymphocyte counts, namely mild, 1500-1800; moderate, 900-1500; and severe, <900.

When the body does replenish protein, lymphocytes are affected first within 24 hours. The next to be replenished is albumin (vascular protein) within 30 days. The last to be helped is cellular protein which takes 30 to 60 days, depending on the severity of PCM malnutrition.

Total lymphocyte count is the most quantitative parameter for protein deficiency and can be monitored daily. Albumin is the most consistent indicator of protein deficiency. Of special note, transferrin is the earliest indicator of protein deficiency and should be monitored weekly.

Lean body mass can be expressed by using the creatinine height index (CHI). The amount of creatinine produced and excreted in the urine over a 24-hour period is proportional to the muscle mass of the body. The ideal urinary creatinine for given heights in males and females is taken from standard tables.

Nitrogen balance is a reflection of protein metabolism and net protein utilization by the body. Calorie expenditure is determined by using the Harris-Benedict equations which calculate basal energy expenditure. Caloric intake can be expressed, therefore, as a percentage of BEE by dividing caloric intake by BEE and multiplying by 100.

In addition to nutritional parameters, electrolytes, blood urea nitrogen, serum creatinine, liver function tests, a complete blood count, serum glucose, serum cholesterol, serum triglycerides, magnesium, calcium, prothrombin time and serum amylase are required for baseline assessment. In the HHC setting, these laboratory tests may need to be repeated every other day or at least twice weekly until parenteral nutrition patients are stabilized. Laboratory data is then needed only once weekly for stabilized patient on short-term parenteral nutrition. Long-term TPN patients, as in Crohn's disease or short bowel syndrome, may only require laboratory tests once a month when stabilized.

A newer diagnostic technique is now being employed to predict body composition - total body water, extra-cellular fluid, fat-free mass, and total body fat. This is a non-invasive technique developed on the principal that the impedance of a biological conductor to the flow of a high frequency alternating electrical current is a function of its geometry and composition. Impedance is the result of two components, resistance and reactance. Measurement of bioelectrical resistance have been demonstrated to correlate highly with the total body water. Reactance is a measure of the quantity of cell membrane capacitance and an indication of the quantity of intracellular or body cell mass. Body fat, total body water, and extra-cellular water offer resistance to electrical current, only cell membranes offer reactance. In theory, the cell membrane will offer little or no resistance and the total resistance will reflect both intra-and extracellular fluid volumes and their ionic concentrations. All bio-impedance data is generated via a computer management system. However, the ability of the current multifrequency devices to accurately differentiate extracellular from total body water remain to be proven.[24]

ENERGY SOURCES

As discussed earlier, basal energy expenditure is calculated from the Harris-Benedict equation. To preserve energy balance is to maintain body weight. This balance is essentially that caloric intake must equal total energy expended (TEE). And TEE is equal to the sum of the resting energy expenditure (REE = BEE plus hypermetabolic factors) plus dietary thermogenesis (DT) plus energy expended with activity (EEA). The degree of hypermetabolism is one variable which may make it most difficult to achieve energy balance. This one variable differs from one cancer to another, in the presence of infections, in HIV positive patients with, as well as without, the diagnosis of opportunistic infections,[17] and other severely ill patients.

With parenteral nutrition therapy, the total caloric intake for adults should be in the range of 25-45 Kcal/kg/day. This represents the total of carbohydrate (glucose) kilocalories plus lipid kilocalories infused per 24 hours. The following types of parenteral nutrition patients have specific calorie requirements:[25]

Pregnancy = 36 Kcal/kg/day
(or use Harris-Benedict Equation + 300 Kcal/day for 2nd and 3rd trimester)

Pediatrics[11]
< 1 year of age = 90-120 Kcal/kg/day
1-11 years of age = 60-90 Kcal/kg/day
> 11 years of age = 30-60 Kcal/kg/day

AIDS = 35 Kcal/kg/day[26]

Carbohydrate in the form of dextrose is the most common source of non-protein calories in parenteral nutrition. In peripheral parenteral nutrition the final concentration of dextrose should not exceed 12%. A higher concentration can cause phlebitis and/or venospasm with a peripheral line. With central lines, the final dextrose concentration can be as high as 45%. Glycerin is an alternate carbohydrate source. However, it provides less Kcals per Gm as compared with dextrose. Calories provided by dextrose are calculated by multiplying the volume of dextrose to be used times grams of dextrose per 100 ml of solution times 3.4 Kcal per Gm of dextrose.

Fats are concentrated providers of calories. Lipids which are infused (fat emulsions) contribute 9 Kcal/Gm. These products are composed mainly of either soybean or safflower oils with emulsifiers including lecithin plus glycerin. Infused lipids remetabolize in the body the same as triglycerides. Triglycerides are metabolized to free fatty acids. They are needed as pulmonary surfactants, as factors in blood coagulation and for prostaglandin synthesis. A 10% fat emulsion provides 1.1 Kcal/ml; a 20% emulsion provides 2 Kcal/ml. Fat emulsions can be infused by peripheral vein or central line. At least 4% of the non-protein caloric intake should be from fat as linolenic acid to prevent essential fatty acid deficiency. This deficiency may not manifest itself for up to a month, Both linolenic acid and linoleic acid are fatty acids which the human body cannot synthesize and must be provided via fat emulsions to prevent this deficiency. Fat emulsions should not constitute more than 60% of the total caloric intake per day for most adult patients. Specific lipid requirements are also imposed for the following types of patients:

Pregnancy [27] = should never exceed 40% of total calories

Pediatrics[11]
0-1 year = 0.5 - 3.0 Gm/kg/day
1-11 years = 1.0 - 4.0 Gm/kg/day
> 11 years = 1.0 - 2.5 Gm/kg/day

AIDS = 100 Gm/day[28]

Protein is a necessary ingredient in parenteral nutrition to preserve the body's protein or restore what has been lost. Unlike carbohydrate and fats, the body cannot store protein. In actuality, non-protein constituents (dextrose and fat emulsions) divert amino acids from being used as an energy source for gluconeogenesis and into protein synthesis. In addition, protein requirements are dependent on the patient's nutritional status before parenteral needs, hepatic and renal function, as well as size and age of patient. For most adult patients the range of protein requirement is 0.8 to 3.0 Gm/kg/day. In pregnancy, the usual protein requirement is 1Gm/kg/day. Up to 2 Gm/kg/day may be needed for moderate to severely stressed patients.[25] For pediatric cases, the protein needs are in the same range as for adults; except for less than 1 year of age, the daily intake should be 2 to 3 Gm/kg. With the limited number of studies showing positive outcomes for TPN-treated AIDS cases, the required protein should be 100 - 114 Gm/day.[26,28]

Requirements may increase with the underlying disease state, as in thermal injury or with coexisting organ dysfunction (hepatic and renal). Whatever the protein needs are, there is growing evidence that branched-chain amino acids may be a better source of protein due to their anticatabolic effects on skeletal muscle and stimulation of protein synthesis. However, more study is needed to determine the optimal ratio of non-protein calories to Gm of nitrogen (from protein) to promote anabolism. With the current products available as amino acid sources, 1 Gm of nitrogen is equal to 6.3 Gm of protein. In an unstressed patient, the optimal calorie-to-nitrogen ratio is 150:1; for a stressed patient, the ratio may be as high as 250:1.

Another way to determine optimal nitrogen assimilation is to estimate nitrogen loss. This is basically used in conjunction with the known amount of nitrogen supplied by the infusion of amino acids to calculate the patient's nitrogen balance. A 24-hour urinary urea nitrogen is measured, since most nitrogen is lost via the urine as urea. The 24-hour nitrogen total plus a correction factor of 4 Gm gives the complete sum of nitrogen loss from all routes. When this loss is subtracted from the total amount of nitrogen ingested plus infused, the resultant value translates into anabolism (+ value) or catabolism (- value). One gram of nitrogen equates to 30 Gm of lean body mass. A patient in positive nitrogen balance should gain lean body mass, heal wounds, regain immune function and strength. It is still controversial whether special amino acid formulations for patients with renal failure are of added benefit. In renal failure, it is important to watch for laboratory changes in potassium, magnesium, phosphorus, and protein. In hepatic dysfunction, patients should not receive more than 50 Gms daily of protein in order to prevent serum ammonia imbalance, metabolic alkalosis, pre-renal azotemia, and hyperammonemia.

Fluid needs will vary depending on the underlying diagnosis for parenteral nutrition. Fluid balance is essential since over hydration can result in congestive heart failure, pulmonary edema, elevation of intracranial pressure, as well as hypervolemia, leading to falsely low values for specific blood chemistries including electrolytes.[29] Fluid overload in infants has been associated with an increased incidence of bronchopulmonary dysplasia, necrotizing enterocolitis and intravascular hemorrhage.[30] Fluid restriction is desirable for patients with renal disease. However, for most other patients, inadequate fluid intake can produce dehydration, hypernatremia, hyperosmolality, and possibly acute renal failure. For most adult patients requiring parenteral nutrition, the daily amount of fluid infused should be 30-35 ml/kg.

FORMULATIONS

Most parenteral nutrition formulations consist of dextrose, amino acids, and lipids. When mixed together in a single TPN container, it is known as 3 in 1 mixture. Electrolytes, minerals and certain other additives can be mixed at the same time in one TPN container. Multivitamins, containing fat soluble vitamins, and certain additives should be added to the parenteral admixture at the time of infusion. Certain additives are stable for short periods of time. The additives which lose significant potency within 24 hours include riboflavin, ascorbic acid,[31] and vitamins A, D, E.[32]

It is very rare today that parenteral nutrition is compounded without adding the lipids. Most 3 in 1 products are stable for a 1-week period. Some modifications in the basic 3 in 1 formulation are routinely made based upon the patient's medical conditions. (See Table 20-1.)

Micronutrients, Vitamins, Other Additives

Additives such as electrolytes, minerals, and trace elements are known as micronutrients. All additives to parenteral nutrition are necessary components and metabolic complications can arise as a result of inappropriate inclusion of these additives. Table 20-2 includes a listing of the more common micronutrients with their normal serum values as well as appropriate concentrations per liter of TPN for adult patients, including pregnant patients and AIDS patients. Table 20-3 lists the ranges for micronutrient additives in pediatric cases.

Sodium

The tendency to retain sodium and water is emphasized, particularly in the elderly and those patients with a past history of cardiovascular or pulmonary problems. Electrolyte needs will vary according to the history of the patient's illness. In the average adult patient, about 100-200 mEq/day can be given. If a past history of cardiac, pulmonary or renal problems are present, this figure would have to be adjusted downward.

Potassium

Potassium is the main intracellular cation, only 2% of the potassium is found extracellularly. Because potassium is found in abundance inside tissue, when this tissue is lost due to trauma or malnutrition, much of the potassium is also lost. Potassium deficiency is an integral part of malnutrition and upon delivery of protein and carbohydrate calories, potassium must be provided to assimilate

Table 20-1 Formulations for Selected Medical Conditions

Hyperglycemia	**Normoglycemia and/or Hypertriglyceridemia**
Dextrose 12 - 15%	Dextrose 25 - 35%
Amino Acids 4 - 6%	Amino Acids 4 - 6%
Lipids 3 - 6%	Lipids 100 Gm/week.
Fluid Restriction	**Renal Disease**
Dextrose 40%	Dextrose 35%
Amino Acids 4.25%	Amino Acids 3.5%
Lipids 100 Gm/week	Lipids 100 Gm/week with decreases in P, Mg, Na, total fluid
Liver Disease	**Pulmonary Disease**
Dextrose 35%	Dextrose 12 - 16%
Amino Acid 3.5%	Amino Acid 3 - 4.25 %
Lipids 150 Gm/week	Lipids 6%
increases in Vit B complex	increase in P
and K, decrease Na	decrease in Na

Table 20-2 Usual Adult Micronutrient Requirements

Electrolyte	Conc./Liter	Normal Serum Levels
Sodium	20-50 mEq	135-145 mEq/L
Potassium	10-50 mEq	3.5-5.0 mEq/L
Chloride	20-50 mEq	98-106 mEq/L
Calcium	5-10 mEq	8.4-10.2 mEq/L
Phosphorus	10-15 mM	2.7-4.5 mg/dL
Magnesium	5- 8 mEq	1.3-2.1 mEq/L
Acetate	10-40 mEq	NA
Zinc	3-10 mg	NA
Copper	1-1.5 mg	NA
Chromium	10-15 g	NA
Manganese	150-800 g	NA
Selenium	40-120 g	NA

Table 20-3 Parenteral Micronutrients in Pediatrics

Sodium	2-5 mEq/kg/day
Potassium	2-5 mEq/kg/day
Chloride	2-5 mEq/kg/day
Calcium	1-2 mEq/kg/day
Phosphate	1-2 mmol/kg/day
Magnesium	0.5 mEq/kg/day
Zinc	
(premature neonate):	300g/kg/day
(infants, children):	100g/kg/day
Copper	20 g/kg/day
Manganese	2-10 g/kg/day
Chromium	0.14-0.2 g/kg/day

glucose in the presence of insulin and to utilize amino acids efficiently. Around 3 mEq of potassium are retained per gram of nitrogen. On the average, 80 to 120 mEq are needed daily for adults on TPN regimens.

Magnesium

This ion is found primarily intracellularly and is a necessary ingredient in TPN formulations. Magnesium is an integral part of many enzyme systems in the cell. It becomes a particularly important ion in patients with histories of alcoholism, malnutrition, malabsorption and parathyroid disease. Commonly, 10 to 30 mEq/day are given, and adjustments upward are made to account for additional losses in patients experiencing diarrhea or draining gastrointestinal fistulas.

Phosphorus

Often overlooked in its importance, phosphorus plays a prominent role in many intracellular activities. Among these are the storage of energy, formation of cell membranes and oxygen transfer. If phosphorus is overlooked during TPN therapy, serious hypophosphatemia can result. Initial symptoms of impaired mentation and tingling of extremities (paresthesia) should alert the clinician to impaired oxygen delivery. As phosphate levels decrease, there is less phosphate in the red blood cell which means less likelihood of oxygen exchange at the capillary and tissue level. These symptoms are more likely to occur in a purely glucose based energy system than the glucose/fat energy mixture. The dual substrate system (glucose/lipid) would appear safer in severely malnourished patients. This is probably due to the fact that fat emulsions contain egg yolk phospholipids. In addition, if lipids are used for a significant portion of the non-protein calorie needs of the patient, there is less likelihood of excessive insulin secretion, a condition which otherwise would drive circulating phosphate ions into the cells.

Calcium

Calcium is the most abundant cation and functions in neuronal transmission, as a co-factor in blood coagulation, enzyme functions and assists hormone secretion. Almost half is bound to protein and 15% is in salt form. The remainder is free ion, which is the active form. Calcium has acidifying effects. With hypocalcemia, a patient can experience malaise, weakness, mental retardation, muscle cramps, tetany, convulsions, stridor and dyspnea, diplopia, abdominal cramps, urinary frequency, stunted growth (pediatrics) and cataracts. Hypercalcemia presents with hypotonia, hypertension, dehydration, tachycardia, fever, abdominal tenderness, muscle weakness, gastrointestinal distress, weight loss, disorientation, bone pain, abdominal pain, polyuria, constipation, coma, thirst and renal colic. Serum calcium measurement includes both ionized and protein bound forms. Usually, as serum calcium levels rise, serum phosphate levels fall.

Chloride

This extracellular anion is often overlooked

in the prescription for TPN. It is sometimes assumed the pharmacist will balance the anion/cation equation and chloride is one of the most common anions available in electrolyte salts. The usual admonition is not to use excessive chloride ions. It is wise to keep the chloride ion around 1:1 or 0.75:1 ratio with the sodium ion being used. This is done to prevent eventual problems associated with hyperchloremic metabolic acidosis which can be an iatrogenic and preventable phenomenon.

Acetate

Acetate is an important anion responsible for metabolic acid-base balance. The acetate indicator by blood measurement is the bicarbonate value. An increase in the bicarbonate level signals an inadequate acetate amount (low H+). Clinically, this can manifest as metabolic alkalosis, weakness, and anxiety. More than adequate amounts of acetate present as decreased bicarbonate levels. Clinically, signs and symptoms include metabolic acidosis, weakness, dyspnea, dry skin and mucous membranes. Both the chloride ion and acetate work together to assist in acid-base balance. For most adult patients the ratio of micronutrient additives of chloride to acetate should be 2:1. If the chloride blood level is elevated, the ratio is 1:1.

Vitamins

Patients on TPN therapy should receive water and fat soluble vitamins as necessary components. Optimum dosages have not been completely defined, but most clinicians use the multiple vitamin infusion solutions on a daily basis. Since some of the ingredients are light sensitive and of short to moderate stability, patients or caregivers are taught to add this daily prior to TPN administration.

Vitamin additives in parenteral nutrition admixtures serve as coenzymes in absorptive and metabolic processes, transfer energy, catalyze formation of nucleic acids and a variety of other endogenous chemicals, as well as assist in wound healing, bone growth and protection of subcellular components. See Table 20-4 for a listing of commonly used vitamins with daily requirements, their functions, and hypovitaminosis status for each. A typical multivitamin formulation for parenteral use is listed in Table 20-5.

Vitamin K is not included in the formulation due to instability. However, this vitamin can be administered at a dose of 10 mg intramuscularly once weekly, to meet its requirement. Insulin may also be needed in parenteral formulations if endogenous insulin secretions cannot adjust to large loads of infused glucose.

Insulin

Regular human insulin is used for patients who are diabetic or when random blood sugar levels rise above 200 mg% while on PPN/TPN. Insulin does bind to glass and plastics, as well as IV tubing. Adsorption is usually around 20 to 30% of the dose administered and maximum contact is within the first 30 to 60 minutes. If a parenteral nutrition patient requires insulin, increasing amounts are added daily and titrated against finger stick blood sugar levels measured on a daily basis. It is advisable to add insulin to the TPN bag at the time of administration. Ideally, the blood glucose level should remain between 100 to 180 mg%.

Trace Elements

The micronutrients known as trace elements (zinc, copper, chromium, manganese, iodine, selenium, molybdenum, and iron) are less than 0.01 % of the body mass. Their functions include enzyme activity, protein synthesis, mitochondrial energy, membrane transport, nerve conduction and muscle contraction. Table 20-6 provides a detailed summary about trace elements, their functions, symptoms with deficiency, time elapsed before deficiency is noted, recommended IV dose, and body content.

Formulation Concerns

Some general principles are adhered to when compounding parenteral nutrition. There are guidelines to follow with regard to the order of mixing micronutrients and also an order for mixing together macronutrients - dextrose, amino acids and lipids. In the dextrose solutions all salts of sodium and potassium (excluding phosphates) calcium, magnesium and trace elements can be added. Sodium and potassium phosphate are added to the amino acid solution. Calcium will precipitate out with higher amounts of phosphate (greater than 30 mEq); that is why each is added to separate macronutrients. A variation to this order of mixing is to add all micronutrients to the dextrose solution, excluding the calcium. This variation may be more desirable, since calcium and magnesium sulfate may precipitate in concentrations over 100 mEq per liter. The order of addition for macronutrients should be dextrose,

Table 20-4 Vitamins in Deficiency States

Nutrient	Deficiency	Toxicity	Recommended Dose
Thiamine (B1)	beriberi, edema, ataxia, neuritis, cardiomegaly	nausea, anorexia, lethargy, gut tone at levels > 400 mg	3 mg/day
Riboflavin (B2)	Conjunctivitis, glossitis, dermatitis, keratosis, cheilosis	none reported	3.6 mg/day
Niacin	pellagra, dermatitis, dementia, diarrhea, death	flushing, pruritus, peptic ulcer, hyperuricemia	40 mg/day
Pyridoxine (B6)	anemia, polyneuritis, dermatitis	peripheral neuropathy and convulsions, dependency	4.0 mg/day
Ascorbic Acid (C)	scurvy, bleeding gums, weakness, petechial hemorrhages, irritability	calcium oxalate stones, false + urine glucose	100 mg/day
Retinol (Vit A)	Bitot's spots, xerophthalmia, night blindness, keratinization, infections	teratogeneses, nausea, vomiting, vertigo, bone pain, edema, inc. CSF pressure, fatigue, fever	3,300 IU/day
Calciferol (Vit D)	rickets, osteomalacia, tetany	hypercalcemia	200 IU/day
Tocopherol (Vit E)	hemolytic anemia, neuronal degeneration	none known	10 IU/day
Pantothenic Acid	irritability, tachycardia, hypotension, burning feet syndrome	diarrhea	15 mg/day
Folic Acid	Macrocytic anemia	masks pernicious anemia, convulsions at high doses	400 mcg/day
Vitamin B 12	pernicious anemia, neuropathy	none known	5 mcg/day
Vitamin K	hemorrhage		
Biotin	dermatitis, neuritis, alopecia, anorexia, depression	none known	60 mcg/day

Table 20-5 Parenteral Multivitamin Formulation

A, IU	3,300	Riboflavin, mg	3.6
D, IU	200	Thiamin, mg	3.0
E, IU	10.0	B6 (pyridoxine), mg	4.0
Ascorbic acid, mg	100.0	B12 (cyanocobalamin), mcg	5.0
Folacin, mcg	400.0	Pantothenic acid, mg	15.0
Niacin mg	40.0	Biotin, mcg	60.0

amino acids, lipids, and water, if necessary, or the reverse order. To prevent excessive local pH effects, the acidic dextrose solution should not be combined with fat emulsion alone. The admixture should be inspected carefully for breaking of the emulsion or "oiling out", as well as for particulate matter or discoloration. If the TPN is not to be used immediately after preparation, it can be stored in a refrigerator for up to seven days. Infusions must be completed within 24 hours.

Flow Rates and Cycles

For peripheral vein infusion of parenteral nutrition, the infusion rate should be between 50 to 100 ml/hour. If a central line is employed, the initial rate should be 50 ml/hour so that the usual quantity of dextrose infused can be metabolized by the available insulin. If the rate of the TPN is too fast, the patient may become hyperglycemic and/or dehydrated. The rate can be increased at a rate of 25-50 ml/hour until the desired rate of infusion is reached. Once it is reached, a constant rate of infusion must be maintained. Usually, the parenteral nutrition rate of infusion has been stabilized by the time a patient is on home infusion service.

Rarely is a home infusion service asked to initiate parenteral nutrition in the home. It can be done for patients diagnosed with hyperemesis gravidarum or for any case where short-term parenteral nutrition can be infused via a peripheral line. A cycling of parenteral nutrition can also be accomplished in the HHC setting for those patients without glucose intolerance or an abnormal fluid imbalance. Parenteral nutrition can usually be cycled beginning with an 18-20 hour infusion period with a goal cycle of 12 hours. Bennett and Rosen[33] described how this can be accomplished over a 4-day period. So as not to produce abrupt changes in glucose levels with cyclic TPN, a taper-up period at the onset of infusion and a taper-down at the end is used. This taper period is usually for one hour at one half the maintenance rate. The maintenance rate is the total volume to be infused within a 24-hour period divided by the total infusion time (hours) minus 1 hour. Blood glucose levels should be tested one hour after the infusion has been finished. Most cyclic TPN metabolic problems can be alleviated by lengthening the infusion period. The only exception is in the case of dehydration where the amount of TPN fluid provided should be reassessed. Although there obviously are more manipulations with the central line with cyclic TPN, there is little evidence of increase in sepsis as long as good technique is utilized.

PATIENT MONITORING

Home infusion pharmacists are in unique positions to assume clinical responsibilities for TPN patient outcomes. It begins with patient assessment. Certain underlying medical conditions may require specific modifications in type of macronutrient or micronutrient infused. A review of the patient's drug and nutrition history can uncover intake of certain foods or drugs which may falsely negate or compound problems. For example, some parenteral antibiotics have significant sodium contents. If needed for a period of time, the sodium content of these antibiotics must be considered when formulating sodium concentrations for PPN or TPN. Nutritional assessment and drug histories need to be thoroughly reviewed so as to avoid problems commonly seen with parenteral nutrition. Once these issues are clarified, the infusion pharmacist outlines a care plan and a prescription with measurable goals of therapy.

The essential elements in a pharmaceutical care plan is to recognize drug-related or therapy-related concerns, assess their causes and severity, and identify approaches for their resolution. Most of the care plan is obtained from information and data taken from the patient's medical history, present medical status, nutritional assessment, and from the patient's drug profile. Gold and Fedder[34] have thoroughly

Table 20-6 Summary of Selected Trace Elements[40]

Element	Physiological Function	Deficiency Symptoms	Time On TPN before Deficiency Noted	Recommended Daily Intravenous Dose	Body Content and Primary Concentration	Dietary Sources
Zinc (Zn)	Metalloenzyme function, protein metabolism, lipid metabolism, vit. A metabolism	Poor growth and sexual development. Impairment of sensory perception (hypogeusia and hyposmla). Impaired wound healing, acrodermatitis entero-hepatica	2 wks to 7 mos (usually 4-8 wks)	Adult: 3 mg, (increase in patients with diarrhea and high output ileostomy) Pediatric: 100-300 mcg/kg	1-2.3 g. present in almost all tissue, highest concentration is intracellular	Meat, liver, eggs, seafood (esp. oysters)
Copper (Cu)	Hemoglobin synthesis, bone mineralization enzyme function	Anemia, defective connective tissue formation, growth retardation, imperfect keratinization and pigmentation of the hair	5 wks to 18 mos (usually 2-4 mos)	Adult: 0.3 mg (increase to 0.5 mg in diarrhea) Pediatric: 15-20 mcg/kg	80-120 mg, liver, brain, heart and kidneys	Nuts, shellfish, raisins, dried legumes, liver
Chromium (Cr)	Glucose metabolism, mediates effect of insulin on membranes	Impaired glucose clearance, peripheral neuropathy, ataxia	5 mos to 3-1/2 yrs	Adult: 20 mcg Pediatric 0.14-0.2 mcg/kg	60 mg, kidney, mainly in combination with transferrin	Animal protein, grain, Brewer's yeast
Manganese (Mn)	Bone structure, reproduction, activator ofenzymes, function of CNS	Impaired growth, skeletal abnormalities ataxia,convulsion fat metabolism abnormalities nausea and vomiting	4 mos on oral chemically defined diet	Adult:0.7 mg Pediatric: 2-10 mcg/kg	12-20 mg, kidneys, pancreas, liver	Green leafy vegetables, nuts, grain, tea
Iodine(I)	Synthesis of thyroid hormones, regulation of basal metabolic role, growth, reproduction and cellular metabolism	Goiter	Unknown	Adult: 120 mcg Pediatric: 0.15 mcg/kg	8 mg, Thyroid gland	Seafood, iodized salt
Selenium (Se)	Muscle metabolism, function of cardiac and skeletal muscles glutathione oxidase, antioxidant	Congestive cardiomyopathy muscle pain, weakness, growth retardation, aspermato-genesi	4 wks to 2 yrs	Adult 20 mcg Pediatric: 0.15 mcg/kg	As low as 1.5 mg, liver, kidney, heart, spleen	Onions, grains, sources vary depending on content in soil
Molybdenum	Component of metallo-enzymes aldehyde oxidase, sulfite oxidase, xanthine oxidase	Tachycardia, tachypnea, and mental changes leading to coma	1 yr	Adult: 25-75 mcg Pediatric: 20-50 mcg	Unknown	
Iron (Fe)	Constituent of hemoglobin, myoglobin, and several enzymes	Anemia, disturbance of bone marrow function	Variable depends on underlying disease state frequency of phlebotomy and iron stores	No formal recommendation can be made, depends on iron stores and other factors	45 mg/kg body weight, hemoglobin, myoglobin, ferritin, hemosiderin	Liver, turkey, veal, oysters, clams, raisins

outlined the specifics for providing quality pharmaceutical care plans.

The information for the actual nutrition prescription is usually gathered from the hospital pharmacy service from which the patient is discharged. It is reviewed and authorized by the prescribing physician or the physician in charge of the patient's home care. The important elements of the prescription include the start time and date, the total time of infusion with specific flow rates, including tapering, and the total volume of parenteral nutrition. In addition, each macronutrient and micronutrient is listed with appropriate concentrations, milliequivalents or millimoles and number of milliliters per liter of PPN/TPN. The specific route of infusion should be listed, whether it be a peripheral, midline or central access with the specific catheter name. Other additives should be listed and how much is to be added per bag. All laboratory samples needed are also specified, including the time of day and which day(s) per week. The types of medical supplies and flushing procedures are outlined on the prescription, along with instructions for replacing the infusion line, if necessary, as well as catheter care procedures. To complete a parenteral nutrition prescription, it is advisable to total and list the non-protein calories provided by dextrose and lipids as well as the grams of protein. And finally, the calories to nitrogen ratio is calculated and listed.

For consistency in patient monitoring, laboratory data should be reviewed by the pharmacist within 24 hours from the draw time. Changes in parenteral nutrition formulations are based on these lab values as well as the patient's clinical status and goals for therapy. A laboratory flow sheet, as well as prescription and non-prescription drug profile are monitored by the pharmacist on an ongoing basis. Each HHC provider, including the pharmacist, must draw upon the interdisciplinary team and their expertise. The team must be somewhat flexible in policies and procedures so as not to make the home environment nonconducive to the care of the patient. On the other hand, the treatment environment should not be so lax as to compromise any part of patient care. There is no substitute for continuous assessment and intervention by the HHC team. At times, the pharmacist assesses complex complications which are secondary to parenteral nutrition. Some of the more common complications are outlined below in Table 20-7. Recognition, prevention, and treatment of these complications are also reviewed.

ENTERAL NUTRITION

The use of liquid formula diets by tube or mouth into the gastrointestinal (GI) tract is known as enteral feeding. This form of nutritional support has been utilized for over 400 years. The recent increase in use is due to a variety of reasons: 1) more clinician awareness; 2) availability of nutritionally complete diets; 3) variations in compositions to fit nutritional demands of specific disease states; and 4) improved delivery systems. Enteral feeding is preferred, when possible, since it does preserve the physiologic sequence of nutrition absorption, metabolism and utilization. Indications of enteral feedings are clearly defined. If the patient is unable to ingest adequate nutrients by mouth and the GI tract is intact (no loss of function), then enteral nutrition is the treatment of choice. ASPEN has clearly outlined the guidelines for use of enteral nutrition:[35]

1. Patient has greater than 10% weight loss or an albumin level less than 3.5 G/dl with little to no oral intake for five days.
2. Patient has normal nutritional status with less than 50% of the required nutrient intake orally for the previous 7-10 days.
3. Patient has severe dysphagia.
4. Patient has major full thickness burns.
5. Patient has massive small bowel resection with the administration of TPN. (Up to 90% resection).
6. Patient has a low output enterocutaneous fistula (less than 500 ml/day).

Enteral nutrition is not indicated in patients with partial to complete gastric or intestinal obstructions, intractable vomiting, acute upper GI bleeding, hypomotility, severe diarrhea, high output external fistula, and severe acute pancreatitis.

The enteral prescription for HHC patients should include the name of the enteral product with the number of calories per milliliter. The directions for use should include any dilutional directions with water as well as whether it is administered by continuous versus bolus feeding. The rate of administration with specific type of tubing and size must also be written. Rates of administration per hour must be stated and whether this is by gravity or pump delivery. The specific type of pump should also be listed. The total calories/day must be stated. The prescription also includes enteral supplies needed plus whether a pole is required. And, finally, specific measurable goals must be stated with the parameters to be evaluated.

Table 20-7 Common Complications Secondary to Parenteral Nutrition

Complication	Signs/Symptoms	Prevention	Treatment
Hyperglycemia with diuresis	incr. urine/blood glucose, incr. urinary output, low urine specific gravity. If rapid increase in blood sugar or temperature, suspect sepsis.	Accurate input and output (I&O), urine specific gravity daily.	Add or increase insulin; may need to decr. infusion rate. D/C PPN/TPN; get blood cultures.
Hypoglycemia (< 60 mg%)	hunger, nausea, lethargy, confusion, agitation, sweating and tremor.	Maintain constant infusion rates; if DM, check blood sugars daily and change insulin dosage accordingly.	Incr. PPN/TPN infusion rate. May need to decr. insulin or incr. dextrose amount in PPN/TPN
Dehydration	weight loss, poor skin turgor, sunken eyes	Accurate I&O's, regulation of IV fluid, Report to MD	Adjust intake accordingly (provide IV hydration); or add more fluid to PPN/TPN
Hypokalemia (< 3 mEq/L)	Usually seen within 1st few days of TPN - weakness, resp. insufficiency, EKG changes	Monitor K+ level regularly, especially in DM patients	Add or incr. K+ in PPN/TPN Do not infuse faster than 10 mEq/hour.
Hyponatremia	Anorexia, fatigue, cramps, diarrhea, hypotension, lethargy	Monitor Na+ level regularly (for true salt depletion).	Increase Na+ in PPN/TPN.
Hypernatremia	increased weight, peripheral edema, pulmonary edema, ascites.	Accurate I&O's, serum albumin and wts daily (for dilution condition)	No Na+; decrease or restrict fluids, maintain serum albumin > 3 Gm%.
Hypophosphatemia	paresthesia, heartblock, mental confusion, weakness, hypertension, cardiac arrhythmias	Check P+ level regularly; limit use of phosphate binders	Add or increase phosphates in PPN/TPN (for normal RF, should be 15 mM phosphate per liter).
Hypocalcemia	paresthesias, tetany, bronchial constriction, CHF, mental changes, convulsions	Check Ca and albumin levels regularly.	Increase Ca in PPN/TPN, if active Ca form is calculated to be low. May need to decr. amount of amino acids.
Hypertriglyceridemia	Moderate elevation in liver enzymes	Monitor liver function test regularly	Decrease rate of fat administration or infuse less often per week.

Administration of enteral nutrients is by mouth when feasible. Alternate routes include nasogastric, nasoduodenal, nasojejunal, or enterostomy, esophagostomy, gastrostomy, and jejunostomy. Feeding by enterostomy is used in patients needing long-term enteral nutrition or in patients who have undergone an intra-abdominal operation. Traditionally, nasogastric tube feeding has been preferred. The stomach does tolerate a variety of formulas, even with high osmotic loads. However, there may be a greater risk of reflex and aspiration versus feeding into the small intestine. Patients with an intact gag reflex and no pulmonary disease do well with nasogastric feeding. Patients with gastroparesis, delayed gastric emptying, or increased chances of aspiration do better with duodenal or jejunal feeding.

Formulations of enteral nutrition are based on nutrient composition. Carbohydrate is the usual source of calories. Some of the common carbohydrates include vegetable oil, corn starch, maltodextrin, sucrose, fructose, and glucose oligosaccharides. The source of protein is from pureed beef, caseinates, whey, soy or free amino acids. Fat is provided from long-chain fatty acids (corn oil, safflower oil, soy oil). Medium-chain triglycerides are available and may offer some advantage since they do not require pancreatic lipase for absorption into the portal circulation. The one drawback is that medium chain triglycerides do not supply essential fatty acids.

Polymeric formulas are lactose free diets. These diets require some digestion ability for protein, carbohydrate and fat. Osmolarity is low and the caloric content is 1 to 2 Kcal/ml. These are the least expensive diets and are considered the initial choice for enteral nutrition.

Oligomeric formulas are known as elemental diets. Fat content can be as high as 30%. With these formulas, there seems to be greater ease of absorption of the peptide-type protein moiety. These formulas are used for periods of digestive or absorptive insufficiency as in gut recovery following major surgery or when polymeric diets are not tolerated.

Modular diets consist of single or multiple nutrients that can be combined to meet specific needs, e.g., individuals needing protein or other component supplementation. Silk and Grimble[36] reviewed the specialty formulas which are necessary for specific underlying conditions.

The two delivery methods of enteral nutrition are bolus and continuous feedings. The more critically ill the patient, the more continuous feeding is utilized. The advantages of bolus feeding are that it is more convenient, does not require an infusion pump, and simulates the normal feeding pattern. The advantages of continuous feedings are improved patient tolerance, as well as less abdominal distention and aspiration. There is rarely a need today to start with diluted enteral formulas. It is safe to start with full strength isotonic or hypertonic formulas at a rate of 25 ml/hour. Increasing the rate by 25 ml/hour every 12 - 24 hours is acceptable until desired volume is attained.[37]

Continuous infusion by mechanical pump offers the lowest risk of complications, reducing nursing time, allows a greater degree of accuracy and can be used in patients with gastric or transpyloric tube placement. Enteral products come in ready-to-use liquid (in cans) or powder (in pouches). There are a multitude of different feeding bags with or without their own tubing sets (including connectors and clamps). Closed enteral feeding systems are also available. The most common complications in enteral feeding are gastrointestinal diarrhea, cramping, distention, bloating, nausea, and vomiting. Of those symptoms, diarrhea is the most prevalent, as high as 68% in the critically ill patient. Diarrhea is due to a variety of reasons including use of antibiotics, hyperosmolar drug solutions, magnesium containing antacids and bacterial infections such as C. difficile.[38] In most cases, slowing the rate of the enteral feeding administration by continuous infusion, and use of a lactose-free formula may prevent or lessen the diarrhea. Overall, treatment of diarrhea is based on its etiology.

Other complications are mechanical - pharyngeal irritation, tube displacement, and obstruction of the tube lumen, as well as metabolic changes which were discussed previously. Obstruction of the tube is many times due to administration of tube-fed medications. The home infusion pharmacist should provide monitoring for these drug and nutrient interactions.

Factors to monitor include physical incompatibilities, thus possibly altering drug bioavailability, stability, and action. When the drug cannot be given by mouth or other non-tube routes, the drug should be added slowly to the nutrient. The final mixture should be inspected for physical incompatibilities. Since these mixtures could be breeding grounds for bacterial growth, the mixture should be infused within eight hours or discarded. A position paper has been developed that clearly outlines which medications can be mixed and how they are to be mixed with enteral formulas.[35] (See Appendix 20-B.) Lehmann and Barber[39] describe a common procedure of giving drugs by nasogastric tube. Aspiration is a serious complication of enteral nutrition with an incidence as high as 44%. It is difficult to determine the risk factors associated with an increased rate of aspiration. Increasing patient age is the only common factor in most studies. Location of the tube is not a related risk factor. Elevating the head of the patient to 30 degrees, periodic measuring of gastric residuals, and inflating endotracheal tube cuffs will decrease the risk of aspiration.

TOTAL QUALITY MANAGEMENT (TQM)

No part of a home infusion service can exist outside the domain of a comprehensive quality management program. The monitoring of patient care and patient outcomes must be evaluated objectively and systematically. Each aspect of the parenteral and enteral service is evaluated with regard to the quality and appropriateness of care, review of identified problems, evaluation of patient outcomes, and evaluation of patient and customer satisfaction. Avenues should be researched and plans outlined to improve the care and services provided. (See also Chapter 4.)

The monitoring and evaluation process should focus on high risk and problem-prone areas. Indicators may include process-oriented criteria, for example, adhering to the numerous steps in aseptic admixture technique required in the proper dispensing of parenteral and enteral infusions. Laminar air flow equipment should be located in a clean, low traffic area. Sink and refrigeration equipment should be nearby, along with solutions, syringes and other necessary supplies for compounding. Procedures must be adopted for batch testing of finished product and accurate records must be kept. Avoid touch contamination during all compounding procedures. Laminar air flow equipment should be certified annually by qualified personnel. Inspection should include air velocity and flow patency of the HEPA filter. Prefilters should be changed at regular intervals to ensure that proper air flow is not compromised.

More emphasis is now placed on outcome indicators. One such indicator is whether treatment goals are reached. For example, if one of the objective goals in TPN therapy is to gain one pound of weight per week, then this would be monitored and evaluated as an outcome indicator. TQM can only be as effective as its team members. However, an unbiased audit team is oftentimes employed to review and audit day-to-day service activities, completeness of charts, infection control in parenteral admixture products, depth of staff knowledge in policy and procedures, as well as clinical skills in state-of-the-art infusion therapies. Reports completed by the audit team become valuable learning tools for improving the overall service to the community served. All components of TQM fall under standardized policies and procedures developed by governing bodies, the Joint Commission on Accreditation of Healthcare Organizations.

CONCLUSION

Home parenteral and enteral therapies can be very complex, requiring exceptional clinical skills by the pharmacist. The gamut of pharmacist's activities, with the multitude of clinical responsibilities, clearly requires the highest level of quality in caring for these patients.

Appendix 20-A Formula for Calculating Basic Nutritional Parameters

% ideal body weight $= \dfrac{\text{actual weight}}{\text{ideal body weight}} \times 100$

Arm muscle circumference (cm) = Arm circumference (cm) - [0.314 x tricep skinfold (cm)]

% standard $= \dfrac{\text{actual measurement}}{\text{standard}} \times 100$

Serum transferrin = (0.8 x TIBC) - 43

Total Lymphocyte Count $= \dfrac{\%\ \text{lymphocytes} \times \text{WBC}}{100}$

Creatinine Height Index $= \dfrac{\text{actual urinary creatinine (mg)}}{\text{Ideal urinary creatinine (mg)}} \times 100$

Nitrogen Balance $= \dfrac{\text{Protein intake}}{6.25} - (\text{urinary urea nitrogen} + 4)$

Harris Benedict Equations:

males: BEE = 66 + (13.7 x Wt.) + (5 x Ht.) - (6.8 x Age)
females: BEE = 65.5 + (9.6 x Wt.) + (1.7 x Ht.) - (4.7 x Age)

Appendix 20-B Position Paper on Medication/Enteral Formula Interactions[35]

The combination of a medication with an enteral feeding product raises the potential for physical and or chemical interactions between the drug and the formula. For this reason, combining or coadministering these two products should only be ordered by appropriately trained health care professionals who are familiar with the drug package insert and have duly considered the following potential medication/formula interactions:

A. General Considerations:

1. As directed by the drug package insert, medications that should not be taken with foods should not be mixed or coadministered with enteral formulas.
2. Medications which might be mixed with foods may adversely affect the bioavailability of certain nutrients and or the taste acceptability of orally consumed formulas. Additionally, if GI intolerance to the mixture is observed, the cause of the intolerance is obscured.
3. The therapeutic effects of some medications depend on rapidly achieving high blood levels. If these medications are combined with a formula, chemical interactions with the mixture may reduce the effective amount of the drug provided. Further, if the mixture is slowly fed, drug administration is protracted and peak blood levels may be blunted.

B. Preparation and Feeding Considerations:

1. The addition of medications to enteral feeding products should be conducted in a clean, controlled environment to minimize the risks of microbiological contamination and the accidental administration of an incorrect medication. Enteral formulas that have been mixed with medications should be appropriately labeled.
2. The distal end of the feeding tube must be appropriately positioned for administering the medication being considered. Drugs that should be delivered to the stomach may not be effectively utilized if directly administered into the duodenum or the jejunum.
3. Administer the prescribed medication during, before, or after a feeding as recommended for the drug in use. If the preferred route of medication delivery is direct administration through a feeding tube, first rinse the feeding tube with a small amount of water to wash out residual formal, administer the medication via the tube and then rinse the tube with water to assure complete-drug delivery.
4. Although water-soluble medications offer more flexibility in mixing than do non-water soluble medications or tablets, consideration must be given to the pH of the drug being administered and the osmolality of the resulting combination product.
    a. Strongly alkaline or acidic drugs will measurably affect the pH of the formula and may cause protein denaturation (curdling).
    b. Medications which contain or consist of salts in solution or are highly concentrated, can be hypertonic. When hypertonic materials are rapidly administered, nausea, abdominal cramping, and diarrhea may result.
5. When non-water-based medications are added to enteral feeding products there is a high probability that the active drug will precipitate or separate from solution and inadvertently become highly concentrated. Under these circumstances, a portion of the drug may remain as a residue in the feeding container or may block the feeding tube. Further, the patient may receive irregular doses of the intended medication.
6. Viscous medications and thoroughly crushed tablets may be diluted or mixed with water provided there are no contraindications known and the drug is soluble in water. Enteric coated tablets and time-released capsules should not be crushed.

REFERENCES

1. OASIS, Home Nutrition support patient registry, Annual Report 1989. The Oley Foundation, Albany, NY. 1991.
2. Hiyama DT. The current role of small-bowel transplantation in intestinal failure. Nutr. Clin. Practice. 1993; 8:5-11.
3. Heber D, Byerley LO, Chi J, et.al. Pathophysiology of malnutrition in the adult cancer patient. Cancer (Suppl.) 1986; 58:1867-1873.
4. American College of Physicians. Parenteral nutrition in patients receiving cancer chemotherapy. Ann. Intern. Med. 1989; 110:734 - 6.
5. Howard LJ, Heaphey L, Fleming CR, et.al. Four years of North American registry home parenteral nutrition outcome data and their implications for patient management. JPEN. 1991; 15:384-393.
6. Foulks CJ, Goldstein DJ, Kelly MP, et.al. Indications for the use of intradialytic parenteral nutrition in the malnourished hemodialysis patient. J. Renal Nutr. 1991; 1:23-33.
7. Wolk R. Intraperitoneal nutrition. Hospital Pharmacy. 1992; 627:893-904.
8. Hurley RS, Campbell SM, et.al. Outcomes of cancer and non-cancer patients on hpn. Nutr Clin Practice. 1990; 5:59-62.
9. Ingoffo RJ. Parenteral nutrition support in patients with cancer. Pharmacotherapy. 1992; 12(4):353-357.
10. Hanigan MJ and Walter GA. Nutritional support of the child with cancer. J Ped Onc Nursing. 1992; 9:110-118.
11. MacFarlane K, Bullock L and Fitzgerald JF. A usage evaluation of total parenteral nutrition in pediatric patients. JPEN. 1991; 15:85-88.
12. Raiten DJ. Nutrition and HIV infection. A review and evaluation of the extant knowledge of the relationship between nutrition and HIV infection. Nutr. Clin. Pract. 1991; 6(Suppl.1):1S-94S.
13. Grunfeld C and Feingold KR. Metabolic disturbances and wasting in the acquired immunodeficiency syndrome. NEJM. 1992; 327:329-337.
14. Kotler DP, Tierney AR, et.al. The magnitude of body cell mass depletion determines the timing of death from wasting in AIDS. Am J Clin Nutr. 1989; 50:444-447.
15. Feingold KR, Adi S, Staprans I, et.al. Diet affects the mechanisms by which TNF stimulates hepatic triglyceride production. Am J Physiol. 1990; 259:E177-E184.
16. Hellerstein MK, Kahn J, Madie H, and Viteri F. Current approach to the treatment of human immunodeficiency virus-associated weight loss: pathophysiologic considerations and emerging management strategies. Seminars in Oncology. 1990; 17:17-33.
17. Grunfeld C, Pang M, Shimizu L, et.al. Resting energy expenditure, caloric intake and short-term weight changes in human immunodeficiency virus infection and the acquired immunodeficiency syndrome. Am J Clin Nutr. 1992; 55:445-60.
18. Greenson JKL, Belitsos PC, Yardley JH, Barlett JG. AIDS enteropathy; occult enteric infections and duodenal mucosal alterations in chronic diarrhea. Ann Inter Med. 1991; 144:366-372.
19. Sharkey SJ, Sharkey KA, Sutherland LR. Nutritional status and food intake in human immunodeficiency virus infection. J. Ac. Immune Def Syn. 1992; 5:1091-1098.
20. Mildren D, Machado SG, Wilets I, et.al. Endogenous interferon and triglyceride concentrations to assess response to zidovudine in AIDS and advanced AIDS-related complex. Lancet 1992; 339:453-456.
21. Aloia RC, Jensen FC, Curtain CC, et.al. Lipid composition and fluidity of the human immunodeficiency virus. Pro Natl. Acad Sci. 1980; 85:900-904.
22. ASPEN Board of Directors. Guidelines for use of home total parenteral nutrition. JPEN. 1987; 11:342-346.
23. Blackburn GL, Bistrian BR, Maini BS. Nutritional and metabolic assessment of the hospitalized patient. JPEN. 1977; 1:11-22.
24. Heymsfield SB, Waki M, Kehayias J, et.al. Chemical and elemental analysis of human in vivo using improved body composition models. Am J Physiol. 1991; 261:E190-E198.
25. Wolk RA, and Rayburn WF. Parenteral nutrition in obstetric patients. Nutr Clin Practice. 1990; 5:139-152.
26. Kotler DP, Tierney AR, Culpepper-Morgan JA, et.al. Effects of home total parenteral nutrition on body composition in patients with acquired immunodeficiency syndrome. JPEN. 1990; 14:454-458.
27. Rayburn W, Wolk R, Mercer N, et.al. Parenteral nutrition in obstetrics and gynecology. Obstet Gynecol Surv. 1986; 41:200-14.
28. Singer P, Rothkopf MM, Kvetan V, et.al. Risks and benefits of home parenteral nutrition in the acquired immunodeficiency syndrome. JPEN. 1991; 15(1):75-79.
29. Kerner JA, Sunshine P. Parenteral alimentation. Semin. Perinatol. 1979; 3:417-34.
30. Goldberg RN, Chung D, Goldman SL, et.al. The association of rapid volume expansion and intraventricular hemorrhage in the preterm infant. J Pediatr. 1980; 96:1060-3.
31. Van der Horst A, Martens H, de Goeda P. Analysis of water soluble vitamins in total parenteral solutions by high pressure liquid chromatography. Pharm Week Sci Ed. 1989; 11:169-74.
32. Gillis J, Jones G, Pencharz P. Delivery of vitamins A, D, and E in total parenteral nutrition solutions. JPEN. 1983; 7:11-14.
33. Bennett KM and Rosen GH. Cyclic total parenteral nutrition. Nutr Clin Practice. 1990; 5 163-165.
34. Gold ML, Fedder DO. Developing a pharmaceutical care plan. US Pharmacist. 1992; 17:53-60.
35. ASPEN Board of Directors. Guidelines for the use of enteral nutrition in the adult patient. JPEN. 1987; 11:435-439.
36. Silk DBA and Grimble GK. Relevance of physiology of nutrient absorption to formulation of enteral diets. Nutrition. 1992; 8:1-12.
37. Kudsk KA, Croce MA, Fabian TC, et.al. Enteral versus parenteral feeding. Effects on septic morbidity after blunt and penetrating abdominal trauma. Am Surg. 1992; 215:503-13.
38. Edes T, Walk B, Austin J. Diarrhea in tube-fed patients.

Feeding formula not necessarily the cause. Ann J Med. 1990; 88:91-93.
39. Lehmann S, Barber JR. Giving medications by feeding tube. How to avoid problems. Nursing. 1991; 43:58-61.
40. Roarty SLP, Muller RJ. Metabolic complications in long-term parenteral nutrition patients. Hosp Pharm. 1986; 21:641-642.

21 Home Chemotherapy

Jane W. Kwan, B.S. Pharmacy, M.P.H.

The diagnosis of cancer imposes on the patient a devastating sense of loss of control over one's life. Home chemotherapy allows patients to become active participants in administering their own therapy, providing an opportunity to regain some of that control. Patients who receive chemotherapy at home enjoy greater independence and are often able to carry on with the routine activities of daily living, to remain at home, or return to work. The familiar environment of the home setting and the emotional support of family and friends contribute to a greater sense of well-being, an improved tolerance to drug-related side-effects, and an overall improved quality of life.[1]

Approximately one million new patients will be diagnosed with cancer every year according to estimates by the National Cancer Institute.[2] As recently as fifteen years ago, a patient receiving chemotherapy would expect to be hospitalized for the administration of that drug regimen. Advances in both vascular access devices and infusion pumps have enabled an ever growing number of patients to receive chemotherapy at home safely and reliably. While chemotherapy represents only 4% of the total home infusion market, the annual growth rate of the home chemotherapy market is estimated to be 19.2%. The chemotherapy market is expected to reach a value of $152.2 million in 1993, according to estimates by Biomedical Business International.[3]

The role of the home health care (HHC) pharmacist in a home chemotherapy therapy program can be defined in terms of many functions and responsibilities, but the overall responsibility of the pharmacist is to optimize patient outcomes. Outcomes can be optimized by ensuring the safe and appropriate use of all drugs used in the HHC setting. (See also Chapter 23.)

BASIC CONCEPTS OF CHEMOTHERAPY

The pharmacist must have an understanding of the basic concepts of chemotherapy to be able to develop a comprehensive and appropriate role in home chemotherapy. Although the term chemotherapy refers generally to the use of drugs to treat any medical condition, the term is widely used to refer to the use of antineoplastic drugs for the treatment of cancer.

The goal of chemotherapy is to selectively kill cancer cells. While recent research efforts have focused on targeting drug delivery to tumor cells, chemotherapy still exerts cytotoxic effects on normal cells. The systemic effects of chemotherapy on normal cells are demonstrated by the toxicities and side effects associated with chemotherapy. Such side effects include nausea, vomiting, bone marrow suppression, alopecia, and neuropathy.

Chemotherapy regimens are generally administered as a course of therapy. A course of chemotherapy may consist of a single dose of drug or multiple doses over a specified time period that might be repeated at specified intervals, typically 21 to 28 days. The duration of the interval between courses of chemotherapy is primarily dependent on the time required for recovery of normal cells, particularly blood components, e.g., bone marrow suppression, neutropenia.

When more than one chemotherapeutic agent is administered, the regimen is termed combination chemotherapy. Combination chemotherapy regimens are designed to maximize cell kill while minimizing drug toxicity by combining different drugs. The selection of the drugs is generally based on three criteria:

1. Each drug in the combination has demonstrated single agent activity against the specific tumor.
2. The drugs have different mechanisms of action to enhance efficacy.

3. The drugs have different toxicities to avoid cumulative toxic effects.

Continuous Infusion Chemotherapy

Chemotherapy can be administered by a variety of routes, including oral, topical, subcutaneous, intramuscular, intrathecal, intra-arterial, and intravenous. Intravenous chemotherapy may be administered either as continuous infusions or bolus injections, although home chemotherapy is often administered as a continuous infusion.

Continuous infusions have been shown to improve the therapeutic index of certain antineoplastic agents and to improve patient tolerance to the course of chemotherapy. As an example, continuous infusion of doxorubicin has been shown to be less cardiotoxic than bolus injections and permits a larger cumulative dose to be administered.[4] Some cytotoxic agents, such as cisplatin, are more emetogenic with bolus injections, and continuous infusion can reduce both the occurrence and severity of nausea and vomiting.[5]

The rationale upon which continuous infusions has been based is an attempt to take advantage of both pharmacokinetic characteristics of antineoplastic drugs and cytokinetic characteristics of tumor cells. Cytotoxic drugs with short half lives benefit from prolonged exposure of drug to the tumor cells. Drugs that show activity in specific phases of the cell cycle benefit from the prolonged exposure of drug to a greater proportion of the tumor cell population.

Use of Infusion Technology in Home Chemotherapy Patients

The development of infusion technology has facilitated the treatment of chemotherapy patients in the home with both continuous infusion and bolus injections in the home.[6] Home chemotherapy patients may also require concurrent therapy for other conditions, such as total parenteral nutrition, patient controlled analgesia, antibiotics, and antiemetics. While administration of intravenous doses may be accomplished in the home by the patient or nurse using a standard minibag via gravity, technology is now available to permit the use of infusion pumps to deliver these doses. Patients can be taught to manage infusion pump systems and self-administer these therapies at home.

Chemotherapy was one of the earliest therapeutic options for which infusion pumps were first developed. Both electromechanical pumps and disposable pumps have been developed to deliver either bolus intermittent doses or continuous infusions of a single or multiple day duration. Electromechanical pumps typically offer the user more sophisticated programming capabilities than disposable devices, although there are longer term expenses to the HHC provider such as distribution, tracking, maintenance, and service. The advantages of disposable pumps typically include ease of use, low acquisition costs, and no maintenance costs. (See also Chapter 19.)

Stability and Compatibility Information

The use of infusion devices to deliver home chemotherapy requires an expanded knowledge base of drug stabilities and compatibilities by the pharmacist. When a drug is delivered in an infusion pump system, the compatibility of the drug with pump system components must be determined.[7] Examples of pump system components include the medication reservoir, administration set, or pump materials wherever the drug comes into direct contact with the pump.

One of the primary benefits of infusion pumps is the ability to deliver multiple doses of drug from a single reservoir, if drug stability allows. Reducing the number of reservoir changes by the patient decreases the potential for contamination of system components during the change and therefore the opportunity for patient infection. This benefit must be weighed against the potential for microbiological proliferation of an inadvertently contaminated medication reservoir that is stored at room or body temperature over multiple days. It cannot be assumed that cytotoxic infusions are bactericidal.[8]

Preparation of Home Chemotherapy Doses

The preparation of home chemotherapy doses must meet the same guidelines and standards for sterility assurance and quality control as the preparation of any aseptically prepared sterile product. Most home chemotherapy programs are established as part of a total home infusion therapy program. The home infusion therapy program is generally licensed as a community pharmacy by the state board of pharmacy, although a few states have adopted specific guidelines for the licensure of pharmacies preparing sterile products. In Texas, the state board of pharmacy has adopted regulations which include both operational requirements of such pharmacies and new guidelines for patient care and clinical services.[9] The Joint Commission for the Accreditation of Healthcare Organizations has also promulgated standards of practice for pharmaceutical services for HHC organizations.[10] The American Society of Hospital Pharmacists is currently drafting guidelines on the pharmacist's role in home infusion therapy, with particular emphasis on the provision of pharmaceutical care to the patient receiving injectable drug therapies in the home setting. The United States Pharmacopoeia has also published an informational chapter on the preparation of sterile drug products intended for home use.[11]

In addition to the guidelines that apply to all sterile products, guidelines specifically for the preparation of cytotoxic doses have also been developed. The primary goal of such guidelines has been to limit the exposure of personnel preparing and administering cytotoxic doses. Although the long term risks to personnel involved in the preparation, administration, and handling of cytotoxic and hazardous agents are unknown, some increased short term adverse effects associated with the handling of antineoplastic drugs have been documented.[12]

Guidelines for the handling of cytotoxic agents have been developed by several organizations, such as the American Society of Hospital Pharmacists,[13] the National Study Commission on Cytotoxic Exposure,[14] and the Federal Occupational Safety and Health Administration.[15] Using these guidelines, the home infusion therapy pharmacy should develop policies and procedures for the handling of cytotoxic agents.[16] The guidelines are primarily directed toward the work environment and address methods by which personnel preparing and administering cytotoxic agents should be protected. These include use of a Class II or III Biological Safety Cabinet, wearing of appropriate protective garb, use of techniques and procedures to minimize potential exposure during the preparation process, storage and transport, cleanup of spills, and disposal of hazardous drug waste. Although none of these guidelines addresses precautions to be taken in the home environment, the HHC provider should develop procedures for nursing staff administering chemotherapy doses, as well as for patients and/or family members in the home.

Disposal

Although cancer patients in the home may receive therapeutic doses of cytotoxic drugs, they and family members should also be considered at risk to accidental exposure when preparing or administering cytotoxic drugs. Guidelines for education of home patients should be developed to include instruction on potential risks, proper storage, administration, and disposal of these drugs, all with the intent of minimizing the risk of exposure to the patient, family members, or nurse administering the drug in the home.[17] Although OSHA guidelines are directed toward occupational exposure, adaptation of these guidelines for home use would be prudent, particularly as it relates to administration and disposal of cytotoxic waste.

Syringes, needles, tubing, and other waste generated during the preparation and administration of cytotoxic agents should be placed in specially labeled disposal containers which are leak and puncture proof. These containers should be provided to the patient and upon completion of therapy or when full, picked up and replaced by the home infusion therapy provider. A spill kit, containing supplies to use in case of an accidental spill, should also be provided when chemotherapy is administered in the home. The spill kit should contain such items as a protective gown, gloves, spill towels, plastic bags, and other supplies as appropriate.

Administration

The first dose of a cytotoxic agent may be administered in the home only if the safety and conditions of such administration have been decided upon by the physician, nurse, and pharmacist.[18] While many patients receive chemotherapy directly through a peripheral vein, drugs delivered by an infusion pump, particularly those that are vesicants, should be administered through a central venous catheter access line.

A growing number of venous access devices are now available, and the pharmacist should be knowledgeable of the characteristics of the various systems and how the system impacts drug delivery. Some general categories of devices include silicone elastomer central catheters, implanted infusion ports, and peripherally inserted short term catheters.[19] Although venous access devices are widely and successfully used in the HHC setting, there are potential complications associated with their use. These include catheter occlusion, air embolism, phlebitis, infiltration, and infection.[20] Policies and procedures should be developed that address the prevention, monitoring, and management of potential complications.[21]

Extravasation of vesicant agents can result in permanent tissue damage. Nurses administering vesicant drugs and patients receiving them should be taught to monitor for signs of extravasation and to take immediate action in response to an extravasation. A treatment plan for the management of extravasation should be developed and in place whenever a vesicant agent will be administered in the home.[22] The components of the plan should include a list of agents categorized as vesicants, irritants, or non-vesicants, as well as the steps to be taken in the case of a suspected extravasation for specific vesicants.

Investigational Drugs

The administration of investigational drugs is usually initiated in the hospital or other institutional setting, although administration can continue into the home setting, typically with agents classified as Phase II or Phase III. When investigational drugs are provided by the home infusion therapy pharmacy, specific requirements for their use are imposed, including recordkeeping, adherence to protocol guidelines, and monitoring.

Investigational drugs may, in some cases, be initiated in the HHC setting. The review and approval of the protocol prior to dose preparation and administration is often performed by the medical advisory board of the HHC provider. A copy of the investigational protocol and patient informed consent should be included in the patient's medical record. Documentation of prescribed monitoring, e.g., lab tests, patient assessment, and outcome criteria, should also be reported.

If the HHC provider will be responsible for obtaining investigational drugs, additional procedures must be developed. The American Society of Hospital Pharmacists has published guidelines for the use of investigational drugs in institutions[23] that can be adapted for HHC providers.

PATIENT SELECTION CRITERIA

Careful patient selection is crucial to the success of a home chemotherapy program.[24] Criteria for home chemotherapy patients are, in many ways, similar to those of other home therapies:

1. The patient, family member(s), and other caregiver(s) must have the ability to learn the necessary skills for home infusion.
2. The patient must have the motivation to assume that responsibility. A supporting environment in which there is a willingness to learn the required procedures contributes to a successful therapeutic outcome.
3. The patient must have basic environmental requirements in the home. The preparation of a drug dose for administration requires a clean area in which to perform aseptic procedures, and drug storage often requires refrigeration. Telephone access for the patient to obtain emergency help when problems arise and to enable communication between the home patient and the home care provider is a critical requirement.

Home chemotherapy patients differ from patients with diagnoses other than cancer. Primary differences include:

1. The chemotherapy patient has a need for more frequent and prolonged venous access, requiring multiple courses of therapy over an extended time period. In addition, many antineoplastic agents are vesicants and can be irritating to the vein, necessitating the use of central venous access catheters for home chemotherapy administration.
2. A common side effect of many antineoplastic agents is leukopenia. Patients receiving such agents become more susceptible to infection due to chemotherapy administration.
3. The patient may receive multiple therapies, e.g., antibiotics, pain control, total parenteral nutrition, hydration, and antiemetics, in addition to chemotherapy, requiring more intense monitoring of the therapeutic regimens by the pharmacist.

Multidisciplinary Communication

The provision of home chemotherapy requires a coordinated effort among health care professionals, the patient, and family members. Each member of the health care team should be assigned defined responsibilities, but the critical component required for successful patient outcomes is effective communication among the various disciplines.

In many HHC settings, it is the pharmacist's responsibility to assure that communication takes place. The pharmacist is responsible for communication of the pharmaceutical care plan to other members of the HHC team. The pharmacist typically receives laboratory values and then is responsible for interpreting those results and making recommendations to the physician for any adjustments in dose, continuation, or discontinuation of the drug regimen. Communication with the nurse or technician making the home visit is necessary to determine patient utilization of doses in order to prepare the doses or send needed supplies to the patient's home.

Pharmaceutical Care Plan

Care plans have typically been developed from a nursing perspective for home infusion therapy patients. In conjunction with the nursing care plan, the pharmaceutical care plan helps to ensure that the patient receives safe and appropriate therapy. A pharmaceutical care plan should be developed and documented in the medical record when the patient is accepted into home care services and updated regularly as long as the patient remains on service. (See also Chapter 9.)

The purpose of the pharmaceutical care plan is to optimize the drug regimen by identifying, monitoring, preventing, and treating chemotherapy-induced toxicities. Components of the plan include identification of the desired outcome of drug therapy, potential problems and their solutions, monitoring parameters by which to measure those problems and outcomes, and a schedule for conducting that monitoring.

The first step in the development of a pharmaceutical care plan for the chemotherapy patient is assessment of the patient's initial status. The assessment provides information that will serve as a baseline reference for drug therapy monitoring and determination of patient outcomes. Such information includes patient diagnosis, physical assessment, medical history, medication history, drug allergies, most recent laboratory test results, goals of therapy, desired outcome indicators, and extent of patient education already received.

The next step in developing the pharmaceutical care plan is to identify expected potential problems that might occur during chemotherapy, actions to be taken when problems occur, and a scheduled plan for monitoring the occurrence of problems and outcomes of therapy. The pharmaceutical care plan should address the most frequent and the most serious types of toxicities that might be encountered with the drug being administered. Examples of such toxicities that can cause negative patient outcomes include drug induced renal dysfunction, nausea and vomiting, dehydration, neutropenia, and uncontrolled pain. Documentation of treatment should include the dose for each regimen, the cumulative dose received, the response to the regimen, the toxicity of treatment, and the results of routine monitoring.

MANAGEMENT OF TOXICITIES

Dose reductions or treatment delays can compromise the success of a therapeutic regimen, so that a plan to prevent, minimize, and manage predictable toxicity should be developed. Potential problems that might occur in patients most often are due to predicted side effects of antineoplastic agents. Side effects occur because antineoplastic agents affect normal cells, as well as cancer cells, and depending on the severity of toxicities, can also be the dose limiting factor in chemotherapy regimens. Among the cells most likely to be affected are bone marrow, gastrointestinal tract, reproductive system, and hair follicles. Resultant side effects can include nausea, vomiting, stomatitis, lowered sperm count, amenorrhea, alopecia, and decreases in blood counts, including red blood cells, white blood cells, and platelets.

Nausea and Vomiting

Patients should be encouraged to take small, frequent meals, particularly with low acid and low residue foods. Cold foods, such as popsicles and ice chips, and bland foods, such as toast or crackers, are generally more tolerable to chemotherapy patients. Chemotherapy can also change the taste of food, so patients might be told not to eat favorite foods while on chemotherapy, since a dislike to that food could occur. Patients should be encouraged to increase their fluid intake if they become nauseous during the course of chemotherapy. Patients should be taught to monitor their weight and report substantial (e.g., 3-5 pound weight loss in a week or an overall 10 pound change) weight loss/gain to their physicians.

Mouth Sores

Patients can help prevent the occurrence of mouth sores by using a soft toothbrush, avoiding commercial mouthwashes which are usually high in alcohol content, keeping lips moist using a lubricant, and avoiding tart acidic foods. Swabs may be substituted for toothbrushes. If mouth sores develop, patients should be encouraged to maintain a soft bland diet and avoid both acidic mouthwashes and bristled toothbrushes. An example of an alternative mouthwash is:

Salt	One Teaspoon
Soda	One Teaspoon
Warm Water	q.s. One Quart

Diarrhea

Patients should be encouraged to drink lots of fluids and to avoid roughage, spicy foods, coffee, and alcohol. In cases of severe diarrhea, the physician should be contacted.

Constipation

Increasing both fiber and fluid intake can decrease the potential for the development of constipation. According to physician advice, the use of natural laxatives, e.g., prunes, and the use of commercial stool softeners or laxatives might also be recommended.

Bone Marrow

Bone marrow suppression is an expected consequence of certain antineoplastic agents. Although in these cases, bone marrow suppression cannot be prevented, patients can be taught to manage the effects of bone marrow suppression. Bone marrow suppression may result in lowered red blood cells, white blood cells, or platelets. Anemia is the result of decreased red blood cell counts, and patients should be advised to take rest periods as needed and to report signs and symptoms of weakness and pallor to their physician. Leukopenia is the result of lowered white blood cell counts, and patients should avoid potential sources of infection, e.g., persons with infections, large crowds, etc. Patients should be taught to take their temperature regularly and to report other signs and symptoms of infection, e.g., sore throat, cough, burning on urination. The introduction of hematopoietic growth factors, e.g., G-CSF and GM-CSF, has led to their administration in an effort to shorten the duration of neutropenia following chemotherapy and thus reduce the incidence of infection. With lowered platelet counts, patients should avoid sources of trauma, e.g., use of an electric razor instead of a blade, avoid aspirin, and report any unusual signs of bleeding or bruises.

Alopecia

While hair loss may occur with the administration of some drugs, the loss is usually reversible. Hair growth will resume after discontinuing chemotherapy, usually within two to three weeks. In some patients, the new hair may be different in color and/or texture from what it was before. Patients may choose to wear wigs, scarves, or hats during the period of hair loss.

Reproductive System

Females on chemotherapy may experience decreased sexual desire, amenorrhea, or in near menopause women, premature menopause. Males may experience decreased sexual desire, reduced sperm count, and sterility may occur. Contraception is recommended, since the effects of chemotherapy on the fetus is unknown.

PATIENT TEACHING

Patient teaching is a shared responsibility of the HHC team, and is a critical factor in the success of a home infusion therapy program. Patient teaching should be comprehensive and include topics such as aseptic technique, catheter care, procedures for drug administration, use of equipment and supplies, expected side effects, and management of complications that could occur.

Although the nursing staff is most often responsible for patient teaching, pharmacists in home chemotherapy programs are taking more active roles in performing the teaching. Teaching content for chemotherapy patients should include general information on chemotherapy and specific information on the drugs the patient will receive. General information should include a discussion of what chemotherapy is, the role that chemotherapy plays as one of four treatment modalities for cancer, how chemotherapy works, an explanation of a course of chemotherapy, the rationale for drug selection, and why combination chemotherapy might be used. Resources for this information include the National Cancer Institute[25] and the American Cancer Society.

Specific drug information on the agent(s) the patient will receive should be provided prior to drug administration. Such information includes an explanation of how each drug works, a description of early side effects that might occur during or immediately after administration, late side effects that might occur three to four weeks after administration, storage instructions, and any other special precautions the patient might need to take, such as drinking plenty of fluids for certain drugs to prevent bladder irritation. Good resources for drug specific information include publications from the National Cancer Institute[26] and the USP DI.[27]

Patient teaching should be both structured and documented to ensure standardized content and method of teaching.[28] The development of teaching plans ensures standardization. Components of a teaching plan include identification of the instructor, e.g., nurse, pharmacist; the objective to be met; the content to meet that objective; the teaching action to be used, and the outcome criteria against which the instructor should be able to assess the success of the teaching.

Documentation of patient teaching should be included in the home care record and should include identification of the learning needs of the patient and/or significant other; the specific topic(s) taught; an indication of the patient's readiness to learn and any learning barriers, e.g., handicaps, acuity of illness; the specific teaching tool(s) utilized; the patient outcome to teaching, e.g., demonstrated skills, verbalized understanding, requires additional teaching; and signature of the person taught.

QUALITY IMPROVEMENT

Assessment and improvement of performance is achieved through a quality improvement program. The development of a program to improve quality in a home chemotherapy program focuses on patient satisfaction and desirable patient outcomes. Such a program involves a multidisciplinary approach and the development of indicators to measure system performance. Outcome indicators for home infusion therapy are in development by the Joint Commission on Accreditation of Healthcare Organizations and include unscheduled inpatient admissions, discontinued infusion therapy, interruption of infusion therapy, development of infection, adverse drug reactions, and interventions based on patient monitoring of medication use.[29] The indicators are intended to be further categorized by type of therapy, so that application of the general indicators can be focused on the chemotherapy patient. (See also Chapter 4.)

CONCLUSION

The delivery of chemotherapy to the HHC patient offers a challenging opportunity to the HHC pharmacist. The selection, preparation, and delivery of a compounded product has served as the basis for pharmacist roles in HHC. Today, the pharmacist has the opportunity to expand participation in the management of the chemotherapy patient to optimize therapeutic outcomes.

The provision of home chemotherapy is one in which the pharmacist utilizes both pharmaceutical and clinical skills. Such a role requires a sound knowledge base in the principles of chemotherapy to develop a strategy to provide the product, to ensure compliance to the therapeutic regimen, and to develop the pharmaceutical care plan to ensure the optimum outcome.

REFERENCES

1. Schlag P, Schwarz A, Frohmuller S. Drug Delivery to cancer patients in home care: Experience with intraarterial and intravenous chemotherapy. In Drug Delivery in Cancer Treatment II. Domellof L, ed. New York; 1989.
2. Holleb AI, Fink DJ, Murphy GP. American Cancer Society Textbook of Clinical Oncology. American Cancer Society, Inc. 1991.
3. Increase in market for home infusion product and services predicted. Am J. Hosp Pharm. 1990; 47:958,960.
4. Robert J. Continuous infusion or intravenous bolus: What is the rationale for doxorubicin administration? Cancer Drug Delv. 1987; 4:591-9.
5. Vokes EE, Ackland SP, Vogelzang NJ. Cisplatin, carboplatin, and gallium nitrate. In Cancer Chemotherapy by Infusion. Lokich JJ., ed., Chicago. 1990; 176-96.
6. Shaw HL. Treatment of the patient with cancer using parenteral electronic drug administration. Cancer. 1992; 70(4S):993-7.
7. Kowaluk EA, Roberts MS, Polacy AE. Interactions between drugs and intravenous delivery systems. Am J Hosp Pharm. 1982; 39:460-7.
8. Wilson JP, Solimando DA. Aseptic technique as a safety precaution in the preparation of antineoplastic agents. Hosp Pharm. 1981; 15:575-81.
9. Texas State Board of Pharmacy. Texas Pharmacy Rules. 2/29/92: Title 22, Part 15; 98-99.
10. Joint Commission on Accreditation of Healthcare Organizations. Accreditation Manual for Home Care, Volume 1 Standards. Pharmaceutical Services. Oakbrook Terrace, Illinois. 1993; 35-43.
11. Dispensing practices for sterile drug products intended for home use. Pharmacopeial Forum. 1992; 18(2):3054-5.
12. Valanis GB, Vollmer WM, Labuhn KT, et al. Association of antineoplastic drug handling with acute adverse effects in pharmacy personnel. Am J Hosp Pharm. 1993; 50:455-62.
13. Anon. ASHP technical assistance bulletin on handling cytotoxic drugs in hospitals. Am J Hosp Pharm. 1990; 47:1033-49.
14. Recommendations for handling cytotoxic agents. Providence, RI: National Study Commission on Cytotoxic Exposure. 1987.
15. Yodaiken R. Safe handling of cytotoxic drugs by health care personnel. Washington, DC: Occupational Safety and Health Administration. 1986; 1,29:(Instructional publication 8-1.1).
16. Mayer DK. Hazards of chemotherapy. Implementing safe handling practices. Cancer. 1992; 70(S4):988-92.
17. Barstow J. Safe handling of cytotoxic agents in the home. Home Health Nurse. 1986; 3:46-7.

18. Parker GG. Chemotherapy administration in the home. Home Health Nurse. 1992; 10:30-6.
19. Goodman MS, Wickham R. Venous access devices: an oncology nurse overview. Hosp Pharm. 1985; 20:495-7,501-3,506-8, 511.
20. Hayward SR, Ledgerwood AM, Lucas CE. The fate of 100 prolonged venous access devices. Am Surg. 1990; 56:515-9.
21. Richardson D and Bruso P. Vascular access devices: management of common complications. J Intravenous Nurs. 1993; 16:44-9.
22. Hirsh JD, Conlon PF. Implementing guidelines for managing extravasation of antineoplastics. Am J Hosp Pharm. 1983; 40:1516-9.
23. ASHP guidelines for the use of investigational drugs in institutions. Am J Hosp Pharm. 1983; 40:449-51.
24. Reville B, Almadrones L. Continuous infusion chemotherapy in the ambulatory setting: The nurse's role in patient selection and education. Oncol Nurs Forum. 1989; 16:529-35.
25. U.S. Department of Health and Human Services, National Institutes of Health, National Cancer Institute. Chemotherapy & You, A Guide to Self-Help During Treatment. NIH Publication No. 88-1136. Bethesda, Maryland. 1987.
26. U.S. Department of Health and Human Services, National Institutes of Health, National Cancer Institute. Chemotherapy & You, A Guide to Self-Help During Treatment. NIH Publication No. 88-1136. Bethesda, Maryland. 1987.
27. United States Pharmacopeial Convention. USP Dispensing Information, Advice for the Patient Volume II. Rockville, Maryland. 1993.
28. Lynch M, Yanes L. Flowsheet documentation of chemotherapy administration and patient teaching. Oncol Nurs Forum. 1992; 18:777-83.
29. Regenstein M. JCAHO reports field testing of six indicators for home infusion therapy. Nutr Clin Pract. 1992; 7:44-5.

22 Pain Management

Patricia New, Pharm.D.
Richard Bulich, Pharm.D.

The management of acute and chronic pain presents many challenges to the home health care (HHC) provider. Increasing economic pressures are forcing health care providers to utilize outpatient management of acute pain associated with surgery and chronic pain related to such diseases as cancer or AIDS. This chapter will describe the methods for providing parenteral pain therapies outside the traditional acute care setting.

DEFINITIONS RELATED TO PAIN MANAGEMENT [1-3]

Before a clinician can begin to manage pain of any type, it is first necessary to understand the pain symptoms presented by many patients. The five major types of pain are:

- Acute pain: pain of short duration, with an expected resolution within days or weeks, usually associated with trauma, surgery, or an infectious process;
- Chronic pain: pain of long duration, usually months to life, usually without the hope of resolution, usually associated with cancer or other catastrophic illness such as AIDS, debilitating arthritis, or major injury;
- Somatic pain: pain originating from muscle, bone, or other skeletal regions;
- Visceral pain: pain originating from an organ, such as the liver, stomach, or pancreas; and
- Neuropathic pain: pain involving nerves, or the nerve plexus, that is usually described as sharp, burning, or stabbing pain; sometimes referred to as deafferentation pain. Neuropathic pain is the most difficult pain syndrome to manage in any setting.

When dealing with narcotic analgesics it is extremely important to understand the terminology associated with their use as well as many of the misconceptions and misunderstandings. The following definitions and terms assist in overcoming some of the barriers associated with pain management. A clear understanding of these concepts is vital to all health care professionals involved in pain management and is needed to avoid giving sub-therapeutic doses to patients in severe pain.

Drug Tolerance: A physiologic effect that requires increasing doses of a narcotic analgesic to produce the same or continued pharmacologic effect or pain relief. This term should not be confused with progression of disease in terminal cancer patients usually seen at the end stage of the disease. Drug tolerance is usually first identified by a decrease in the time interval between doses of narcotic analgesic due to recurrence of pain prior to the next scheduled dose. The most effective method of management of drug tolerance is to change to a sustained release form of narcotic or to continuous infusion of narcotics. Another method is to switch the patient to another class of narcotic, being careful to adjust the dose to compensate for incomplete cross tolerance between narcotic analgesics.

Drug Dependence: A physiologic effect that occurs when a patient has been receiving a narcotic analgesic for a prolonged period of time (weeks to months), in which sudden cessation of the drug will cause withdrawal symptoms of muscle aches or twitching, perspiration, anxiety or pain. This effect is somewhat analogous to the physical dependence that develops after long term use of caffeine, nicotine, or alcohol. Drug dependence is often confused with addiction by patients and health care providers.

Drug Addiction: A psychological phenomena of drug seeking behavior associated with obtaining a drug for reasons other than relief of physical pain. A select group of patients that are seen for chronic pain may have addictive behavior, but the majority of patients with severe pain utilize their medications for the relief of their physical pain.

GENERAL PRINCIPLES OF PAIN MANAGEMENT

The goal of management of pain in any setting is to use the simplest, least expensive, and most effective modality possible. Even though pharmacologic management is the most common and often most effective method for the management of the majority of pain syndromes, other non-pharmacologic interventions should be utilized as part of a treatment plan. Examples of these non-pharmacologic modalities include direct application of heat or cold, relaxation techniques, hypnosis, distraction, visualization and the use of TENS (transcutaneous electrical nerve stimulation). Use of these interventions may provide an important component in the management of complicated pain problems, as an adjuvant to more sophisticated pharmacologic interventions.[2,3]

The World Health Organization has established basic guidelines for the pharmacologic approach to pain. A standard stepladder approach to the control of pain is recommended. [4] This approach divides pain into three levels of severity: mild, moderate, and severe. Mild pain can be treated with aspirin, acetaminophen or non-steroidal anti-inflammatory drugs (NSAIDs) by the oral route whenever possible. As pain becomes more severe and aspirin, acetaminophen, or NSAIDs no longer provide adequate relief, the second level of pharmacologic management is the use of weak opiates such as codeine or oxycodone. It is important to continue the first level of analgesics, if possible, especially if inflammation or bone pain is being treated. The synergistic effect of the NSAID can potentiate the weak opiates, thus allowing for lower opiate doses. More severe pain may necessitate the use of more potent opiates such as morphine. These agents may be given orally, rectally or via the transdermal route initially. If these methods no longer provide acceptable pain relief, injectable narcotics would be indicated. Parenteral narcotics may be administered by subcutaneous or IV intermittent injections, continuous infusion with or without patient controlled analgesia capability, epidural or intrathecal injections or infusions.

Assessing Pain

Clinicians involved in pain management for both acute and chronic pain syndromes should understand the issues that relate to pain assessment that can at times provide barriers to delivering adequate pain relief. The issue of assessing pain is laden with many psychosocial components. It is a subjective report by the patient and is often difficult to measure. In some cases, patients may actually understate their pain when asked to report to a clinician or family member. It is most important to utilize a method of evaluation of pain that is consistent, especially when multiple caregivers (family members, nurses, pharmacists) are interacting with the patient. Many systems for categorization of pain exists.[2,3]

Numerical systems categorizing pain from zero to five or zero to ten are most commonly used. Zero represents no pain while five or ten represents the most severe pain ever experienced or imagined by the patient. It is essential to recognize that a pain level of three for one patient may not equal the same number for another patient with a similar source of pain. Utilization of a standardized measurement of pain allows the caregiver to assess pain for the specific patient and is vital for the accurate evaluation of the treatment plan. Another useful way to assess pain management interventions is to ascertain from the patient what specific activities would be desirable to do if the pain was not present. By identifying a goal that is not just attached to a specific number on the pain rating scale, it often becomes easier to the patient and caregivers to see progress. The objective of pain management can not be to eliminate all pain but rather decrease the level of pain a patient perceives and improve the quality of life.[2,3]

TREATMENT OF ACUTE PAIN SYNDROMES

As previously described, acute pain is usually associated with surgery, trauma, or acute illness of short duration. The focus of this section will be on the management of acute postoperative pain management, because economic pressures are directing more surgeries to outpatient surgery centers and HHC pharmacies. Since the outpatient surgery centers are usually staffed for day procedures only, prolonged postsurgical pain management is provided in the home setting. The advent of both parenteral NSAIDs and more effective oral

NSAIDs has helped dramatically improve the effectiveness of treatment for this patient population. Patients should be treated initially with both non-narcotic and narcotic oral drugs. If the oral route fails or is not feasible due to other medical reasons, the use of other forms of analgesia may sometimes be required. Intramuscular ketoralac in doses of 60 mg initially followed by 30 mg every 6 hours after surgery may be given by HHC nurses or family members for short periods of time to manage the acute pain. Transdermal delivery of fentanyl is not generally indicated in this patient population due to variability of response and the length of time needed to stabilize the patient on a given dose.

It may become necessary in some patients who are unable to swallow oral medications or obtain relief from other routes of administration, to utilize small doses of narcotics by patient controlled analgesia (PCA).[5] This method of delivery of narcotics for the postsurgical patient is safe and effective in the hospital setting[6] and is also utilized for this patient population in the outpatient setting. The advent of computerized programmable ambulatory infusion pumps allows for controlled and accurate delivery of narcotic analgesia by the subcutaneous or intravenous rote. This technology allows the initiation of analgesia in the recovery room setting, and continues when the patient returns to the home environment. If the patient has appropriate presurgical teaching and HHC follow-up, PCA is an effective way to manage postsurgical pain. It is recommended in this setting to utilize "bolus only PCA" without the continuous infusion, due to the risk of oversedation during sleeping hours immediately following surgery. If patients are alert enough to activate a bolus dose of narcotic analgesia, they will usually not be at risk for overdosage or oversedation. In patients requiring some type of basal infusion due to severe pain or prevention of clotting an IV line, a very low basal dose is recommended, with lockout intervals of 15 to 30 minutes for rescue doses of narcotic.

Morphine and meperidine are the most frequent postsurgical narcotics used with bolus doses ranging from 2-5 mg for morphine and 10-25 mg for meperidine and continuous infusion doses of 0.5-1 mg for morphine. It is important to note that the concepts used in treating postsurgical acute pain with PCA are very different from those used in chronic pain syndromes that will be described below.[3,5,6]

TREATMENT OF CHRONIC PAIN SYNDROMES

As previously described, chronic pain is usually associated with cancer, other catastrophic illness, or major injury. The treatment of chronic pain for non-malignant pain versus malignant pain requires very different approaches. The treatment of non-malignant pain frequently utilizes lifestyle changes and non-pharmacological interventions as part of the treatment plan. Since the majority of chronic pain patients that are managed by the HHC clinician are related to malignant pain, the focus of this section will be on this type.

It has been reported that at least two thirds of cancer patients in the final stages of their disease will report significant pain.[7] Clinical experience has shown that most cancer patients can initially be treated with oral medications, however alternate routes of administration are required as the disease progresses.[8] Alternate routes of administration may become necessary due to uncontrolled nausea and vomiting, bowel obstruction, malabsorption, mucositis or inadequate pain relief with large doses of oral narcotics. Other methods of narcotic administration may include sublingual/buccal, rectal, transdermal, intermittent subcutaneous or intravenous, continuous subcutaneous or intravenous with or without bolus capability, epidural or intrathecal injections or infusions. Each of these alternatives may have an appropriate role in a specific patient's pain management regimen. It is important that the clinician be aware of the advantages and disadvantages of each, and include the patient and caregiver in the decision making process. Patient/caregiver acceptability for the use of the rectal or sublingual route can be low due to inconvenience and inadequate response. The use of transdermal fentanyl may be appropriate in patients with stable pain syndromes. However, patients with inadequate pain relief or a progressing disease will often be difficult to titrate with this modality, because it may take up to six days to stabilize a patient on fentanyl.

Patient Controlled Analgesia

In most recent years, due to technological advances in the area of ambulatory infusion devices, it has become well accepted that the continuous infusion of narcotics with bolus capability can be administered safely and effectively in the home setting.[5,9] Using this method of administration, the chronic cancer patient receives a continuous infusion of narcotic (basal rate) with the ability to receive a bolus dose (on demand) for breakthrough pain. Lockout intervals between bolus doses are programmed into the infusion device and can only be altered by someone that knows the programming sequence.

Most PCA patients can be maintained on the subcutaneous route of administration. Various subcutaneous needles are available and usually utilize a 25 gauge or 27 gauge needle. Since many of these patients are immunocompromised they have an increased risk for development of subcutaneous site infections. A strict skin care protocol is recommended for sterilization of the area with changing of the site one to two times weekly. The subcutaneous route can be used indefinitely in these patients as long as they have adequate tissue, and the doses of narcotic do not require that the rate of infusion be greater than 2 ml/hr. At rates higher than 2 ml/hr, patients may experience site irritation and erratic drug absorption. For patients that are having site irritation even on low volumes of morphine, it is possible to add dexamethasone in concentrations ranging from 0.02 mg/ml to 0.08 mg/ml.[9] The combination of low dose dexamethasone and morphine is stable for 7 days at room temperature and has been shown to improve subcutaneous site tissue.[5,9]

There are various ambulatory infusion devices available to provide PCA.[10] The following criteria should be used in the selection of the device for home use: 1) adaptability to continuous infusion with or without bolus capability, 2) ease in programming, 3) security of the drug reservoir, 4) range of dose and lockout parameters, 5) easily identifiable bolus button, 6) adequate safety alarm system, 7) lock out features that allow for some selected patient or family ability to adjust basal or bolus doses within programmed limits. (See also Chapter 19.)

PCA may be started in the inpatient or outpatient setting. However, it is recommended that, unless a clinician has significant experience with pain management, patients should not receive home PCA until their pain is under adequate control. It is important to have detailed policies and procedures outlining the role of each member of the team prior to trying to manage a complicated pain patient in the outpatient setting. It is also vital to have adequate 24 hour nursing and pharmacy support for these patients.

PCA Infusions

The initial infusion rates, bolus doses and frequencies should be calculated based on the patient's prior narcotic history. Doses can be calculated by using an equal analgesic conversion chart (Table 22 - 1) to convert the prior 24 hours of narcotic use into the parenteral equivalent with dose adjustments made for cross tolerance.[9] Dividing the value by 24 yields an appropriate initial hourly continuous infusion rate. The bolus dose can generally be about 25% of the initial hourly infusion, but should then be adjusted based on the patient's response after a bolus dose. Initial physician orders should include the hourly infusion rate, the bolus dose and frequency, a range for the continuous infusion rate and bolus, as well as increments to increase the continuous infusion rate and bolus. An example of an appropriate order may be to start a patient on a continuous infusion of

Table 22-1 Equianalgesic Doses of Narcotics[1-3]

NARCOTIC	PARENTERAL DOSE (mg)	ORAL/RECTAL DOSE (mg)
Morphine	10	30
Hydromorphone	1.5	7.5
Oxycodone	-	15
Oxymorphone	-	10
Meperidine	75	300
Methadone	10	20
Levorphanol	2	4
Codeine	130	200

morphine sulfate 5 mg/hr with a 2 mg bolus every 60 minutes with a continuous infusion range up to 10 mg and a bolus dose up to 5 mg. Increases in continuous infusion and bolus doses should be no greater than 1 mg per hour.

Once a patient is stabilized on a given dose, the number of bolus doses the patient uses in a 24 hour period should be the determining factor for dosage adjustments. In general, if a patient requires more than 25% of their available boluses to control their pain on a daily basis, then a dosage adjustment may be indicated. In one report of 117 patients,[9] narcotic dosages ranged from 1 mg/hr for subcutaneous morphine up to 180 mg/hr for intravenous morphine (Table 22-2). Patients may require daily or twice daily nursing visits until the patient is stabilized, followed by weekly or twice weekly visits for ongoing pain assessment, drug reservoir change, and maintenance of subcutaneous site or intravenous vascular access.

EPIDURAL ANALGESIA

In the event of inadequate response to systemic pain therapy or unacceptable side effects of sedation and mental confusion, regional or intraspinal analgesia may be considered. Epidural analgesia is indicated for pain unrelieved by systemic narcotics and concomitant adjunctive therapies; pain relief accompanied by side effects due to systemic narcotic administration, which limit the patient's desired activity level; and localized pain syndromes, particularly pelvic abdominal tumors and bony lesions of the hip, spine or leg. Due to a wide variation in the terminology associated with intraspinal analgesia, the following glossary of terms should serve as a guide to understanding the concept of intrathecal and epidural analgesia. The focus of this section will be epidural analgesia, with a differentiation of intrathecal administration and the intraspinal route of administration.[5,12]

Types of Injections

Intraspinal analgesia is a general term that refers to both epidural and intrathecal administration of narcotics and local anesthetics. More specific terms include the following.

1. Epidural Analgesia is the administration of narcotics and local anesthetics into the epidural space, separated from the central spinal fluid by the membrane. The epidural space contains fat and connective tissue but no fluid. An infection in this space does not represent life threatening meningitis, but manifests as localized infection, easily treated by removal of the catheter and systemic antibiotic therapy. Doses of narcotics into this space are usually 1/10 of the systemic dose delivered in volumes up to 20 ml/hr.
2. Intrathecal Analgesia is the administration of narcotics and rarely local anesthetics into the intrathecal space or central spinal fluid. Doses are 1/5 to 1/10 the dose of epidural administration and volumes are usually 0.5 to 2 ml per day. This volume difference is a significant and distinguishing characteristic between the intrathecal and epidural delivery system. Infections in the intrathecal space represent life threatening meningitis-like syndromes, thus limiting the use of exteriorized catheter systems.

Types of Catheters

The temporary epidural catheter is a very thin and relatively stiff cannula used primarily for

Table 22-2 Typical Narcotic Dosages for HHC Patients

Narcotic	Basal Infusion (mg/hr)		Bolus Dose (mg)	
	RANGE	MEAN	RANGE	MEAN
Morphine SQ	1 to 33	6.5	0.5 to 1.5	4
Morphine IV	2 to 180	24	2.0 to 12	4
Hydromorphone SQ	0.3 to 21	3	0.5 to 15	1

postoperative epidural administration of narcotics and local anesthetics for acute care use for periods of 24 to 72 hours. The permanent exteriorized epidural catheter is a siliconized, soft internal catheter threaded into the epidural space, connected to a subcutaneously tunneled portion which exits at a convenient location, usually in the abdominal area for ease of use by the patient and caregivers. The subcutaneous tunnel provides an infection barrier to bacteria on the skin. The epidural port is a siliconized internal epidural segment tunneled and connected to a subcutaneously implanted port. This port is then accessed through the skin with a special non-coring huber point needle for intermittent injection or continuous infusion.

Implanted Pump For Intrathecal Pain Therapy

Surgically implanted infusion pumps are designed to deliver intrathecal narcotics for patients requiring pain therapy for long duration, usually six months or longer. The pump reservoir is filled with 24 to 28 days supply of medication via a Huber needle through the skin. Infrequent entry into the closed system lessens the chance for infection and requires minimal care.

Initiating Therapy

The usual epidural bolus dose of preservative free morphine sulfate ranges from 2 to 10 mg every 12 to 24 hours. Each dose is usually diluted to final volumes of 5 to 15 ml per dose in the hospital setting. Preservative free morphine is used most often. Although morphine is the most commonly used and least expensive, in some cases fentanyl or hydromorphone may be used if morphine causes nausea or sedation.

Once a permanent catheter system has been implanted by the physician, a 0.22 micron filter should be placed in-line at the hub of the catheter or Huber needle extension set and changed usually every 72 hours or twice per week. This filter will prevent particles from injection caps and rubber stopped vials from entering the epidural space and provide bacterial protection from possibly contaminated injectate.

Although some patients can be managed with intermittent bolus injections, others require continuous infusion of drug as their disease progresses. The addition of local anesthetics to potentiate the analgesic action of narcotic may be used in severe chronic pain syndromes. The addition of local anesthetics however, requires a continuous infusion delivery system in the outpatient setting to prevent hypotension associated with bolus dosing of these drugs.

Because of the risk of toxicity, the addition of local anesthetic to opiate infusions should be initiated in the acute care setting, to allow proper management of hypotension associated with initial doses of local anesthetics.

The use of preservative free narcotics and local anesthetics is an issue of continued debate and should be evaluated on a patient by patient basis. Factors involved in the decision include diagnosis and prognosis of the patient, economic impact, physician preference and experience, and informed consent of the patient and family members. Neurotoxic preservatives such as formaldehyde and phenol are known to cause toxicity and possible injury to nerve tissue.[11,12] Other neurosafe preservatives (methyl paraben, sodium bisulfite, chlorbutanol) may be infused in the epidural space.[11] Even though preserved products are significantly less expensive than preservative free products, the preserved products are not FDA approved for epidural use. Preservative containing products should not be used for intrathecal use, another distinguishing difference between the two intraspinal delivery systems.

Monitoring For Side Effects And Catheter Infections

Although respiratory depression and death have occurred in patients receiving epidural opiates for acute pain management, [9,11] severe respiratory depression has not been reported in cancer patients who are accustomed to long term narcotic administration. If oversedation occurs, a reduction in the dose of narcotic with the addition of local anesthetic should be considered. If nausea and vomiting occur, use of a different opiate, such as hydromorphone or fentanyl should be considered. The additional cost factor in the chronic pain setting should also be considered.

Catheter related problems are a significant factor in patients with indwelling epidural catheters. Nurses should monitor for catheter leakage, dislodgment and infection. Signs of leakage are obvious with moisture at exit site or fluid accumulation at the spinal cord insertion site. Epidural catheter infections, however, are more difficult to diagnose and often go unnoticed for long periods of time. The epidural space will often conceal infections so that common manifestations of infection, such as fever and white count elevation, are absent. Common clinical signs of infection are pain on injection or change in pain control or increased pain despite increased dose of analgesic.

Epidural catheter infection should be confirmed by culturing the epidural space by aspirating injectate from catheter and by epiduragram, showing thc location of dye around the catheter tip and retrograde pooling of injectate. If epidural infection is confirmed, the catheter should be removed and systemic antibiotics administered for 7 to 10 days directed at the cultured organism, if isolated. The catheter can be reinserted when the infection has cleared.

CONCLUSION

Parenteral administration of narcotics and local anesthetics may be safely and effectively managed in the outpatient setting if a multidisciplinary team approach is employed, directed by an experienced physician and assisted by qualified nurses and pharmacists. Proper protocols for catheter care and patient teaching are vital. Selection of the proper drug, dose, and infusion rate is necessary to control pain in HHC patients.

REFERENCES

1. Maciewicz R, Martin JB. Pain in Wilson, et al. Harrison's Principles of Internal Medicine. McGraw-Hill, New York, 1991.
2. Baumann TJ. Pain Management in DiPiro, et al. Pharmacotherapy. Appleton and Lange, Norwalk, 1993.
3. Lipman AG. Pain Management in Herfindal, et al. Clinical Pharmacy and Therapeutics. Williams and Wilkins, Baltimore, 1988.
4. World Health Organization: Cancer Pain Relief. Geneva, World Health Organization, 1986.
5. Smythe M. Patient Controller Analgesia. Pharmacotherapy. 1992;12:132.
6. White PF. Patient-Controlled analgesia: A new approach to the management of postoperative pain. Seminoanesth. 1985; 4:255-266.
7. Daut RL, Cleveland CS. Prevalence and severity of pain in cancer. Cancer. 1982; 50:1913-1918.
8. Coyle N, Adelhardt J, Foley KM. Changing patterns in pain, drug use, and routes of administration in the advanced cancer pain patient. Pain. 1987; 28:S339,(suppl 4).
9. Swanson G, Bulich R, New P, et al. Patient-Controlled Analgesia for Chronic Cancer Pain in the Ambulatory Setting: A Report of 117 Patients. J Clin Onc. 1989; 7:1903.
10. Kwan JW. High Technology IV Infusion Devices. Am J Hosp Pharm. 1989; 46:320-52.
11. DuPen SL, Ramsay DH. Compounding local anesthetic and narcotics for epidural analgesia in cancer outpatients. Presented as Poster, ASA Annual Meeting, October 1990.
12. Smith J, Bulich RG, and New PB. High-Tech Advances in the Treatment of Chronic Cancer Pain. Caring. 1989; 10:8.

23 Newer Parenteral Therapies

Norm Enriquez, Pharm.D.

The home infusion therapy (HIT) industry has grown over the past 10 years at a consistent 20-30% rate per year. For example, in 1991 home infusion revenues were $2.8 billion as a result of servicing over 350,000 patients. Tables 23-1 and 23-2 outline the demographics of the rapidly growing industry and the various factors that have contributed to this continued exponential growth shared by few other markets.[1,2] Continued widespread growth is expected, with the industry projected to reach $6 billion by 1995.[3] The result has been the development of an industry that is complex in character, served by clinicians engaging in a wide variety of therapies requiring keen clinical judgment. A few of the stimuli contributing to HIT's continued expansion are discussed briefly below.

First, economic pressures in America have had significant influence on the HIT market. Managed care providers, health maintenance organizations (HMO), preferred provider organizations (PPO), and provider networks have flourished, while the patient with pure indemnity insurance has dwindled. The evolution of these managed care groups has encouraged the rapid growth of HIT as each of the above entities seeks the most price efficient alternative to hospitalization.

Second, significant technological advances have contributed to an HIT armamentarium that is

Table 23-1 Profile of the U.S. Home Infusion Market (1992)[1]

Home health care agencies, total	12,000
Medicare certified home health care agencies	5,831
Home health care agencies providing drug infusion services	7,000
Patients treated by home IV therapy	350,000
Home health care revenues, total	16 billion
Home drug infusion services revenues	3.2 billion

Table 23-2 Factors Stimulating Growth of Home Infusion Services in the U.S.[1]

Earlier discharge
Pressures to contain upward spiraling hospital costs
Advances in technology (e.g., better venous access devices and pumps)
New drugs relevant to home care
Improved methods of disease detection
Increased survival of chronically ill patients
The AIDS crisis
Demographic shift toward an older population
Increased awareness and acceptance of home infusion by physicians, discharge planners, payers and patients

both diverse and eccentric. Specialized infusion devices engineered to specifically support the home-bound patient provide sound mechanical support to insure a safe home situation, guarantee compliance, and assist with complex infusion regimens.

Third, pharmacologic advances have resulted in the use of intravenous (IV) drugs that were once thought of as pharmacologic and biotechnologic dreams. Chronic disease states that were previously untreatable, are now candidates for treatment at home. Examples of disease states with this characteristic include Gaucher disease, various carcinomas with poor prognosis (e.g., hairy cell leukemia and metastatic ovarian cancer), and the various co-morbidities associated with the acquired immune deficiency syndrome (AIDS). These newer agents, along with a brief reflection on HIT's economic growth and the advances in an area referred to as traditional therapies are discussed below.

HISTORICAL PERSPECTIVE

Various investor industry reports have predicted the continued growth of HIT.[4] The projected cumulative growth rate for HIT is approximately 15% following nearly ten years where growth was estimated to be between 20-30% per year. In 1991 the bulk of the therapies (on a dollar basis) consisted of antibiotics contributing 48%; total parenteral nutrition (TPN), 32%; and enteral nutrition, 15%. The industry profile for 1996 is predicted to reflect an erosion in the contribution to the overall TPN market, decreasing to 20% with a concomitant rise in antibiotics to 54%. It is important to note that the changes in dollar percentages are a function mostly of the overall increases of other therapies which were not possible in the 1980's as well as shifts in attitudes and methods of treating various disease states.

Overall, the future health of HIT remains robust. Pressures of a pending economic reform platform proposed by the Clinton administration contribute to the speculation that HIT may realize a windfall as millions of previously uninsured Americans may have access to the clinical advantages of home health care (HHC). Additionally, as cost-benefit studies continue to be published, the case managed segment of health care payers will surely funnel a larger number of patients to the HIT arena.

NEW ANGLES TO TRADITIONAL THERAPIES

Table 23-3 lists a variety of therapies historically thought of as the traditional therapies in HIT. These therapies are important from a clinically historic perspective since they established the clinical track record for HHC clinicians.[5] As a result payers and physicians acknowledged that HIT was not a compromise in therapeutic efficacy. The end result was heightened physician confidence in the HHC concept. Equally important is the fact that traditional therapies helped provide the economic basis for insurance payers to recognize the financial advantages of caring for patients in venues other than hospitals. Both factors were important stimuli to the rapid growth of HIT in the period from 1982 to 1992.

Despite the rather routine appearance of the list in Table 23-3, new clinical insights and mechanical devices have made feasible the more frequent use of older therapies once thought too cumbersome for the HHC patient. Also, a willingness on the part of the HHC pharmacist to participate in critical therapies and test new horizons has contributed greatly to the added spectrum of new therapies.

Parenteral Nutrition

The provision of electrolytes, carbohydrates, lipids, protein and other micronutrients was first made possible following the perfection of the central venous catheter by Hickman.[5,6] Patients requiring long-term nutritional support for a variety of gastrointestinal maladies found their life-span prolonged, resulting in a substantial gain in quality of life. Also, nutritional failure was no longer the greatest contributor to death in patients with Crohn's disease, inflammatory bowel disease, infarcted bowel, or cancer. (See also Chapter 20.)

Table 23-3 Traditional Parenteral Therapies at Home

Total parenteral nutrition	Chemotherapy regimens
Parenteral antibiotics	Hydration
Enteral feedings	Anticoagulation therapy

Short term parenteral nutrition has been made possible via soft, pliable catheters that may be inserted in the antecubital space, eventually being threaded to the axillary region or superior vena cava (using peripherally inserted central catheters, PICCs) to provide the dilution factor necessary to reduce the phlebitic nature of the hypertonic nutrition solution. The true PICC insertion, with its end-point in the superior vena cava, is identical in utility to a Hickman®, Groshong®, or Port-A-Cath® device because of its final location. This group of catheters is generically referred to as central lines. Midline catheters, Landmark® catheters or other heparin lock devices are referred to as peripheral lines. Nurses specializing in the insertion of these devices place the catheters at the patient's hospital bedside, physician office, home care office or patient's home. The importance of these catheters cannot be overemphasized since the primary historic deterrent to patient's receiving TPN was the requirement of a surgically inserted central catheter. (See also Chapter 19.)

One patient type in particular that is in need of nutrition support is the pre-operative and post-operative patient. The American College of Physicians support the use of TPN in surgical patients.[6] Further support for optimal nutritional status during the operative period is found in other studies.[7,8]

In addition to the surgical candidate, parenteral nutrition in the 1990s can be expected to find great clinical utility in several disease states in patients who would benefit from brief intensive nutritional support. Examples of these conditions include the patient with hyperemesis gravidarum (where prolonged nausea and vomiting could possibly lead to premature and/or low-birth weight infants); patients with AIDS (where the ravages of opportunistic infections prohibit the absorption of nutrients or prevent intake secondary to painful mouth and esophageal ulcers); cancer patients; or patients with anorexia secondary to end stage renal disease (ESRD).

Some adjustment in the electrolytes, vitamins, and trace elements may be needed to account for differences in pregnant versus non-pregnant patients. For example, calcium, phosphorous, zinc, and iron may be needed in higher concentrations. Clear recommended daily allowances have not been established for these individuals. The majority of data concerning TPN in the pregnant patient comes from case studies.[9-11]

AIDS. Many patients with AIDS experience weight loss that can be so severe that patients become significantly debilitated and require complete nursing care. (See also Chapter 25.) Inadequate intake and malabsorption are readily corrected with TPN, whereas malnutrition secondary to overwhelming infection leading to a hypermetabolic state is more difficult to resolve. The morbidity associated with malnutrition, particularly in AIDS patients, remains significant and potentially correctable.[12-16]

Cancer. The use of TPN in the cancer patient continues to be a hotly contested issue. Historic arguments against TPN have centered on the inability of TPN to halt the cancerous process by increasing the patient's tolerance to chemotherapy and/or radiation, or the speculation that TPN may feed the rapidly dividing tumor cells.[17-19] Sufficient data to refute the arguments against the use of TPN in cancer patients has accumulated. More difficult to pinpoint has been the defined patient population that would benefit most from nutritional supplementation.[20] (see also Chapter 21)

End Stage Renal Disease. Parenteral nutrition has been used with increasing frequency in the patient with end stage renal disease (ESRD). Patients with uremia often suffer severe bouts of anorexia, in addition to the hypoalbuminemia secondary to chronic dialysis. Intradialytic parenteral nutrition (IDPN), or the infusion of concentrated amounts of protein and dextrose during the dialysis period, has been shown in a variety of studies to maintain visceral proteins, contribute to positive nitrogen balance, promote weight gain, increase lean body mass, as well as heighten the quality of life in the ESRD patient.[21,22]

Parenteral Antibiotics

Intravenous parenteral antibiotics have continued to be a mainstay of the HIT market, constituting 48% of the 1991 market and $1.8 billion in 1991 revenue.[4] Continued growth of this market segment will be a result of many disease states that are reaching colossal proportions, including AIDS (and its many complications), Lyme disease, and chronic fatigue syndrome.[23,24] Past studies have centered on the definite cost-efficiency of treating the long-term infectious disease patient outside of the hospital. Various cost analyses and models have been developed to support the outpatient approach.[25] Clearly, the contribution of drugs with longer half-lives to the growth of this segment should not be minimized. Equally important though, has been the significant benefits derived from the newer pump and microprocessor technology.[26] By utilizing this new technology, patients previously incapable of being treated at home now complete their therapies with an added measure of compliance contributing to their treatment success. Reductions in the treatment costs and treatment failures secondary to non-compliance can be achieved by combining exceptional technology with financially economic antibiotic regimens. (See also Chapter 24.)

With the advances in pump technology, patient participation in self-infusions has been minimized or eliminated altogether. Once per day cassette changes (cassettes containing an entire day's worth of drugs are used) and catheter flushes have obviated the need for patient participation and/or frequent nursing visits. A variety of pumps exist that infuse the drug automatically at predetermined intervals, over a pre-set infusion period. (See also Chapter 19.)

Chemotherapy

Outpatient chemotherapy, while not a major segment of the HHC market, has had its growth affected by several new techniques and agents. (See also Chapter 21.) Regimens such as 6 week courses of 5-fluorouracil (5FU) with or without leucovorin (to potentiate the effect of the 5FU) demonstrated increased patient tolerance, while achieving good clinical response.[27] Newer agents such as mitoxantrone, etoposide, and carboplatin, soon found themselves in the home environment, along with the supportive hydration and anti-emetic regimens required to support patients receiving these drugs. Again, the diligent clinician was forced to contend with the severe mucositis, nausea, marrow nadirs and reduced blood counts that are inherent to these powerful medications. Herein lies the most powerful tool of HHC. Ten years ago, patients receiving these toxic cytotoxic agents would have had to be re-admitted to the hospital usually between 7-14 days post-chemotherapy for infectious complications, hypercalcemia as a result of bone metastases or tumor lysis syndrome, severe nausea and/or weight loss, or anemia requiring transfusion of packed cells or platelets. The complete HHC service now monitors and anticipates the adverse sequelae from the chemotherapy and uses several pre-emptive approaches: growth factors (e.g., erythropoietin, filgrastim, sargramostim) obviate the need for repeated transfusions and help avoid the devastating (and often potentially lethal) infectious complications; and parenteral antibiotics active against gram positive, gram negatives and pseudomonas are often used prophylactically to provide systemic sterilization during the nadir. Additionally, anti-fungals are often employed in patients who remain febrile past one week.[28] Overall, the attempt is made to keep the neutropenic patient out of the hospital, where nosocomial infections may prove more difficult to treat because of more virulent pathogens in hospitals.

Newer supportive regimens have been added that address the problem of hypercalcemia of malignancy. Two such agents, gallium nitrate (Ganite®) and pamidronate (Aredia®) are successful in achieving normo-calcemia for longer periods of time as well as the added benefit of a reduced toxicity profile as compared to older regimens such as calcitonin, plicamycin, etidronate, hydration or diuretics.[29,30]

Patients suffering from severe, continuous nausea may derive great clinical benefit from ondansetron, a relatively new potent 5-HT3 blocker. Ondansetron is often used in combination with dexamethasone resulting in greater than 90% control of nausea related to chemotherapy.[31] A regimen consisting of a 5 mg dose 30 minutes prior to chemotherapy, then 6 and 12 hours after chemotherapy (e.g., cisplatinum) has found a place in HHC.

Parenteral Narcotic Analgesics

Narcotic analgesics have long had a place in the HHC armamentarium. The 1991 contribution from pain management is estimated at 5% ($191 million) of the total home care market.[4] The use of parenteral narcotics have continued to be one of the founding blocks of the HIT industry. Traditionally, parenteral narcotics have been reserved for the terminally ill patient with intolerable pain unresponsive to oral or rectal narcotics. (See also Chapter 22.)

Recently, intrathecal or epidural administration (with the placement of a catheter into the intrathecal or epidural space with the remaining portion of the catheter threaded to the abdominal wall) has gained popularity.[32] Another option for HHC patients suffering from the debilitating pain associated with reflex sympathetic dystrophy (RSD) is the use of parenteral or intrathecal morphine, meperidine, or hydromorphone.[33] Special "outpatient surgery" or "post-op" programs have also been specifically designed to educate the surgery center staffs, train the patient (usually prior to the procedure), and transition the patient home after initiating therapy for the patient in the recovery room.[34]

NEWER CHEMOTHERAPY OPTIONS

In addition to the various support regimens, several new agents are being used frequently in the home. Interleukin-2 (IL-2), cladribine, and paclitaxel have all been infused in the home. Below are brief descriptions of some of these newer agents. (See also Chapter 21.)

Interleukin-2 (Proleukin®) indicated for renal cell carcinoma has provided promising results. The vigilant HHC clinician must be wary of the potential for hypotension, capillary leak syndrome, peripheral and pulmonary edema as a result of increased vascular permeability. Patients with a history of previous cardiac, renal or pulmonary disease have typically not been good candidates for IL-2 infusion because of higher rates of toxicity.

One recent study has analyzed the subcutaneous method of administering IL-2 in an attempt to avoid the significant dose-related toxicity associated with IV bolus or continuous IV infusion.[35] IL-2 doses of 9-18 x 10^6 IU were given five days per week for 6 weeks subcutaneously with only acetaminophen given to prevent pyrexia. Patient tolerance was exceptional with partial remission or stable disease response rates similar to higher dose IV protocols. Additionally, special mixing considerations for the IV route must be adhered to (i.e., the use of albumin to reduce binding of the drug to the delivery system) which contributes to the higher cost and complexity of the IV regimen. Finally, the significant cost of the medication for a typical 9-18 x 10^6 IU regimen x 60 days can prove to be formidable (approximately $10,000/treatment cycle).

Cladribine (Leustatin®) as a continuous IV infusion[36] and subcutaneously[37] for hairy cell leukemia, childhood acute myeloid leukemia,[38] chronic lymphocytic leukemia[39] and various lymphomas[40] has had promising results. Leustatin's toxic profile does not appear to be dissimilar from other chemotherapeutic agents. Usual monitoring guidelines include an assessment for nausea, weight loss, and infectious episodes. Like IL-2, the cost of cladribine can be staggering: $2,100 for a 0.09 mg/kg/day x 7 days regimen. The recommended regimen is a seven day course of therapy, but several patients have undergone repeated regimens at 28 day intervals.

Paclitaxel (Taxol®) has provided great hope for those patients with metastatic ovarian carcinoma unresponsive to traditional chemotherapy. The typical regimen varies according to tumor type and ranges between 135-250 mg/m^2 over 24 hours every 21 days. The cost associated with this dosage is $1500-2500 per regimen. Like Interleukin-2, Taxol® has a unique side effect profile that warrants special attention by the home care clinician. Phase III studies demonstrated a hypersensitivity to the cremaphor component resulting in dyspnea, hypotension, flushing or rash. From this data, the NCI has recommended that Taxol® be given over a 24 hour period. However, newer data have demonstrated that a 3 hour infusion may be better tolerated than the 24 hour rate. No greater incidence of neuropathy or neutropenia was experienced.[41] Regardless of the dosing regimen and treatment length, premedication with an antihistamine (e.g., diphenhydramine), H_2 blocker (e.g., cimetidine or ranitidine) and steroid (dexamethasone) have been recommended, but are not fully protective. The potential for hypersensitivity does decrease with each subsequent dose of Taxol®.

A novel HHC therapy has recently been initiated as a result of the toxicity associated with Taxol®. Many third party payers have opted to recommend home infusion of Taxol® in order to avoid the hospitalization costs needed for a 24 hour admission (realistically about 36 to 48 hours, given the time associated with pre-medications). From this, some HIT pharmacies have devised specific, cautious protocols designed to accommodate both the 24 hour and 3 hour infusion of Taxol®.[42] Special protocols have been designed, along with premedication profiles and clinical follow-up registry data collection forms in order to outline and document HHC patient tolerance to this new agent.[42]

Pediatric oncology cases have always presented a dilemma for both patient and clinician. Difficulty in getting the patient to the treatment center as well as unique family dynamics have prompted many hospitals to promote the outpatient treatment concept. One study in this particular area of practice evaluated the outpatient treatment of febrile neutropenic episodes in children with cancer.[43] Twenty-two episodes of infection in thirteen children were handled successfully outside of the hospital. Distinct advantages cited were patient and family convenience and overall cost reduction.

NOVEL HOME CARE THERAPIES AND INNOVATIONS

Significant pharmacologic advances in the past 10 years have contributed to the continued growth of HHC. One such example has been the development in the area of recombinant biotechnology that has resulted in a plethora of new products.[44] The perfection of biotechnology techniques, in addition to the significant contributions from the infusion pump and vascular access industries, have designed specific systems to accommodate the patient who would have been difficult to treat at home. Below are descriptions of various techniques and therapies that are new to the HHC environment.

Colony Stimulating Factors

The perfection of recombinant technology has allowed for the development of specific growth factors designed to stimulate the growth of either specific blood elements (by acting at a lower point in the hematopoietic process), or whole groups of blood elements (by acting less selectively, or higher up in the hematopoietic process). Recombinant technology involves the use of various expression systems (e.g., murine, yeast) to clone nearly identical, naturally occurring stimulating factors that influence the growth, maturation and efficacy of various blood elements. The end result has been the rapid proliferation of various white cells (e.g., rGM-CSF), neutrophils (specifically using rG-CSF), or red cells (specifically after the use of erythropoietin). Clinically, the benefit of this rapid proliferation is seen in many patients recovering from devastating chemotherapy and radiation, drug induced anemias (e.g., zidovudine), or anemias as a result of various disease states (e.g., chronic renal failure).

Trillet-Lenoir and colleagues[45] in a series of patients documented the significant reduction in febrile neutropenia (53% vs. 26%), requirement for antibiotics (58% vs. 37%), infection-related hospitalization, reduction of chemotherapy dose by 15% or greater (61% vs. 29%), and treatment delays of 2 days or greater (47% vs. 29%) in the placebo versus rG-CSF groups. The reduction in these morbidities, although dramatic, was not reflected in increased tumor response or patient survival.[45]

Miles and colleagues demonstrated the outstanding benefit of erythropoietin and rG-CSF in AIDS patients suffering anemia secondary to AZT.[46] Both erythropoietin and rG-CSF were titrated in a manner to achieve specific neutrophil and hemoglobin levels. AIDS patients were able to tolerate continued AZT treatment, and maintained a neutrophil count of 6 x 10^6/L x 2 weeks and the hemoglobin had increased by at least 15 g/L over the baseline value. Prompt increases in circulating neutrophils were noted as was the ability to raise the dosage of zidovudine which resulted in a rise of CD4 count.

Clinically, rG-CSF has provided tremendous utility to those patients suffering neutropenia as a result of chemotherapy. Several studies have documented the distinct benefits in those patients receiving this colony stimulating factor in the post-chemotherapy phase in order to accelerate neutrophil recovery. Patient response in neutrophil counts are often several times faster resulting in less frequent bacterial infections, lessened severity of neutropenia, less frequent hospitalization, and fewer antibiotic treatments. From a HHC perspective, chemotherapy patients now have a means of avoiding the devastation of prolonged neutropenia that often results in hospitalization (and perhaps, nosocomial infections). Additionally, the HHC relationship allows for significant interaction between the pharmacist, nurse and physician in order to reemphasize the benefits of sterile technique of other infusions, and catheter maintenance in addition to avoiding the potential complication of virulent hospital pathogens.

Finally, rG-CSF could prove to be a significant therapeutic gain in those individuals suffering neutropenia due to AIDS or bone marrow transplantation. Further studies will help define the role and significance of rG-CSF in these disease states.

Similarly, sargramostim (rGM-CSF) has demonstrated clear benefits in patients needing a wider spectrum of stimulation of the blood elements. By acting higher up in the maturation scheme, GM-CSF is able to cause proliferation of monocytes, neutrophils, and eosinophils. Patients undergoing chemotherapy, or in the post-bone marrow transplant period have demonstrated clear benefit from this product.[47]

Colony stimulating factors hold significant promise to the HHC patient by assisting them in avoiding repeated hospitalizations. Unfortunately, the recombinant products are not without significant financial penalty. Table 23-4 charts the average monthly cost of a regimen of rG-CSF, epoietin and rGM-CSF. Recognize, too, that the clinical decision to initiate a patient on the lengthy therapy is costly since the patient's blood elements may decline to baseline once the therapy is discontinued. As a last caution, the HHC clinician is confronted with the dilemma of using these potential life-sustaining products in disease states where the products still have not received FDA approval. The end result may be substantial financial losses if claims for off-label uses are denied by the payer.

The numbers of products as well as the spectrum of uses will continue to escalate. 1993 industry estimates reflect over 100 biotechnology products in development. Many will probably be used in combination to help salvage the patient in the ambulatory environment who had just undergone therapies such as bone marrow transplantation.[44]

Tocolytics

The primary prognostic indicator of fetal well-being is linked inextricably to the ability of the mother to carry the child to full term. However, in approximately 8% of pregnancies premature uterine contractions result in either prolonged hospitalizations to enforce bedrest and infuse betamimetics or magnesium sulfate. The usual course of treatment is then followed by oral betamimetics (e.g., terbutaline sulfate). In 40-50% of women with premature uterine contractions, though, breakthrough contractions will reoccur resulting in readmission or premature birth.

Accordingly, techniques have been developed to support the expectant mother with premature uterine contractions. Included in these are the subcutaneous use of terbutaline sulfate delivered through a micro-processor pump that delivers a basal rate low enough to not affect heart rate or serum blood sugars, in addition to pre-programmed boluses that are based on documented circadian increases in uterine contractions. The two dosing programs used together are able to control the majority of contractions. To insure compliance and clinical success, the patient usually monitors once to twice per day with an electronic monitor that senses uterine contractions. This information is then down-loaded via phone modem to a central monitoring center where trained OB-GYN nurses interpret the strip, and then decide whether or not to alert the primary physician, have the patient re-monitor (after a brief rest and/or hydration period) or consult with the HHC pharmacist regarding altering the dosing pattern of the terbutaline. Clearly, this patient population requires exceptional coordination.

Cytokines

Recent discoveries in this field have resulted in the development of recombinant cytokines that identically mimic the endogenous product. IL-2, as previously discussed, is currently being used as an anti-tumor agent. IL-1 and IL-3 may be good candidates for the home environment because of their infusion and treatment protocols. The HHC

Table 23-4 Hematopoietic Hormones Used in AIDS[74]

Generic names	Erythropoietin, epoietin	GM-CSF, sagramostin	G-CSF, filgastrim
Expected results	Increase in Hb	Increase in WBCs (neutrophils, eosinophils, monocytes)	Increase in WBCs (neutrophils)
Time to response	2-8 weeks	2-3 days (longer if marrow suppressed)	Same as GM
Estimated monthly wholesale cost of treatment	\$720 - \$1,200 (12 x 100 u/kg)	\$6,000 (30 x 500 mcg vial)	\$4,000 (30 x 300 mcg vial)
Alternative treatment	Transfusion	Avoid marrow suppressive treatments	Same as GM

clinician's clinical acumen and monitoring talents will certainly be tested because these products, in addition to their positive clinical benefit, have potentially lethal toxicities.

Inotropic Agents

Patients with chronic congestive heart failure have typically resided in the coronary care unit receiving continuous infusions of inotropes while they awaited either death or the availability of a new heart. Several studies have documented the beneficial effects of brief periodic infusions of inotropes such as dobutamine or amrinone in the outpatient setting as a means to achieve maximal "exercise effect" on the myocardium.[48,49] Patients undergoing these regimens do not seem to experience the tachyphylaxis associated with continuous infusions of inotropes, nor the ineffectiveness of oral inotropes. An increase in quality and quantity of life has been documented.

Similarly, a number of treatments and procedures related to pediatric heart transplantation previously undertaken in a hospital setting have been safely moved to the home. Dobutamine for congestive heart failure, steroid pulses for treatment of rejection and the prophylactic use of OKT3 (Orthoclone®) in order to promote early discharge have been described.[50]

UNIQUE DRUGS FOR CHRONIC DISEASE STATES

A host of medications have been developed for disease states of a chronic nature that were previously untreatable, or had only supportive management available. Examples of these disease states include growth hormone deficiency, alpha-1-antitrypsin deficiency, glucocerebrocidase deficiency, hormone (e.g., GnRH) deficiency resulting in primary amenorrhea and infertility, multiple sclerosis and hepatitis B and C.

Pediatric patients suffering from a deficiency of growth hormone will have retarded growth. Biotechnology techniques have produced two human growth hormone products (Humatrope® and Protropin®) that can be administered parenterally to achieve or approximate normal growth patterns.[51] These products differ in minor respects, and both achieve the same clinical goal. Patients or family members are taught to administer a subcutaneous injection. Dosage is adjusted to approximate a normal growth pattern. Typically, insurance payers will cover the cost of medication, administration supplies and nursing support until the patient reaches the 50th percentile for growth pattern. Additionally, pediatrician interest in human growth hormone has centered on its use in precocious puberty.

Alpha-1-antitrypsin (AAT) deficiency results in a chronic obstructive pulmonary disease-like condition (i.e., congenital emphysema) punctuated by frequent infectious complications. Prolastin® is derived from pooled human plasma. Patients receiving Prolastin® infusions on a weekly basis remain symptom-free for extended periods of time as a result of raising the AAT levels that serve as protection against the destructive enzyme elastase.[52] Historically, patients have had to receive this product over 1-2 hours in an emergency room, short stay ward or physician's office on a weekly basis. The weekly infusions, obviously, were cumbersome not only to the physician or hospital, but also the patient in pursuit of a normal lifestyle. To accommodate their needs, HIT pharmacies have established strict infusion protocols and patient instruction techniques so that the patient with congenital emphysema can stay at home for as long as possible. In an effort to guarantee that this life-sustaining procedure is available to those patients unaware of their disease state, HHC companies in association with local pulmonologists often hold screening clinics where patients suspected of having this condition can have their alpha-1-antitrypsin levels measured.

Glucocerebrocidase Deficiency

Patients with a deficiency of this enzyme have a disease state known as Gaucher disease and clinical symptoms such as hepatomegaly, splenomegaly, bone pain and neurologic symptoms as a result of a buildup of glucocerebrocide in the reticuloendothelial system.[53] Gaucher's patients are classified in one of three conditions depending on level of symptomatology. Until the release of Ceredase®- Genzyme in 1992, patients with Type-1 Gaucher's disease only had splenectomy or gene-transfer as available treatment options. Neither procedure was curative. Doses used have been 60 IU/kg every two weeks, and at a cost of $14,700 per treatment. A 70 kg patient will spend in the neighborhood of $380,000 per year and possibly as high as $765,000 per year in a very ill patient receiving weekly infusions. Newer low dose protocols (e.g., 30 IU/kg/month) have reduced the cost to approximately $95,000 per year.[54]

Primary Hypothalamic Amenorrhea

Primary hypothalamic amenorrhea (HA) results from deficient hypothalamic pulsatile secretion of gonadotropin-releasing hormone (GnRH). In this disorder, pulsatile gonadotropin release is either absent or severely reduced, follicular maturation is arrested, and patients become anovulatory and amenorrheic.

Characteristically, women with primary HA are infertile because of an inherent deficiency in GnRH secretion from the hypothalamus.[55-58] In the past, numerous techniques including clomiphene citrate and human menopausal gonadotropin have been attempted, often with a substantial failure rate. Exogenous GnRH (gonadorelin acetate- Lutrepulse®) in the physiologic dose of 5 mcg every 90 minutes IV (15-20 mcg/pulse SQ) is capable of stimulating follicle growth and release, while still preserving the negative feedback cycle necessary to prevent multiple births and ovarian hyperstimulation.

Ovulation in response to Lutrepulse® usually occurs within two to three weeks after therapy initiation. Lutrepulse® should then be continued for another two weeks. Patients failing previous clomiphene therapy have had reasonable success after undergoing two to three treatment cycles of 21 day duration. This particular treatment regimen has added an extra treatment option for patients wishing to have children.

Multiple Sclerosis

Approximately 300,000 patients in the U.S. suffer from the chronic demyelinating effects of multiple sclerosis (MS). The symptoms associated with this disease, although varied, may reflect the site of demyelination or inflammation in the central nervous system. They include periodic exacerbations manifested by decreasing visual acuity, muscle weakness fatigue, spasticity and reduced cognitive function. Previous theories of this disease have centered on possible viral, or immune etiologies.[59] However, new approaches center on our ability to influence the immune system exogenously via cytokines such as the interferons. Interferon, in fact, may be able to blunt the effects of an over-active immune component (i.e., T-cells) that turn on the myelin sheath, destroying the insulating and conducting capacity of this fatty layer. The replacement of myelin with scar tissue or placques is pathognomonic to MS patients. The scar tissue eventually resolves, which is associated with the periodic symptom-free state. Resolution of the acute attack may occur with or without treatment. Drug therapy may accelerate the rate of recovery from the acute attack, but not necessarily the degree of recovery.

In the past twenty years, only two parenteral medications, adrenocorticotropin hormone (25-60 units infused over an 8 hour period, then tapered over a 10-21 day course) and methylprednisolone (500-1000 mg IV daily for 5 days) have met with varying degrees of success in MS patients. Both have been used in patients with acute exacerbations in the home as patients find this arrangement more conducive to conducting a normal lifestyle. Additional routes of administration include oral, intramuscular and intrathecal.[60,62]

A 1993 FDA advisory panel recently recommended the approval of a novel cytokine, beta-interferon (Betaseron®) for the treatment of patients with moderate to severe MS. Various studies have cited as much as a 40-50% reduction in attacks in patients receiving 45 mU SQ three times weekly.[63] The wholesale cost of this therapy is approximately $5,000 per patient per year. The success of beta-interferon SQ or IV is distinctly positive compared to the negative effects noted with gamma-interferon intrathecally that caused acute exacerbations of MS.

Interferon for Hepatitis

Estimates for the incidence of hepatitis B are up to 24,000 cases per year and 85,000 cases per year for hepatitis C. Interferon alfa-2b (Intron A®) was recently approved for the treatment of these two disease states. Because of the relative infectious nature of these patients, it is critical that they complete their treatment regimens, dispose of infectious waste properly, and know not to discontinue the interferon if they should experience nuisance-like side effects (e.g., fever, fatigue, headache, depression, nausea). A typical dosing regimen of 3 mu SQ 3-7 times per week for 3-6 months is used.[64] HHC practitioners have been instrumental in the initial education and continued follow-up of these patients.

Raynaud's Phenomenon

Patients afflicted with this disease suffer from poor circulation to their extremities causing intense pain, intolerance to cold, and gangrenous digits. Total Pharmaceutical Care recently treated a patient with a potent vasodilator, prostaglandin E_1

(Alprostadil®), in an effort to relieve pain and increase blood-flow.[42] Langevitz and colleagues had previously described this method.[65] The patient received 1.5 mg/hour over a 10 hour period. Rather than be admitted to the hospital three times weekly for the infusion, the patient elected to be infused at home under the supervision of the HHC nurse. The pain, prior to the Alprostadil® infusion, was of such intensity that the patient would screech and writhe with pain in her bed. Her lower extremities were cold to touch without detectable pedal pulses. The pain would subside 30 minutes after starting the infusion, pedal pulses would be present, and the feet would begin to warm. No side effects secondary to the infusion or vasodilator effects were noted.

Migraine Headaches

Migraine headaches affect approximately 10% of the world's population, having a predilection for the adult female population. About a quarter of sufferers experience attacks of such frequency that they require medical attention at some stage in their life.[66-68] Two recently released medications have made possible the immediate relief from this debilitating disease.

Sumatriptan (Imitrex®) has specific action at 5-HT_{1D} receptors resulting in vasoconstriction. A 2-6 mg dose is given subcutaneously with clinical effect realized in 20-60 minutes. Dihydroergotamine (DHE-45) acts at 5-HT_1 receptors to cause vasoconstriction as well as stimulating the chemoreceptor trigger zone. Hence, aside from relief from migraine pain, nausea and vomiting may also occur. In general, the ergot alkaloids should be avoided in patients with severe hypertension, peripheral vascular disease, coronary artery disease, and in pregnant patients.

Special Pediatric Concerns

A growing body of literature analyzing the special concerns in the HHC of the pediatric patient have begun to appear. Kobayashi and colleagues studied the home administration of IVIG in children with primary immunodeficiency.[69] They advise that specific administration and patient selection criteria be adhered to in order to avoid serious complications. Parents were taught to initiate IVs and monitor for side effects. There was no difference in the frequency of illness, antibiotic usage or school absences when comparing the home infusion phase with the previous phase when IVIG was administered in a medical setting by health care professionals.

TREATMENTS ON THE HORIZON

HHC treatments have traditionally been continuations of hospital initiated therapies. Moreover, the techniques, dosing patterns and devices used to deliver these treatments have reflected hospital trends. However, with the success (both cost-efficiency and clinical) that the HIT industry has documented over the past ten years, HIT clinicians are now able to institute novel therapies at home without the patient first being admitted to the hospital.

Theoretically, patients receiving devastating doses of chemotherapy or radiation will have to be supported in the home prior to, during, or immediately following these treatments. Combinations of growth factors, supportive drugs (e.g., anti-emetics, hydration, IVPBs or TPN) will be needed to salvage the patient. Gross evidence of the efficacy of these combined therapies is seen in the bone marrow transplant patient. IL-2[70] and IVIgG[71] may also be used in order to prevent graft-versus-host disease and reduced incidence of post-transplant infection. Additionally, the emerging technique of peripheral stem cell transplants have the advantage of being cost-efficient if performed as an outpatient.

AIDS patients requiring a host of investigational medications will find these treatment alternatives being delivered in the home. Immunomodulators and tumor suppressants (e.g., Ampligen) and drugs targeted against Mycobacterium avium (e.g., gentamicin liposome injection) have been used at home with the HHC clinician being instrumental in the success of the study protocol.

Finally, continued advances in the delivery techniques will allow for the safe administration of medications often occupying tremendous hospital or physician office resources (e.g., intrathecal Baclofen via computerized delivery system for spinal spasticity associated with multiple sclerosis or spinal injury.)[72]

SETTING THE STAGE FOR FUTURE HHC PRACTICE

Donald Graham in his article Nosohusial Infections: Complication of Home Intravenous Therapy makes reference to the paucity of data as it exists on HHC.[73] He is quick to comment that it is in the industry's best interest to document the clinical outcomes of the patients it treats so that expected complication rates can help guide the clinician. The concept of prospective surveillance is outlined as the procedure of choice. For example, Total Pharmaceutical Care,[42] has initiated several nationwide prospective surveillance programs, especially for the more critical drugs such as Taxol® and interleukin-2. Additionally, these programs seek to draw correlations on the success of the home antibiotic patient and the diagnosis, age, sex, type of pump, line, drug and host of other variables that may contribute to the success (or lack of success) in the patient treated at home. These types of prospective surveillance techniques are critical to the future of HHC and must be engaged by HHC practitioners in a cooperative effort in order to generate large bodies of meaningful data.

CONCLUSION

HHC clinicians have developed a specialty practice that has, as part of their career, the anticipation and planning of novel therapies in unique setting. Tremendous pressures from payer sources have established the basis for seeking the most cost effective treatment alternatives. At this time, pending new presidential health plans, the HHC alternative demonstrates cost efficiency and outstanding clinical outcomes. Future developments in treatments at home should continue to bolster this expanding practice.

REFERENCES

1. Anon. Technology & Strategy: Growth in home drug infusion markets. Drug & Market Development. 1993; 3(9):184-189.
2. Anon. Home health care. A shift from acute to chronic illness treatment. MedPRO Month. 1991; 1(11)164-167.
3. Hicks WG, Miner KM. Alternate Site Care. Infusion Services. Cowen Industry Strategies. 1992; 7;20:1-44.
4. Anon. Home and alternate site infusion therapy markets in the U.S. Biomedical Business International. 1992; Report #2822, March.
5. Enriquez N, Akahoshi M. Newer therapies in home care. CJHP. 1990; 2(4):19-21.
6. Health and Public Policy Committee, American College of Physicians. Perioperative parenteral nutrition. Ann Intern Med. 1987; 107:252-253.
7. Askanazi J, Hensle TW, Starker PM. Effect of immediate postoperative nutritional support on length of hospitalization. Ann Surg. 1986; 203(3):236-239.
8. Meijerink WJ, von Meyenfeldt MF, Rouflart MM, Soeters PB. Efficacy of perioperative nutritional support. Lancet. 1992; 340:187-188.
9. Rivera-Alsina M, Saldana L, Stringer A. Fetal growth sustained by parenteral nutrition in pregnancy. Obstet Gynecol. 1984; 64:138-141.
10. Levine M, Esser D. Total parenteral nutrition for the treatment of severe hyperemesis gravidarum: Maternal nutritional effects and fetal outcome. Obstet Gynecol. 1988; 72:102-107.
11. Watson L, Bommarito A, Marshal J. Total peripheral parenteral nutrition in pregnancy. JPEN. 1990; 14:485-489.
12. Kotler DP, Tierney AR, Wang J, et al. Magnitude of body cell-mass depletion and the timing of death from wasting in AIDS. Am J Clin Nutr. 1989; 50:444-447.
13. Kotler DP, Tierney AR, Culpepper-Morgan JA, et al. Effect of home total parenteral nutrition on body composition in patients with acquired immunodeficiency syndrome. JPEN. 1990; 14(5):454-458.
14. Lakshmipathi C, Jastremski M. Incidence of malnutrition in patients with acquired immunodeficiency syndrome. Nutr Clin Pract. 1989; 4:16-18.
15. Janson DD, Teasley KM. Parenteral nutrition in the management of gastrointestinal Kaposi's sarcoma in a patient with AIDS. Clin Pharm. 1988; 7(7):536-544.
16. Singer P, Rothkopf MM, Kvetan V, et al. Risks and benefits of home parenteral nutrition in the acquired immunodeficiency syndrome. JPEN. 1991; 15(1):75-79.
17. Brennan MF. Total parenteral nutrition in the cancer patient. NEJM. 1981; 305(7):375-382.
18. Howard L. Home parenteral nutrition in patients with a cancer diagnosis. JPEN. 1992; 16:93S-99S.
19. Bozzetti F. Effects of artificial nutrition on the nutritional status of cancer patients. JPEN. 1989; 13:406-420.
20. Klein S, Simes J, Blackburn GL. Total parenteral nutrition and cancer clinical trials. Cancer. 1986; 58:1378-1386.
21. Goldstein DJ, Strom JA. Intradialytic parenteral nutrition: Evolution and current concepts. J Renal Nutrition 1991; 1(1)9-22.
22. Foulks CJ, Goldstein DJ, Kelly MP, Hunt JM. Indications for the use of intradialytic parenteral nutrition in the malnourished hemodialysis patient. J Renal Nutrition. 1991; 1(1):23-33.
23. Rahn DW. Antibiotic treatment of Lyme disease. Postgrad Med. 1992; 91(7):57-64.
24. Hassler D, Riedel K, Zorn J, Frbac-Mursic V. Pulsed high-dose cefotaxime therapy in refractory Lyme borreliosis. Lancet. 1991; 338:193.
25. Eisenberg JM, Kitz DS. Savings from outpatient antibiotic therapy for osteomyelitis: Economic analysis of a therapeutic strategy. JAMA. 1986; 255(12):1584-1588.
26. New PB, Swanson GF, Bulich RG, Taplin GC. Ambulatory antibiotic infusion devices: Extending the spectrum of outpatient therapies. Am J Med. 1991; 91:455-461.
27. Erlichman C, Fine S, Wong A, Elhakim T. A randomized trial of fluorouracil and folinic acid in patients with metastatic colorectal carcinoma. J Clin Oncol. 1988; 6(3):469-475.
28. Pizzo PA. Management of fever in patients with cancer and treatment-induced neutropenia. NEJM. 1993; 328(18):1323-1329.
29. Hall TG, Burns-Schaiff RA. Update on the medical

treatment of hypercalcemia of malignancy. Clin Pharm. 1993; 12:117-25.
30. Pochan GM. New medications for the treatment of hypercalcemia of malignancy. Hospital Pharmacy Hotline. 1992; 5(3):1-6.
31. Roila F, Tonato M, Cognetti F, et al. Prevention of cisplatin-induced emesis: A double-blind multicenter randomized crossover study comparing ondansetron and ondansetron plus dexamethasone. J Clin Oncol. 1991; 9(4):675-678.
32. Littrell RA. Epidural analgesia. AJHP. 1991; 48:2460-2474.
33. Smith DL, Campbell SM. Reflex sympathetic dystrophy syndrome: Diagnosis and management. West J Med 1987; 147:342-345.
34. Jones NH. Postoperative pain control: Solving a long-standing problem. Today's OR Nurse. 1988; 10(12):10-16.
35. Sleijfer DT, Janssen RA, Buter J, et al. Phase II study of subcutaneous interleukin-2 in unselected patients with advanced renal cell cancer on an outpatient basis. J Clin Oncol. 1992; 10(7):1119-1123.
36. Piro LD, Saven A, Ellison D, et al. Abstract #846- Prolonged complete remissions following 2-chlorodeoxyadenosine (2-CdA) in hairy cell leukemia (HCL). Proceedings of ASCO. 1992; 11:119.
37. Juliusson G, Liliemark J: Rapid recovery from cytopenia in hairy cell leukemia after treatment with 2-chloro-2'deoxyadenosine (CdA): Relation to opportunistic infections. Blood. 1992;79(4):888-894.
38. Hurwitz CA, Krance R, Schell MJ, et al. Current strategies for treatment of acute myeloid leukemia at St Jude Children's research hospital. Leukemia. 1992; 6(Suppl 2):39-43.
39. Juliusson G, Elmehorn-Rosenburg A, Liliemark J. Response to 2-chlorodeoxyadenosine in patients with B-cell chronic lymphocytic leukemia resistant to fludarabine. NEJM. 1992; 327:1056-1061.
40. Saven A, Carrera CJ, Carson DA, et al. 2-Chlorodeoxyadenosine: An active agent in the treatment of cutaneous T-cell lymphoma. Blood. 1992; 80(3): 587-592.
41. Swenerton K, Eisenhauer E, Bokkel-Huinink W, et al. Abstract #810- Taxol® in relapsed ovarian cancer: High vs. low dose and short vs. long infusion: A European-Canadian Study Coordinated by the NCI Canada Clinical Trials Group. Proceedings of ASCO. 1993; 12:256.
42. Anon. Total Pharmaceutical Care, Inc. Personal Communication, Santa Barbara CA, July 30, 1993.
43. Wiernkowski JT, Rothney M, Dawson S, Andrew M. Evaluation of a home intravenous antibiotic program in pediatric oncology. Am J Pediatr Hematol Oncol. 1991; 13(2):144-7.
44. Sindelar RD. Overview/preview of current and future recombinant DNA-produced pharmaceuticals. Drug Topics (Suppl). 1992; 3-13.
45. Trillet-Lenoir V, Green J, Manegold C, et al. Recombinant granulocyte colony stimulating factor reduces the infectious complications of cytotoxic chemotherapy. Eur J Cancer. 1993; 29A(3)319-324.
46. Miles SA, Mitsuyasu RT, Moreno J, et al. Combined therapy with recombinant granulocyte colony-stimulating factor and erythropoietin decreases hematologic toxicity from zidovudine. Blood. 1991; 77(10):2109-2117.
47. Brandt SJ, Peters WP, Atwater SK. Effect of recombinant human granulocyte-macrophage colony-stimulating factor on hematopoietic reconstitution after high-dose chemotherapy and autologous bone marrow transplantation. NEJM 1988; 318(14):869-876.
48. Haddad A. The risks and benefits of intravenous amrinone therapy. Home Health Nurse. 1992; 10(5):17-18,70.
49. Berger M, McSherry CK. Outpatient dobutamine infusion using a totally implantable infusion pump for refractory congestive heart failure. Chest. 1985; 88(2):295-296.
50. O'Brien P, Hanley FL. New directions in pediatric heart transplantation. Critical Care Nursing Clinics of North America. 1992; 4(2):193-203.
51. Milner RD. Proper use of growth hormone. Archives of Disease in Childhood. 1990; 65(1):70-71.
52. Gibaldi M. Understanding and treating some genetic diseases. Ann Pharmacother. 1992; 26:1589-1594.
53. Beutler E. Gaucher disease: New molecular approaches to diagnosis and treatment. Science. 1992; 256:794-799.
54. Beutler E, Kay A, Saven A, et al. Enzyme replacement therapy for Gaucher disease. Blood. 1991; 78(5):1183-1189.
55. Reid RL, Fretts R, Van Vugt DA. The theory and practice of ovulation induction with gonadotropin-releasing hormone. Am J Obstet Gynecol. 1988; 158:176-185.
56. Schriock ED. Practical aspects of pulsatile gonadotropin-releasing hormone administration. Am J Obstet Gynecol. 1990; 163(5):1765-1770.
57. Gompel A, Mauvais-Jarvis P. Induction of ovulation with pulsatile GnRH in hypothalamic amenorrhoea. Human Reproduction. 1988; 3(4):473-477.
58. Santoro N. Efficacy and safety of intravenous pulsatile gonadotropin-releasing hormone: Lutrepulse for injection. Am J Obstet Gynecol. 1990; 163:1759-1764.
59. Noseworthy JH. Therapeutics of multiple sclerosis. Clin Neuropharmacol. 1991; 14(1):49-61.
60. Rudick RA, Goodkin DE, Ransohoff RM. Pharmaco therapy of multiple sclerosis: Current status. Cleve Clin J Med. 1992; 59:267-277.
61. Heun R, Sliwka U, Ruttinger H, Schimrigk K. Intrathecal versus systemic corticosteroids in the treatment of multiple sclerosis: Results of a pilot study. J Neurol. 1992; 239:31-35.
62. Thompson AJ, Kennard C, Swash M, et al. Relative efficacy of intravenous methylprednisolone and ACTH in the treatment of acute relapse in MS. Neurology. 1989; 39:969-971.
63. Panitch HS. Interferons in multiple sclerosis- A review of the evidence. Drugs. 1992 44(6):946-962.
64. Perrillo RP, Schiff ER, Davis GL. A randomized, controlled trial of interferon alfa-2b alone and after

prednisone withdrawal for the treatment of chronic hepatitis B. NEJM. 1990; 323:295-301.

65. Langevitz P, Buskila D, Lee P, Urowitz MB. Treatment of refractory ischemic skin ulcers in patients with Raynaud's phenomenon with PGE1 infusions. J Rheumatol. 1989; 16:1433-1435.
66. Anon. Optimum treatment of acute migraine and the place in therapy of sumatriptan. Drugs & Therapy Perspectives. 1993; 1(1):1-4.
67. Ensink FB. Subcutaneous sumatriptan in the acute treatment of migraine. J Neurol 1991; 38:S66-S69.
68. Silberstein SD, Schulman EA, McFadden-Hopkins M. Repetitive intravenous DHE in the treatment of refractory headache. Headache. 1990; 30:334-339.
69. Kobayashi RH, Kobayashi AL, Lee N, et al. The home administration of IVIG in children with primary immunodeficiency. Peds. 1990; 85(5):705-709.
70. Nakajima K, Smith CV, Mixon A, et al. In vitro and in vivo effects of recombinant human interleukin-2 in naive miniature swine. J Immunother. 1992; 11(3):169-175.
71. Spitzer TR, Cottler-Fox M, Sullivan P, et al. Continuous infusion intravenous immunoglobulin is associated with a reduced incidence of infection and achieves higher serum immunoglobulin G levels than intermittent infusion following bone marrow transplantation. Semin Hematol. 1992; 29(3 Suppl 2):123-6.
72. Savoy SM, Gianino JM. Intrathecal baclofen infusion: an innovative approach for controlling spinal spasticity. Rehabil Nurs. 1993; 8(2):105-113.
73. Graham DR. Nosohusial infections. Complication of home intravenous therapy. Infectious Diseases in Clinical Practice.1993; 2(2):158-161.
74. McPhedran, P. Using hematopoietic hormones in HIV disease. AIDS Clin Care. 1992; 4:44.

24 Home Parenteral Antibiotics

Michael P. Akahoshi, Pharm.D.

Home parenteral antibiotic therapy (HPAT) is the largest single component of home infusion therapy.[1] With this therapy, patients receive their infusions via peripheral or central veins depending on the estimated length of treatment. Infusions are usually administered intermittently, making this therapy more labor-intensive then other types of therapy. Because of the sophisticated nature of home IV antibiotic therapy, patients and caregivers are taught to be active participants rather than just recipients of treatment. In patients who are clinically stable and whose diseases require prolonged IV antibiotic therapy, early discharge from the hospital can result in important savings to the institution, third party payers, and patients.

Home health care (HHC) pharmacists provide HPAT services to patients recovering from infectious illnesses, who require antimicrobial therapy by IV administration. Hospitalized patients with infectious diseases are candidates to receive HPAT. Patients who traditionally received seven to ten days of parenteral antibiotic therapy in the hospital, now may receive several days of that therapy at home. Patients with relatively simple infections, such as urinary tract infections, infected wounds, and respiratory infections may be referred to HPAT. Patients with Lyme disease, cystic fibrosis, bacterial endocarditis, osteomyelitis and septic arthritis routinely receive HPAT. These conditions are briefly reviewed below. Home IV antibiotic therapy for AIDS patients is discussed in Chapter 25.

PATIENT SELECTION

Regardless of the disease to be treated, patients should meet established acceptance criteria. A successful course of HPAT may be achieved if appropriate criteria are used. See Table 24-1. By using the patient selection criteria, decisions to accept patients who have been referred to the HHC pharmacist may be made on a rational basis. The home of the patient should be evaluated to insure the safe use and proper storage of the HPAT.

The potential pitfalls in using the patient selection criteria may be restated as exclusion criteria. For example, poor venous access, immaturity, inability to maintain heparin locks, evidence of non-compliance, and other factors may become increasingly important as exclusion criteria. Additionally, complications of existing illness may hamper successful therapy. Examples include compromised vision, poor dexterity due to arthritis, tremors, alcoholism, or a history of drug abuse.

It is extremely important to document that the patient understands and can demonstrate the ability to actively participate in his therapy at home. Failing this, a caregiver (often a family member)

Table 24-1 Patient Selection Criteria for Home IV Antibiotic Therapy[3,17]

- Patient is Medically Stable
- Motivation of the Patient to be Treated at Home
- Ability of the Patient to be Trained and Educated
- Technical Ability of Patient/Caregiver to Administer Therapy
- Adequate Family/Caregiver Support System at Home
- Risk of Patient to Abuse IV Access
- Adequate Insurance Coverage for Home Infusion Antibiotic Therapy

must undertake responsibility to assist in this capacity in order to insure the successful completion of the course of therapy. Guidelines for accepting referred patients for home IV antibiotic therapy are included in Appendix 24-A.

TYPICAL INFECTIONS

HPAT is most appropriate for those patients who need extended therapy, who are in relatively stable medical condition, and who have no other needs requiring hospitalization.[1] Some of the typical infectious diseases that may be appropriately treated with IV antibiotics are briefly described below. (See Table 24-2). More complete coverage of these topics is reported elsewhere.[4-6]

Table 24-2 Infections Treated with IV Antibiotics at Home[18]

Infection/Diagnosis	Percent of Sample
AIDS	13.6
Lyme Disease	13.3
Osteomyelitis	6.4
Postoperative Infection	3.3
Cystic Fibrosis	2.5
Bacterial Endocarditis	<2.0
All Other Diagnoses	59.0

Osteomyelitis

Osteomyelitis may be caused by hematogenous spread of bacteria which lodge in the bone, by contiguous spread of bacteria from adjacent tissue, or by direct inoculation of organisms due to trauma or surgery.[7] Childhood osteomyelitis commonly is the result of hematogenous spread, and classically occurs within the metaphysis. The nutrient arteries end in the metaphyses as narrow capillaries which make hairpin turns near the growth plate and form veins with wider diameters. This leads to the slowing of blood flow in the area and presumably allows bacteria to settle and grow. In addition, there is a lack of functioning phagocytes in the metaphysical capillaries. Infections in children usually involve the femur, tibia, and humerus (long bones). In most cases, the causative agent is Staphylococcus aureus although Streptococci and Gram negative bacilli are also known pathogens.[7]

Osteomyelitis associated with the contiguous spread from adjacent tissue is more commonly found in adult patients. A number of cases are the result of infections involving fingers and toes. Less common is mandibular involvement from infected teeth or bone involvement from chronic sinus infections. Once again Staphylococcus aureus is the most common infectious agent in the contiguous spread type of osteomyelitis. The important distinction between this type of osteomyelitis and the hematogenous type is that this one is commonly associated with multiple organism involvement. Gram negative aerobes as well as anaerobes may be found. When vascular insufficiency is present osteomyelitis is often difficult to manage. This is often the scenario in the patient with a past history of diabetes mellitus. In fact, the most common factors which lead to anaerobic osteomyelitis are diabetes mellitus and previous fractures.[7]

Bacteriologic diagnosis is obtained by blood cultures, percutaneous biopsy and/or open wound sampling. In cases of chronic osteomyelitis the presence of draining sinuses may be a source of contamination and give misleading results.

Therapy should be directed at the specific causative organism(s). Commonly, B-lactam drugs (penicillins, cephalosporins), aminoglycosides, and/or clindamycin are selected, depending upon the specific culture report. Because antibiotic concentration in bone may be a function of serum concentration and capillary blood flow to the adjacent tissue, high doses of the appropriate antibiotic(s) administered intravenously are usually required for a successful outcome.[7]

In those instances in which the patient develops recurrent infection or a resistant organism, two or three other antimicrobials may be added to the HPAT to assure eradication. Multiple parenteral drug therapy will add complexity to the management of the patients in terms of drug compatibility, dosing schedules, monitoring parameters, and the logistics of administering several doses each day.

The length of therapy commonly recommended to treat chronic osteomyelitis is four to six weeks of intravenous antibiotic(s) followed by one, two, or more months of oral antibiotic(s). Patients with chronic osteomyelitis have a poorer prognosis than those with acute illness because the dead bone can act as a reservoir for bacteria and can continue to reseed adjacent bone and soft tissue.

Infective Endocarditis

Another important disease requiring aggressive HPAT is endocarditis. Infective endocarditis, also known as bacterial endocarditis, is a microbial infection of the inside lining of the heart (endocardium) and predominantly involves the heart valves. The infection may develop abruptly (acute) or insidiously (subacute). It may pursue a fulminant or prolonged course, and is fatal unless treated.[8]

The most common pathogen causing subacute bacterial endocarditis is Streptococcus viridans, which is part of the normal upper respiratory tract flora. Simple dental procedures can be the event that introduces a sufficient number of bacteria into the blood stream to initiate the infection. Subacute endocarditis occurs most frequently in persons with preexisting cardiac disease, and the most common area involved is the left side of the heart. Valves damaged by rheumatic fever, arteriosclerosis, or previous surgery are also frequently targeted by pathogens. Streptococcus faecalis (enterococcus), found in fecal and perineal flora is also a frequent pathogen in this disease, particularly in older males experiencing prostatism or other urinary tract conditions. Staphylococcus aureus can also be a prominent causative agent.[6]

Infection commonly develops on irregular surfaces of the endocardium. The initial event is an abnormality in the blood flow which results in damage to the endothelium. The body's response to this inflammation is to establish successive layers of fibrin and platelets. Microorganisms introduced into the blood stream may attach themselves to the fibrin and platelets. To compound the insult, vegetations of bacteria sometimes break off, sending emboli to various sites, resulting in a variety of symptoms which may include myalgias, sudden visual disturbances, aphasia, flank pain, hemiplegia, and many others. Fever is present in most cases, but may not always be demonstrated, particularly in the older patient. Abnormal blood flow in the heart resulting in murmurs is frequently found.[8]

The most important consideration in treating bacterial endocarditis is achieving bactericidal concentrations of the appropriate antimicrobial(s) at the site of infection.[9] Bacteriostatic versus bacteriocidal action is often a function of the phenomenon of serum concentration. Bacterial colonies are often found beneath the vegetating surface, where phagocyte activity is nil. Hence, there is a lack of activity by macrophages, neutrophils and lymphocytes. Antimicrobial agents are usually present in sub-optimal concentration at the tissue site. Colony counts of 10 per gram of tissue are seen. Unchecked, this can lead to peripheral embolization, alluded to earlier. Because of this scenario, it is important to emphasize the administration of the appropriate antimicrobial, in an aggressive fashion (intravenously) for an appropriate length of time (six weeks). Relapse and the necessity for retreatment with increased risk of irreversible valve damage, usually are the price paid for shorter courses of therapy.

Patients with endocarditis commonly achieve apparent clinical stability (as measured in terms of vital signs and temperature, restoration of appetite, and general well-being) within days of the start of IV antibiotic therapy. However, the hallmark of the disease is the occurrence of late complications, including aneurysms, clinically significant embolic events, and progressive valvular deterioration, all potentially catastrophic complications sometimes occurring two weeks or more after apparent clinical stability has been achieved.[2]

Because of the nature of this disease (as opposed to the relatively milder nature of osteomyelitis) it is imperative that patient compliance with the drug regimen be assured. This added responsibility in the outpatient setting requires careful coordination of information among the physician, pharmacist, nurse and patient. If the treatment regimen requires antimicrobial dosing on a four hour schedule, patients and caregivers may experience exhaustion from lack of sleep early in the therapy. New technologies involving programmable ambulatory infusion devices are available to address this most important aspect of therapy. (See also Chapter 19.) Short of this fact, it may prove beneficial to use antimicrobials with half-lives that allow less frequent dosing, if it can be demonstrated that the therapeutic outcome will not be compromised. Obviously, patient convenience is never a substitute for less aggressive therapy in this illness.

Septic Arthritis

An example of a third illness that may be treated on an outpatient basis with antibiotics via the IV route is acute bacterial (septic) arthritis. This arthritis differs from rheumatoid arthritis in that usually one joint is involved and chills are frequently a reported symptom. Gout is excluded as a potential diagnosis when hyperuricemia is absent and crystals are not found in synovial fluid.[10]

The illness usually appears suddenly, and more often than not, it occurs in weight-bearing joints and wrists. The involved joint is painful, swollen, and warm to the touch. As stated earlier, chills and fever are frequent findings. If bacteria can be demonstrated in synovial fluid, the diagnosis can be confirmed. Sometimes bacteria cannot be grown, particularly if the infection is in periarticular tissue and there has been no focal ulceration into the joint fluid. The most common pathogens responsible for this illness are staphylococci, pneumococci, gonococci, and Gram negative organisms.[10]

Systemic antimicrobial therapy with the appropriate agent usually provides dramatic improvement. Supplemental warm compresses and joint immobilization early in the recovery phase will lessen pain symptoms. As the infection clears, range of motion exercising is helpful. The need to get bactericidal concentrations of the drug at the actual site of infection for an appropriate period of therapy must be emphasized. The outcome sought is complete functional recovery of the involved joint without articular destruction. Inadequate therapy must be avoided.[6,7]

Infection In Cystic Fibrosis

Pulmonary infection in patients with cystic fibrosis is often treated with aggressive IV antimicrobial agents in the home setting. The major cause of morbidity and mortality in many of these patients results from tenacious secretions, mucous plugs and secondary infections which lead to pneumonia, bronchiectasis and chronic sinusitis. In addition to hydration, aggressive pulmonary percussion and drainage, bronchodilators and expectorants, the use of aggressive antimicrobial therapy at the onset of infection can sometimes obviate the need for frequent hospitalization.[11]

Infections in cystic fibrosis patients become increasingly more difficult to treat as the disease progresses. For most patients that have a progressive type of disease, recurrent pulmonary infections may require higher doses of antibiotics or combination therapy.

Lyme Disease

Lyme borreliosis is a spirochetal illness that is transmitted by ticks. Most of the cases of lyme disease in the United States have been reported in the northeastern U.S., from Massachusetts to Maryland, and in the Midwest, in Wisconsin and Minnesota. Cases of Lyme disease have been reported in 33 states, most commonly in the summer months.[12] The disease is accompanied by flu-like or meningitis-like symptoms (stage 1), followed by meningitis, neuritis, or carditis (stage 2), or by intermittent arthritis, or neurologic or skin abnormalities (stage 3).[12]

For early Lyme disease, tetracycline is effective in adults. In children, amoxicillin or phenoxymethylpenicillin is effective. Later in the illness, parenteral antibiotic therapy may be necessary, especially in patients with meningitis or neuropathies. Up to four weeks of IV therapy with penicillin G or ceftriaxone is recommended.[12-14]

Other Infections

Other diagnoses being treated aggressively in the HHC setting are cellulitis, post-operative wound infection, sinusitis, pelvic inflammatory disease and pyelonephritis. Considering the current economic climate and the emphasis to control escalating health care expenditures, the list of diagnoses being treated with HPAT will probably increase.

ANTIMICROBIAL SELECTION

The most common antimicrobials selected for use in the home environment are the penicillins, cephalosporins, and the aminoglycosides. (See Table 24-3.) Clindamycin, vancomycin and various antifungal agents are also selected where appropriate. Although culture and sensitivity determinations are the primary, initial factor in the selection of the antimicrobial, convenience for the HHC patient is also a priority. Desirable features include favorable pharmacokinetic properties and adequate stability characteristics. The role of newer pump technology is equally important, especially for patients who previously could not be treated at home.[15] Typical selection criteria for antibiotics are listed in Table 24-4.

Table 24-3 Most Frequently Prescribed IV Antibiotics for HHC Patients[18]

Antibiotic	Percent
Ceftriaxone	14.6
Ganciclovir	11.9
Vancomycin	11.8
Cefazolin	10.4
Tobramycin	4.5
Gentamicin	4.3
Amikacin	4.2
Ceftazidime	4.1
Other, not specified	33.0

Table 24-4 Antibiotic Selection Criteria for Home IV Therapy[3,17]

- Antimicrobial Sensitivity
- Long Half-Life
- Relatively Simple Monitoring Parameters
- Few Adverse Drug Reactions
- Extended Drug Stability
- Cost Effectiveness

Stability of IV Drugs

The stability and compatibility of antibiotics for IV administration at home should be considered in the antimicrobial selection process. The effect of infusion fluid (e.g., dextrose 5%, normal saline) and drug concentration upon the expiration date should be determined early in the drug therapy selection process. The effects of storage time and temperature, duration of infusion, and pH may preclude the use of a particular antibiotic at home.

The composition of the infusion container may affect the stability and compatibility of the antibiotic. The varying effects of glass containers versus polyvinyl chloride plastic bags on intravenous admixtures have been reported. Use of a standard reference on IV stability, such as King Guide to Parenteral Admixtures, is recommended.[16] (See also Chapter 5.)

Pharmacokinetic Considerations

The half-life of an antibiotic is an important determinant of the number of times a day that the drug must be administered to the patient.[1] Antibiotics that are administered once or twice a day, are more convenient for HHC patients than antibiotics that must be given every four hours. The other important pharmacokinetic consideration is the manner in which drugs are metabolized and excreted. Dosage adjustments in patients with hepatic or renal impairment are part of the antibiotic selection process.

Monitoring Parameters

As with other drug categories, some antibiotics have fewer adverse effects and warrant less intense monitoring of outcome than others.[1,17] Reactions such as anaphylaxis, leukopenia, neutropenia, severe diarrhea, as well as kidney and liver impairments may occur. Therefore, home administration of these agents must be carefully monitored. For example, cephalosporins with a methyltetrazolethiol sidechain (cephamandole, cefoperaxone, moxalactam) have been associated with certain adverse reactions (e.g., disulfiram-like reactions, hypoprothrombinemia).[17] It should be borne in mind that the HHC patient should abstain from alcoholic beverages while receiving therapy, a circumstance more difficult to control outside the hospital setting. The HHC pharmacist should recommend prothrombin times at regular intervals so that patients are closely monitored for episodes of spontaneous bleeding and darkening of urine and stool must be monitored closely.

Aminoglycoside antibiotics have been the treatment of choice for large numbers of hospitalized patients with gram negative aerobic infections. Patients are also treated with these agents in the home setting, because of their advantages in certain instances over extended spectrum penicillins and cephalosporins. Since these agents interfere with protein synthesis in the cell, there is more tendency to cause insult to human tissue, in particular ototoxicity and nephrotoxicity.[1,17]

Other Dosing Issues

The accuracy of peak and trough levels in the HHC setting requires that special attention be given to the timing of blood sampling, and to the appropriate dosing intervals. Peak and trough levels which indicate toxic concentrations may result from the previous dose being given late. The trough level is indeed elevated, but only because of an inappropriate time interval between doses. The peak level is elevated only because an additional amount of drug was infused in the presence of an already elevated serum through level. Sub-therapeutic levels may not indicate an inappropriate dose or dosing interval, but may indicate the patient has missed the previous dose.[17]

It is extremely important to establish a relationship of confidence and honesty with the patient, such that missed doses or inappropriately timed doses are reported to the HHC team. Without this rapport, erroneous information provided by the patient may lead to incorrect adjustments in the therapy and result in therapeutic failures or toxicities.

Initiating Therapy

An area of concern when starting therapy is the issue of the patient's initial exposure to an antimicrobial. Should this occur in the home setting? The safest option is to give the first dose when the patient is hospitalized where emergency measures can be instituted at the first signs of allergic reaction.

However, as physicians, nurses, and pharmacists have become more familiar and comfortable with administering IV antimicrobials in the outpatient setting, the need for hospitalization in all instances may be questioned. The administration of the first dose of an antimicrobial in the home without the availability of medical supervision and resuscitation capabilities has been reported as a medical risk.[2] If hospitalization is unacceptable, an alternative may be to give the first dose in the physician's office. A thorough and complete medical history may reveal a previous uneventful use of the drug and should always be an initial part of the procedure for accepting a new referral.

ADMINISTERING IV ANTIBIOTICS AT HOME

Training patients and family members to administer IV antibiotics while maintaining good catheter care is challenging. In many instances it is the first time they have been invited to actively participate in their own care using sophisticated and technically advanced devices.

The selection of peripheral or central venous access will be predicated upon the length of therapy, status of peripheral veins, patient motivation, family support and access to HHC personnel. Patients and caregivers must be instructed in their therapy, the drugs being administered, potential side effects, drug storage, aseptic technique, and heparinization procedures.

Antimicrobials may be administered intravenously by several methods. The most common one is the piggyback (small volume parenteral infusion) method. Here, the drug is added to 50 ml or 100 ml of 5% dextrose or normal saline solutions and infused over 30 to 60 minutes into a peripheral IV cannula through a heparin-lock device. Some drugs, such as nafcillin and vancomycin, may require more diluent in order to minimize peripheral vein irritation and avoid phlebitis. Administration sets, needles, alcohol swabs, syringes and heparinized saline are usually supplied along with the premixed drug.

Another cost effective method employs the use of a syringe pump. In this instance, the drug is reconstituted and provided in the form of pre-filled syringes. The volumes may vary depending upon the drug selected. Diluents include sterile water for injection, 5% dextrose solution, or normal saline. Selection of a diluent that allows an osmolarity near that of blood may assist in keeping the peripheral vein patent. Syringe pumps are useful for pediatric patients or patients with fluid restriction.

A third choice employs the use of a programmable infusion device. The ambulatory pump is compact, portable and programmable in a way that allows intermittent infusion of antimicrobials at preset intervals throughout the day and night. Patients are not required to awaken to infuse middle-of-the-night doses. (See also Chapter 19.)

The choice of system will be directed by economic issues, reimbursement constraints, patient learning capabilities, and motivation to participate. As an example, a patient with compromised vision who lives alone may not be able to set the infusion rate of the piggyback system using a roller clamp and gravity drip method. On the other hand, some third party payers only recognize the piggyback system as a reimbursable method to administer these drugs. Issues other than convenience often dictate the choice of system.

One or more members of the HHC team must be available 24 hours a day to respond to the needs of their patients. Patients must be given home telephone numbers of those persons or, at the very least, an answering service number.[17] The availability of pocket paging devices often serves to satisfy this need.

Written step-by-step manuals of instruction must be provided to patients and their families in order to reinforce their knowledge and understanding of the therapy. This is one of the important steps that leads to quality assurance and consistency of care. The most effective programs have methods by which patients, family members, and physicians are afforded the opportunity to evaluate the services rendered, providing another quality assurance technique. Patients or caregivers must be able to verbalize knowledge and to undertake dosing responsibilities.

CONCLUSION

As this nation faces up to an economic climate that calls for more cost-effective medical care, the use of IV antibiotic therapy at home will inevitably increase. The treatment of infections in environments other than hospitals has reduced length of hospital stay and the cost of care for patients who receive HPAT. The future challenge will be to provide this type of high technology service in all community settings where the need exists, without compromising patient care.

Appendix 24-A Guidelines for Accepting Referred Patients for Home IV Antimicrobial Therapy[3]

1. All signs and symptoms of infection will be under control, and the patient's condition will be stable at the time of discharge from the hospital except for the need to continue IV antimicrobial therapy.
2. The patient and his or her family should understand the necessity of continued IV therapy at home and agree with the treatment plan.
3. The patient is willing to receive IV therapy at home.
4. The patient understands and can perform IV infusion techniques to the satisfaction of the pharmacist or nurse after the completion of in-hospital training.
5. The patient's home environment will be safe and the patient will have a telephone, a refrigerator for storage of the drugs, and dependable transportation arrangements.
6. The patient's vein can endure repeated cannulation.
7. Arrangement for regular change of the catheter is made before the patient is discharged for home therapy.

REFERENCES

1. McPherson ML. Monitoring home IV antibiotic therapy. Home Health Care Pract. 1990; 2:69-77.
2. Goldenberg RI. Pitfalls in the delivery of outpatient intravenous therapy. Drug Int and Clin Pharm. 1985; 4.
3. Chattopadhyay T, Catania PN, Mergener MA. Therapeutic outcome of elderly and nonelderly patients receiving home intravenous antimicrobial therapy. Am J Hosp Pharm. 1990; 47:335-339.
4. Job ML and Matthews HW. Bone and Joint Infections. In. Herfindal ET, et al. Eds. Clinical Pharmacy and Therapeutics. Williams and Wilkins Baltimore. 1988.
5. DiPiro JT, et al. Eds. Pharmacotherapy. Appleton and Lange Norwalk CN. 1993.
6. Wilson JD ,et al. Eds. Harrison's Principles of Internal Medicine. McGraw-Hill, Inc. New York. 1991.
7. Armstrong, EP. Bone and Joint Infections . In DiPiro JT, et al. Eds. Pharmacotherapy Appleton and Lange, Norwalk CN. 1993.
8. Kaye D. Infective Endocarditis. In Wilson JD, et al. Eds. Harrison's Principles of Internal Medicine. McGraw-Hill, Inc. New York. 1991.
9. Polk RE, et al. Infective Endocarditis. In DiPero JT, et al. Eds. Pharmacotherapy. Appleton and Lange, Norwalk CN. 1993.
10. Rotrosen D. Infectious Arthritis. In Wilson JD, et al. Eds. Harrison's Principles of Internal Medicine. McGraw-Hill, Inc. New York. 1991.
11. Colten HR. Cystic Fibrosis. In Wilson JD, et al. Eds. Harrison's Principles of Internal Medicine. McGraw-Hill, Inc. New York. 1991.
12. Steere AC. Lyme Borreliosis. In Wilson JD, et al. Eds. Harrison's Principles of Internal Medicine. McGraw-Hill, Inc. New York. 1991.
13. Rahn DW. Antibiotic Treatment of Lyme Disease. Postgrad Med. 1992; 91:57-64.
14. Hassler D, et al. Pulsed high dose cefotaxime therapy in refractory Lyme borreliosis. Lancet. 1991; 338:193.
15. New PB, et al. Ambulatory antibiotics infusion devices. Am J Med. 1991; 91:455-461.
16. King JC. Guide to Parenteral Admixtures. PaceMarq., Inc. San Francisco. 1993.
17. Vickery TR. Home Parenteral Antimicrobial Therapy. In Catania PN and Rosner MM. Eds. Home Health Care Practice. Health Markets Research, Palo Alto. 1986.
18. Winters RW, Parver AK, and Sansbury JD. Home infusion therapy: a service and demographic profile. National Alliance for Infusion Therapy. Washington DC. 1992.

25 Special Requirements for AIDS Patients

Julie Wilson Ganz, Pharm.D.

As the epidemic of Acquired Immunodeficiency Syndrome (AIDS) progresses, home health care (HHC) pharmacists will be caring for these patients in increasing numbers. With its 10-year incubation period, AIDS will unquestionably be a continuing and major focus of clinical practice for decades to come. The role of pharmacists includes ensuring rational drug therapy and management of drug therapy to improve patient quality of life in accordance with acknowledged standards of pharmaceutical care.[1] This chapter describes the syndrome, basic treatment modalities, and the progress achieved in the treatment of AIDS and its manifestations in the HHC setting.

ACQUIRED IMMUNODEFICIENCY SYNDROME

Etiology And Pathology

AIDS was first recognized and reported in the United States in 1981 after clusters of Pneumocystis carinii pneumonia and Kaposi's sarcoma cases were reported.[2,3] The etiologic agent of AIDS is a retrovirus designated as the Human Immunodeficiency Virus (HIV). The CD_4 lymphocyte is the primary target for HIV infection because of the affinity of the virus for the CD_4 surface marker.[4] The CD_4 lymphocyte (inducer, helper) is a subset of T lymphocytes which coordinates a number of important immunologic functions. A loss of these functions results in a progressive impairment of the immune response. After penetrating the nucleus of the cell, the retrovirus integrates its genetic material into that of the cell through the action of a unique enzyme, reverse transcriptase, and begins to replicate itself. The pathogenic life cycle of the HIV has been valuable in identifying potential therapies but exactly how the virus kills T lymphocytes remains an enigma. The virus is also capable of replicating in a limited number of other cells in the human body including macrophages, CNS cells, and gastrointestinal mucosal cells. Studies of the natural history of HIV infection have documented a wide spectrum of disease manifestations ranging from asymptomatic infection to life-threatening conditions characterized by severe immunodeficiency, serious opportunistic infections, and cancers.[5,6] Studies have also shown a direct relationship between the development of life-threatening opportunistic illnesses and the absolute number or percentage of CD_4 lymphocytes.[7-11] As the number of CD_4 lymphocytes decreases, the risk and severity of opportunistic illnesses increases.

Definition

The Centers for Disease Control (CDC) case definition for AIDS was first developed in 1982 and revised three times, in 1985, 1987, and 1993. The primary intent of the AIDS case definition is to assist epidemiologic surveillance of the AIDS epidemic but it is also used for other purposes; for qualifying individuals for entitlement programs, federal funding for AIDS programs, and accessing health care and social services.[12] The revised classification system categorizes the clinical conditions associated with HIV infection on the basis of the CD_4 lymphocyte count. There are three clinical categories, A, B, & C (Table 25-1) and three laboratory categories -1, 2, & 3 (Table 25-2) which result in a matrix of nine mutually exclusive AIDS categories (Table 25-3). Application of the definition for children differs from that for adults or adolescents and is not included in this summary. The 1993 case definition was expanded to include four additional diagnoses: 1) invasive cervical cancer, 2) pulmonary tuberculosis, 3) recurrent bacterial pneumonia, and 4) HIV-infected persons with a CD_4 lymphocyte count $< 200/mm^3$ (previously $400/mm^3$).[13]

Table 25-1 Summary of Clinical Conditions Associated with HIV Infection[13]

CATEGORY A (conditions occurring in documented HIV infected persons; conditions in Categories B and C must not have occurred)

1. Asymptomatic HIV infection
2. Persistent generalized lymphadenopathy (PGL)
3. Acute HIV infection with accompanying illness or history of acute HIV infection

CATEGORY B (symptomatic conditions occurring in documented HIV infected persons not included in Category C. Examples of conditions in Category B, include, but are not limited to:)

1. Bacillary angiomatosis
2. Candidiasis, oropharyngeal (thrush)
3. Candidiasis, vulvovaginal; persistent, frequent, or poorly responsive to therapy
4. Cervical dysplasia (moderate or severe) / cervical carcinoma in situ
5. Constitutional symptoms, such as fever (38.5 C) or diarrhea lasting > 1 month
6. Hairy leukoplakia, oral
7. Herpes zoster, (shingles), involving at least two distinct episodes or more than one dermatome
8. Idiopathic thrombocytopenic purpura
9. Listeriosis
10. Pelvic inflammatory disease, particularly if complicated by tubo-ovarian abscess
11. Peripheral neuropathy

CATEGORY C (AIDS indicator conditions)

1. Candidiasis of bronchi, trachea, or lungs
2. Candidiasis, esophageal
3. Cervical cancer, invasive *
4. Coccidioidomycosis, disseminated or extrapulmonary
5. Cryptococcosis, extrapulmonary
6. Cryptosporidiosis, chronic intestinal (> 1 month duration)
7. Cytomegalovirus disease (other than liver, spleen, or nodes)
8. Cytomegalovirus retinitis (with loss of vision)
9. Encephalopathy, HIV-related
10. Herpes simplex: chronic ulcer(s) (> month's duration); or bronchitis, pneumonitis, or esophagitis
11. Histoplasmosis, disseminated or extrapulmonary
12. Isosporiasis, chronic intestinal (>1 month's duration)
13. Kaposi's sarcoma
14. Lymphoma, Burkitt's (or equivalent term)
15. Lymphoma, immunoblastic (or equivalent term)
16. Lymphoma, primary, of brain
17. Mycobacterium avium complex or M. kansasii, disseminated or extrapulmonary
18. Mycobacterium tuberculosis, any site (pulmonary* or extrapulmonary)
19. Mycobacterium, other species or unidentified species, disseminated or extrapulmonary
20. Pneumocystis carinii pneumonia
21. Pneumonia, recurrent *
22. Progressive multifocal leukoencephalopathy
23. Toxoplasmosis of the brain
24. Wasting syndrome due to HIV

* Added in the 1993 expansion of the AIDS surveillance case definition.
Note: This table summary applies to adult and adolescent patients only (≥13 years of age).

Table 25-2 Summary of Laboratory Categories Associated with HIV[13]

CD4 T-cell Category	CD4 T-cells/uL	CD4 % *
1	>500	>29
2	200-499	14-28
3	<200* *	<14

* The percentage of lymphocytes that are CD4 T-cells

* * Added on the 1993 AIDS surveillance case definition

Table 25-3 1993 CDC Revised Classification system for HIV Infection and AIDS Case Definition for Adults and Adolesents[13]

Laboratory Categories (According to Table 25-2)	Clinical Categories (According to Table 25-1)		
	A	B	C
1	A1	B1	**C1***
2	A2	B2	**C2***
3	**A3***	**B3***	**C3***

*Expanded AIDS surveillance case definition

Transmission

There are three known modes of HIV transmission: sexual contact (homosexual and heterosexual), direct exposure to infected blood or blood products (transfusions, accidental needle sticks, needle sharing amongst intravenous drug abusers) and transmission from an infective women to her fetus. Studies have established that body fluids which provide sufficient quantities of virus or cofactors are limited to blood and infectious body secretions such as semen, vaginal secretions, and breast milk. Although HIV has been isolated from saliva, there is no evidence to date that can demonstrate that transmission occurs through casual contact with an infected person (e.g., kissing, sharing eating utensils) possibly due to the presence of low saliva concentrations of HIV or the necessary cofactors for infection.[14] There are clear high risk factors or activities for contracting HIV infection. Individuals who are at high risk for HIV infection include: sexually active homosexual or bisexual men, intravenous drug abusers, blood recipients from 1981-1985, hemophiliacs, people who engage in unprotected sexual intercourse with several partners, and neonates of HIV infected mothers.[15]

Prevalence

The epidemic proportions of HIV infections has emerged as a leading cause of death in the United States. As of March 1993, the CDC reported the following AIDS statistics:[16]

Total Number	289,320	
Adults	284,840	(98%)
Children	4,480	(2%)
Homosexuals & Bisexual Males	160,345	(55%)
Intravenous Drug Users	65,778	(23%)
Men	252,363	(87%)
Women	32,477	(11%)
Deaths	182,275	(63%)
Heterosexuals	19,178	(7%)
Transfusion Cases	5,384	(2%)

The incidence rate for men is almost eight times that for women. In 1991 alone, 29,850 U.S. residents died from HIV infection; of these, 3% were < 25 years old; 74% , 25-44 years; and 23%, > 45 years. HIV was the ninth leading cause of death overall and the third leading cause of death among persons aged 25-44 years.[17] Based on current levels of HIV infections in the United States, the CDC estimates that the expanded case definition could increase cases reported in 1993 by approximately 75%. This effect on the number of reported cases is expected to be much smaller in subsequent years.

HIV Testing

Current serologic tests for HIV infection are based on the observation that most persons infected with HIV develop specific antibodies within a few weeks, and nearly all persons develop antibodies within a few months. These HIV-specific antibodies persist during the course of latent infection and, to varying degrees, during subsequent progression to overt disease.[18,19] Of the tests available for HIV diagnosis, enzyme-linked immunosorbent assays (ELISA) for HIV-1 antibody are the most widely used. Specimens which are initially reactive are retested in duplicate, then if either of the duplicate tests is positive, the sera are said to be repeatedly reactive and must then be tested by a supplemental assay, such as immunofluorescence or "western blot" (Figure 25-1).[20]

Figure 25-1 Algorithm for HIV Testing[20]

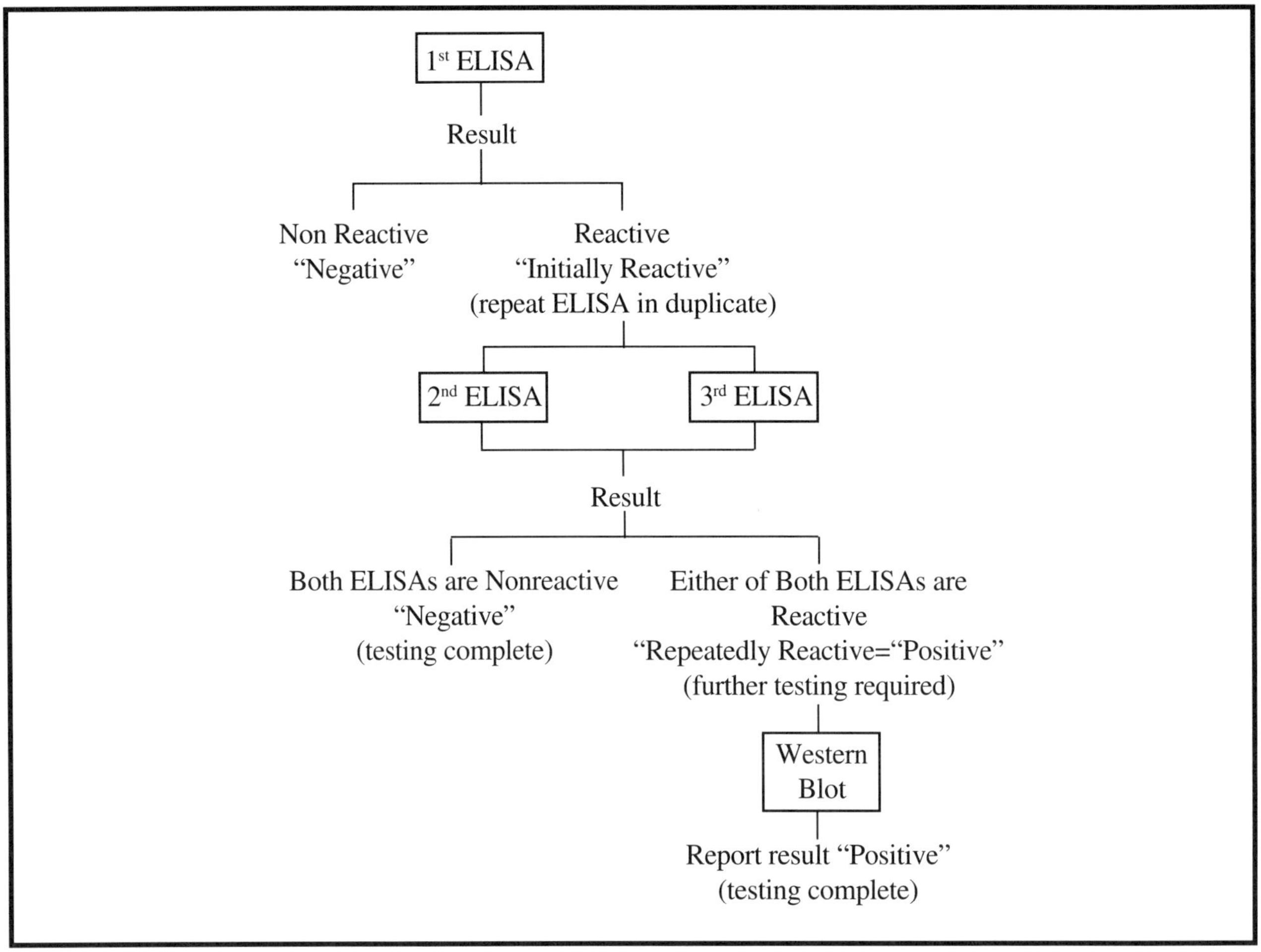

The sensitivity and specificity of commercial ELISAs were found to be between 98.1% and 100% in a study that compared their results to western blot.[21] When properly performed, the average specificity of ELISAs is 99.8%.[21] Patients are informed that they are positive only when they are repeatedly reactive by ELISA and western blot positive. Although assays are capable of identifying HIV infection, infected persons can transmit HIV to others before the antibody tests prove positive. HIV infection is also detectable by cultivating the HIV from T lymphocytes and can prove positive before the antibody test becomes positive, but due to high costs, relative insensitivities, and lengthy time requirements, culture testing is generally not used. The relentless depletion or destruction of T_4 (CD_4) cells characteristic in AIDS patients may be quantified by determining the T_4/T_8 (or CD_4/CD_8) ratio. The T_4 lymphocyte is the helper or inducer cell and the T_8 lymphocyte is the suppressor or cytotoxic cell. The normal ratio for immunocompetent individuals is 2:1, while that of AIDS patients is lower or inverted (i.e., 1:2-1:100).[22] The absolute T_4-cell count is a more specific marker for severe immunodeficiency with clinical complications and is used as a parameter for initiating antiretroviral therapy, assessing response to therapy, and stratifying patient entry into clinical trials.

Antiretroviral Therapy

Treatment may be directed either at the life cycle of HIV or at stimulation of residual immune function. Zidovudine (AZT, Retrovir®) is a thymidine analog indicated as first-line therapy for the treatment of HIV infected individuals with a T_4-cell count < 500. AZT is converted by cellular enzymes to a triphosphate form which is mistaken by HIV's reverse transcriptase for the natural substrate - thymidine triphosphate. It is incorporated into the DNA transcript causing premature chain termination of the retroviral DNA. Adverse reactions reported during the first several weeks of therapy include headache, insomnia, nausea, vomiting, abdominal discomfort, diarrhea, malaise, myalgias, rash, and fever.[23] Symptoms usually subside with ongoing therapy. The major toxicity associated with AZT is bone marrow toxicity including anemia, neutropenia and, less commonly, thrombocytopenia.[23] Dosage recommendations for AZT vary according to the stage of HIV infection. For symptomatic adults the dosage regimen should be 100 mg every 4 hours while awake, 5-6 times/day, (500-600 mg/day). For asymptomatic adults the dosage regimen should be 100 mg every 4 hours while awake, 5 times/day, (500 mg/day).[24]

Didanosine (ddI, Videx®) is a nucleoside analog which inhibits retroviral reverse transcriptase halting HIV replication. Didanosine is reserved as second-line treatment for patients with advanced HIV infection who are intolerant of AZT or who have progressive HIV infection during AZT therapy. Drug induced neutropenia is minimized with ddI versus AZT. The major side effects and toxicities associated with didanosine therapy include peripheral neuropathy, pancreatitis, diarrhea, hyperamylasemia, and increases in serum urate levels.[25] The adult dosage recommendations are based on weight and will range between 250 mg/day (125 mg chew tabs BID or 167 mg buffered powder pckts. BID for wt. of 35-49 kg) to 400-500 mg/day (200 mg chew tabs BID or 250 buffered powder pckts. BID for wt. of 50-74 kg) or 600-750 mg/day (300 mg chew tabs BID or 375 mg buffered powder pckts. BID for wt. of 75 kg.).[26]

Zalcitabine (ddC, Hivid®) is another nucleoside analog which demonstrates an in vitro synergistic inhibitory activity with AZT against HIV.[27] Zalcitabine is FDA approved for the treatment of HIV infection, not as monotherapy, but in combination with AZT for individuals with advanced HIV disease (T_4-cell count <300) who show signs of clinical deterioration despite AZT or ddI monotherapy. Like ddI, ddC does not appear to cause significant bone marrow toxicity but can cause a major dose-limiting toxicity of painful sensorimotor peripheral neuropathy involving predominately the lower extremities. Initial toxicities include rash, esophageal or oral ulcers, and fever during the first 1-4 weeks of therapy but may resolve without interruption of therapy. On rare occasions ddC has been associated with pancreatitis. The recommended adult dosage combination with AZT is 0.75 mg (ddC) with 200 mg (AZT) every 8 hours.

In addition to, or in place of, the "traditional" treatment regimens for HIV infection, patients may choose one or many of the "non-traditional" or alternate therapies which include herbal preparations, manipulative therapies, dietary regimens, religious healing, or non-conventional uses of domestic and imported pharmaceuticals. As some of these alternatives are chemically based, they must be considered for potential drug-drug interactions as well as drug-organ toxicities.

HHC pharmacists must understand the AIDS disease, its sequelae, treatment modalities and complications in order to interact competently with other health care team members and patients when caring for this patient population.

OPPORTUNISTIC INFECTIONS

HIV infected persons are clearly at risk for specific opportunistic infections (OIs) when the CD_4 T-cells are slowly depleted and the count falls to certain levels.[9,28,29] It appears that Mycobacterium tuberculosis can occur early in the course of HIV disease with CD4 counts of approximately 350.[30] As the CD_4 count drops to 200, Pneumocystis carinii pneumonia (PCP) can develop. Between 100-200, toxoplasmosis can occur. When the CD_4 count falls below 100, OIs most likely to develop include cryptococcal meningitis, candidiasis, and Mycobacterium avium complex (MAC). The prevention of OIs may lead to an increase in patient survival and improved quality of life. However, whether the use of prophylactic therapy merits risking the development of resistance that could render later therapy useless must be considered. There are essentially three stages in approaching the treatment of OIs:[31] 1) primary prophylaxis: therapy given prior to clinical infection; 2) acute treatment: therapy administered for active clinical infection; 3) secondary prophylaxis: therapy instituted after completion of acute treatment to prevent relapse. The remainder of this chapter will focus on reviewing the home parenteral therapies used to treat opportunistic infections and neoplasms in patients with AIDS.

VIRAL INFECTIONS

Cytomegalovirus (CMV)

More than 90% of AIDS patients demonstrate evidence of CMV infection and almost one-third of them will experience severe clinical manifestations. CMV is ubiquitous and infection usually occurs with activation of latent virus but can be sexually transmitted between homosexual men.[32,33,34,35] Though ganciclovir has proven significantly effective for treatment of CMV infection, there have been reports of ganciclovir resistant CMV. A new study suggests that combining or alternating ganciclovir and foscarnet for the treatment of CMV retinitis may help fight strains resistant to one or the other drug.

Pathogen: Cytomegalovirus, a member of the Herpes virus family.

Site of infection: Primary site - eye (CMV retinitis), lung (CMV pneumonia) GI tract (CMV stomatitis, esophagitis, gastritis, colitis). Other sites - CNS (CMV encephalitis or polyradiculitis), liver (CMV hepatitis), and the adrenal glands.

Prophylaxis: Not applicable.

Treatment:

Ganciclovir Induction - 5 mg/kg/dose over 60 min., Q 12 hrs., for 10-14 days;

Ganciclovir Maintenance - 5 mg/kg/dose, over 60 min., QD, 7 days/week or 6 mg/kg/dose, over 60 min., QD, 5 days/week;

Foscarnet Induction - 60 mg/kg/dose over 60 min., Q 8 hrs., for 14 days. Recommended hydration NS 500 ml w/each dose; or 100 mg/kg/dose, over 2 hrs., Q 12 hrs., for 21 days.[35] Recommended IV hydration NS 500 ml w/each dose.

Foscarnet Maintenance - 90-120 mg/kg/day, over 2 hrs., QD, 7 days/week. Recommended hydration NS 500-1000 ml w/each dose. Refer to Table 25-4 (ganciclovir) and Tables 25-5a & 5b (foscarnet) for dosage adjustments according to renal function. Dose adjustments should also be made according to weight changes (i.e., > or < 2 kg). Discontinuation or dose change may be necessary according to neutrophil count (<500/mm3) for ganciclovir.

Laboratory monitoring:

Ganciclovir - obtain baseline values then complete blood count (CBC) with differential (w/diff) 2-3 x/week and Platelets (Plts), electrolytes (lytes), blood urea nitrogen (BUN), Creatinine (Cr), weekly during induction; CBC w/diff, Plts, Lytes, BUN, Cr, every 1-2 weeks, and liver function tests (LFTs) monthly, during maintenance therapy.

Foscarnet - obtain baseline values, then BUN, Cr, Lytes, Ca, Phosphate (Phos), Mg, 2-3 x/week, and CBC w/diff, Plts, LFTS, alb, weekly during induction; in patients with borderline renal function a 24-hour urine collection for a real creatinine clearance (CrCl) calculation may be indicated prior to starting therapy; BUN, Cr, Lytes, Calcium (Ca), Phos, Mg, 1-2 x/week and CBC w/diff, Plts, LFTs, albumin (alb), every 1-2 weeks, during maintenance therapy. Note: since foscarnet can chelate divalent ions in vitro, lab samples should be drawn prior to infusion to avoid false low values.

Adverse drug reactions:

Ganciclovir - Neutropenia (dose related), anemia, thrombocytopenia, transient liver enzyme abnormalities, low incidence of nausea, vomiting, and headache.

Foscarnet - Renal toxicity, anemia, hypocalcemia, hypophosphatemia, headache, fever, nausea/vomiting, diarrhea, seizures, genital ulcers (penile ulcers). Phlebitis with peripheral access. Hyperphosphatemia, hypokalemia, hypomagnesemia and nephrogenic diabetes insipidus have also been reported.

Drug-drug interactions:

Ganciclovir - Bone marrow suppressor agents (TMP/SMX, zidovudine, vancomycin pentamidine).

Foscarnet - Renal toxic agents (aminoglycosides, pentamidine has potential additive hypocalcemia effect, amphotericin, vancomycin, TMP/SMX, acyclovir); zidovudine has additive anemic effect.

Infusion device system:

Ganciclovir - Gravity drip, infusion pump, or disposable infusion device.

Foscarnet - Must be administered through infusion pump or disposable infusion device.

Drug dilutions:

Ganciclovir - dose in 100 ml of D5W or

Table 25-4 Ganciclovir Dosing According to Renal Function

Level of Renal Function	Induction Therapy	
	CrCl (ml/min)	Dosage (mg/kg)
Normal	> 80	5.0 BID
Mild Impairment	50-79	2.5 BID
Moderate Impairment	25-49	2.5 QD
Severe Impairment	< 25	1.25 QD

* For maintenance therapy, halve the dosage

$$CrCl = \frac{(140\text{-age})(Wt,kg)}{(72)(SrCr)} \quad (\text{x } 0.85 \text{ for females})$$

NS, in viaflex, stable for 35 days under refrigeration or at room temperature.[36]

Foscarnet - Through central line - undiluted (24 mg/ml); through peripheral line - diluted (1mg/ml and 12 mg/ml in D5W or NS, in viaflex, stable for 35 days under refrigeration).[37]

Herpes Simplex Virus (HSV)

Chronic cutaneous lesions due to HSV in patients with AIDS have been described.[38] HSV infections manifest themselves as vesicular lesions on an erythematous base in oral or genital areas. Destruction of mucosal and cutaneous barriers by progressive HSV infection may increase the risk of bacterial or fungal infection.

Pathogen: Herpes simplex.

Site of infection: Oro-facial, genitals, anorectal area, esophagus, CNS.

Prophylaxis: Acyclovir 400 mg BID or 200 mg TID (PO).

Treatment:

Acyclovir (PO) - 200 or 400 mg 5 x/day, for 7-10 days (standard therapy).

Acyclovir (IV) - 5 mg/kg/dose over 60 min., Q 8 hrs., for 7 days (for severe, non-encephalitis infections); 10 mg/kg/dose over 60 min., Q 8 hrs., for 10 days (for encephalitis).

Foscarnet - 40-60 mg/kg/dose over 60 min., Q 8 hrs., for 14 day[39,40] (for acyclovir-resistance). Recommended hydration NS 500 ml w/each dose.

Table 25-5A Foscarnet Dosing According to Renal Function

Induction Therapy	
CrCl (ml/min/kg)	mg/kg/Dose (Q 8 hrs)
≥1.6	60
1.5	57
1.4	53
1.3	49
1.2	46
1.1	42
1.0	39
0.9	35
0.8	32
0.7	28
0.6	25
0.5	21
0.4	18

$$CrCl = \frac{(140\text{-age})}{72} \text{ x } SrCr$$

(x 0.85 for females)

Table 25-5B Foscarnet Dosing According to Renal Function

Maintenance Therapy	
CrCl (ml/min/kg)	mg/kg/Dose (Q 24 hrs)
≥ 1.4	90
1.2 - 1.4	78
1.0 - 1.2	75
0.8 - 1.0	71
0.6 - 0.8	63
0.4 - 0.6	57
CrCl (ml/min/kg)	mg/kg/Dose (Q 24 hrs)
≥ 1.4	120
1.2 - 1.4	104
1.0 - 1.2	100
0.8 - 1.0	94
0.6 - 0.8	84
0.4 - 0.6	76

Acyclovir and foscarnet doses should be adjusted according to renal function.

Laboratory monitoring:

Acyclovir - obtain baseline values then CBC w/diff, Plts, Lytes, weekly; BUN, Cr 1-2 x/week.

Foscarnet - obtain baseline values, then BUN, Cr, Lytes, Ca, Phos, Mg, 2-3 x/week; CBC w/diff, Plts, weekly. Note: since foscarnet can chelate divalent ions in vitro, lab samples should be drawn prior to infusion to avoid false low values.

Adverse drug reactions:

Acyclovir - Renal toxicity, nausea, phlebitis, transient liver enzyme abnormalities, rash.

Foscarnet - Renal toxicity, anemia, hypocalcemia, hypophosphatemia, headache, fever, nausea/vomiting, diarrhea, seizures, genital ulcers (penile ulcers). Phlebitis with peripheral vascular access. Hyperphosphatemia, hypokalemia, hypomagnesemia and nephrogenic diabetes insipidus have also been reported.

Drug-drug interactions:

Acyclovir - Renal toxic agents (aminoglycosides, pentamidine, amphotericin, vancomycin, TMP/SMX, foscarnet).

Foscarnet - Renal toxic agents (aminoglycosides, pentamidine has potential additive hypocalcemia effect, amphotericin, vancomycin, TMP/SMX, acyclovir); zidovudine has additive anemic effect.

Infusion device system:

Acyclovir - Gravity drip, infusion pump or disposable infusion device.

Foscarnet - Must be administered through infusion pump or disposable infusion device.

Drug dilutions:

Acyclovir - Dose in 100-150 ml of D5W or NS (500 mg/100 ml) in viaflex, stable for 37 days at room temperature or refrigeration[41] (white precipitate forms under refrigeration but dissolves when warmed to room temperature).

Foscarnet - Through central line - undiluted (24 mg/ml); through peripheral line - diluted (1mg/ml and 12 mg/ml in D5W or NS, in viaflex, stable for 35 days under refrigeration).[37]

Varicella Zoster Virus (VZV)

Commonly known as shingles, this herpes virus can occur without demonstrable underlying immunodeficiency in middle-aged individuals. Herpes zoster is usually self limiting even in individuals with relatively advanced HIV infection, although such individuals are at risk of developing chronic progressive cutaneous[42,43] or CNS infection following herpes zoster infection.

Pathogen: Varicella zoster.

Site of infection: Lateral and anterior chest reflecting the radicular nerve distribution, ophthalmic division of the trigeminal nerve. Infection may disseminate viscerally to the lungs, liver, or CNS.

Prophylaxis: Not applicable.

Treatment:

Acyclovir (PO) - 600-800 mg 5 x/day, for 7-10 days for 7-10 days;

Acyclovir (IV) - 10 mg/kg/dose over 60 min., Q 8 hrs., for 7-10 days (for recurrent infection).

Foscarnet - 40 mg/kg/dose over 60 min., Q 8 hrs., for 14 day[44] (for acyclovir-resistance). Recommended hydration NS 500 ML w/each dose.

Acyclovir and foscarnet doses should be adjusted according to renal function.

Laboratory monitoring:

Acyclovir - obtain baseline values then CBC w/diff, Plts, Lytes, weekly; BUN, Cr 1-2 x/week.

Foscarnet - obtain baseline values then BUN, Cr, Lytes, Ca, Phos, Mg, 2-3 x/week; CBC w/diff, Plts, weekly. Note: since foscarnet can chelate divalent ions in vitro, lab samples should be drawn prior to infusion to avoid false low values.

Adverse drug reactions:

Acyclovir - Renal toxicity, nausea, phlebitis, transient liver enzyme abnormalities, rash.

Foscarnet - Renal toxicity, anemia, hypocalcemia, hypophosphatemia, headache, fever, nausea/vomiting, diarrhea, seizures, genital ulcers. Phlebitis with peripheral vascular access. Hyperphosphatemia, hypokalemia, hypomagnesemia and nephrogenic diabetes insipidus have also been reported.

Drug-drug interactions:

Acyclovir - Renal toxic agents (aminoglycosides, pentamidine, amphotericin, vancomycin, TMP/SMX, foscarnet).

Foscarnet - Renal toxic agents (aminoglycosides, pentamidine has potential additive hypocalcemia effect, amphotericin, vancomycin, TMP/SMX, acyclovir); zidovudine has additive anemic effect.

Infusion device system:

Acyclovir - Gravity drip, infusion pump or disposable infusion device.

Foscarnet - Must be administered through infusion pump or disposable infusion device.

Drug dilutions:

Acyclovir - Dose in 100-150 ml of D5W or NS (500 mg/100 ml) in viaflex, stable for 37 days at room temperature or refrigeration[41] (white precipitate forms under refrigeration but dissolves when warmed to room temperature).

Foscarnet - Through central line - undiluted (24 mg/ml); through peripheral line - diluted (1mg/ml and 12 mg/ml in D5W or NS, in viaflex, stable for 35 days under refrigeration).[37]

PARASITIC INFECTIONS

Pneumocystis Carinii Pneumonia (PCP)

PCP is the most common opportunistic infection in AIDS patients. Pneumocystis carinii attaches to alveolar epithelial cells causing degeneration. Aveolar cells injury and loss lead to increased permeability of the alveolar capillary barrier, fluid leaks into the alveolar space, consequent reduction of surfactant content, and intrapulmonary blood shunting with decreased lung compliance. The result is hypoxemia, increased work of breathing, and ultimately, respiratory failure.[45] PCP is thought to be transmitted by the respiratory route. It is also presumed, but not proven, that infection occurs early in life and remains latent until immunodeficiency permits the development of disease.

Pathogen: Pneumocystis carinii.

Site of infection: Lung, other extrapulmonary sites have been reported usually upon autopsy.

Prophylaxis:

TMP/SMX (PO) - 160 mg-TMP/800 mg-SMX, (1 DS tab) BID, 2, 3, or 7 days/week;

Dapsone (PO) - 50-100 mg, QD or 2-3 days/week.

Aerosolized Pentamidine - 300 mg inhaled by Respirgard II® nebulizer every 4 weeks pre-medicated with bronchodilator inhalant (i.e., metaproterenol 2 puffs 10-15 mins. prior to treatment).

Pentamidine (IV) - 4 mg/kg/dose, over 60-120 mins., every 4 weeks.

Treatment: TMP/SMX (PO) - 15-20 mg-TMP/kg/day, divided Q 6-8 hrs., for 14-21 days.

TMP/SMX (IV) - 15-20 mg-TMP/kg/day over 60-90 mins., divided Q 6-8 hrs., for 14-21 days.

Pentamidine (IV) - 3-4 mg/kg/day[46] over 60-120 mins., QD for 14-21 days.

Dapsone + TMP (PO) - 100 mg Dapsone QD + 15-20 mg-TMP/kg/day divided Q 6-8 hrs., for 21 days.[47]

Clindamycin (PO) 300 - 450 mg Q 8 hrs. Primaquine (PO) 15 - 30 mg QD for 14-21 days.

Clindamycin (IV) 600 mg Q6 hrs. or 900 mg Q8 hrs over 30 mins.+ Primaquine (PO) 15 - 30 mg QD 4 14 - 21 days.[48]

Corticosteroid Therapy - recommendations for their use with other drugs follow specific criteria.[49] Dose starts with prednisone 40 mg BID for days 1-5 then tapered from days 6-21.

Laboratory monitoring:

TMP/SMX (IV) - obtain baseline values then CBC w/diff, Plts, Lytes, BUN, Cr, LFTs, 1-3 x/week; LDH weekly

Pentamidine (IV) - obtain baseline values then CBC w/diff, Plts, Lytes, Ca, Mg, Phos, BUN, Cr, Glucose, Amylase, 2-3 x/wk; LDH, LFTs, weekly (fingerstick glucose monitoring pre-, during, and post infusion may be necessary in patients with unstable glucose levels).

Clindamycin (IV) - obtain baseline values, then CBC w/diff, Plts, Lytes, BUN, Cr, weekly.

Adverse drug reactions:
TMP/SMX (IV) - Neutropenia, thrombocytopenia, GI disturbance (nausea, vomiting, anorexia), rash, fever, renal toxicity, hepatic toxicity, azotemia.
Pentamidine (IV) - Neutropenia, thrombocytopenia, hypotension, hypo/hyperglycemia, renal toxicity, hepatic toxicity, azotemia, hypocalcemia, phlebitis, tachycardia, confusion, hallucination, metallic taste, diarrhea, anorexia, abdominal discomfort, and anaphylactic reaction.
Pentamidine (Inh.) - Cough, bronchospasm, metallic taste.
Clindamycin (IV) - Colitis, GI disturbance (abdominal pain, nausea, vomiting, diarrhea), rash, transient liver enzyme abnormalities, azotemia, phlebitis, transient neutropenia.

Drug-drug interactions:
TMP/SMX (IV) - Bone marrow suppressor agents (ganciclovir, zidovudine, vancomycin, pentamidine); renal toxic agents (aminoglycosides, pentamidine, amphotericin, vancomycin, foscarnet, acyclovir).
Pentamidine (IV) - Bone marrow suppressor agents (ganciclovir, zidovudine, vancomycin, TMP/SMX); renal toxic agents (aminoglycosides, TMP/SMX, amphotericin, vancomycin, foscarnet-additive hypocalcemia potential, acyclovir)
Clindamycin (IV) - hepatotoxic drugs.

Infusion device system:
TMP/SMX (IV) - Must be administered through infusion pump or disposable infusion device.
Pentamidine (IV) - Must be administered through infusion pump or disposable infusion device.
Clindamycin (IV) - Gravity drip, infusion pump or disposable infusion device.

Drug dilutions:
TMP/SMX (IV) - 5 ml of drug/75 ml D5W for 2 hr. stability at room temperature; average dose mixed in 250-500 ml D5W; pre-drawn syringes with separate D5W viaflex bags dispensed to home, dose added to bag just prior to administration; drug stable in PVC syringes for 60 hrs.[50]
Pentamidine (IV) - dose in D5W 250 ml; stable for 5 days at refrigeration.[51]

Cryptosporidiosis

Cryptosporidium parvum is the most widely recognized enteric pathogen in AIDS patients. Cryptosporidium is a protozoal parasitic infection of the GI tract which can cause "slim disease,[11] a wasting syndrome described in Africa. Transmission is via the fecal-oral route from animal to person, person to person, or through contaminated water. Symptoms include massive secretory diarrhea, epigastric cramping pain, nausea, vomiting, anorexia, and weight loss. The diarrhea may lead to severe dehydration, electrolyte imbalance, and malabsorption syndrome. No antimicrobial therapy has been shown to consistently improve symptoms or eradicate infection. Spiramycin, an investigational agent, has undergone several clinical trials with disappointing results at a dose of 1 gm TID. The mainstay of supportive care is antidiarrheals, analgesics, and hydration (IV or PO). The use of total parenteral nutrition (TPN) as supportive treatment is prescribed by some clinicians but remains controversial since there is no evidence that weight loss is minimized. Octreotide, an analogue of somatostatin, has been approved for use in secretory diarrheas with anecdotal reports of decrease in the volume of diarrhea.

FUNGAL INFECTIONS

Cryptococcal Meningitis

Cryptococcal meningitis is a potentially life-threatening infection that affects up to 10 percent of AIDS patients. Cryptococcus neoformans is a fungus that grows in pigeon feces and in the soil at lower concentrations. Initial infection occurs via the lungs through inhalation of aerosolized organisms.

Pathogen: Cryptococcus neoformans.
Site of infection: CNS, both the brain and the meninges (pneumonia and fungemia are the most common extraneural infection).
Prophylaxis: Fluconazole 100-200 mg/day.[52]
Treatment: Amphotericin (IV) - 0.3-0.7 mg/kg/day, over 1-4 hrs., 3-7 days/week for a total dose of 1-2 gms. Recommended IV hydration 250-1000 ml NS boluses pre or post infusion (to limit renal toxicity). With Flucytosine (optional) - 150 mg/

kg/day, divided QID or Q 6 hrs.
Fluconazole (PO/IV) - 400 mg (IV-over 120 mins.) for 1st day, then 200 mg (IV-over 60 mins.) QD for 10-12 weeks (reserved for 2nd line therapy to amphotericin).[53] Dosage adjustments must be made for impaired renal function for both amphotericin and fluconazole. Pre-medication regimens are recommended with amphotericin infusions, especially in the faster 1-2 hr. infusion rates (diphenhydramine 25-50 mg with acetaminophen 650 mg; meperidine IV 25-50 mg for patients with a history of shaking chills or rigors). Infusion related phlebitis in peripheral vasculature may be avoided by adding heparin (500-1000) units and hydrocortisone (15-25 mg) directly to the amphotericin dose. Ketoconazole is not indicated for use in cryptococcal meningitis.

Laboratory monitoring:
Amphotericin - obtain baseline values then Lytes, BUN, Cr, Ca, Mg, 1-3 x/week, CBC w/diff, Plts, Alb, 1 x/week, LFTs every 1-2 weeks.
Fluconazole (IV) - obtain baseline values then CBC w/diff, Plts, Lytes, BUN, Cr, LFTS, weekly.

Adverse drug reactions:
Amphotericin - Renal toxicity, anemia, thrombocytopenia, fever, chills, transient hypotension, myalgias, nausea, vomiting (often related to infusion rate), hypokalemia, hypocalcemia, hypomagnesemia, phlebitis.
Fluconazole (IV) - Hepatic toxicity (elevated LFTs), rash, headache, nausea, vomiting, diarrhea, and abdominal pain have occurred at an incidence rate of <1%.

Drug-drug interactions:
Amphotericin - Renal toxic agents (aminoglycosides, pentamidine, foscarnet, vancomycin, TMP/SMX, acyclovir); corticosteroids (enhanced K+ loss).
Fluconazole (IV) - Hepatotoxic drugs.

Infusion device system:
Amphotericin - Must be administered through infusion pump or disposable infusion device.
Fluconazole (IV) - Gravity drip or infusion pump.

Drug dilutions:
Amphotericin - Admix with D5W (only) to a final concentration of 0.1 mg/ml for administration through a peripheral vascular access catheter, and to a final concentration of 0.25 mg/ml for administration through a central line. Both solutions are stable at refrigeration for 35 days.[54]
Fluconazole (IV) - Available in ready to use 200 mg/100 ml and 400 mg/200 ml iso-osmotic solution viaflex bags, stored at room temperature.

Coccidioidomycosis

Coccidioides is a soil fungus. It has not been established whether coccidioidomycosis in AIDS patients represents reactivation of latent infection or primary infection. This infection most frequently involves the lungs due to the inhalation route of infection. Ketoconazole is used to treat focal infections not involving the skin and soft tissue at a high dose of 400-800 mg/day.[55] The information below applies to treatment for coccidioidal meningitis with IV amphotericin.

Pathogen: Coccidioides immitis
Site of infection: Lung (focal and diffuse), cutaneous tissue, CNS (meningitis), lymph node, liver.
Prophylaxis: Uncertain; both ketoconazole 200-400 mg/day and fluconazole 200-400 mg/day[56] are used in clinical practice in patients for several months up to indefinitely.

Treatment:
Amphotericin (IV) - 0.3-0.7 mg/kg/day, over 1-4 hrs., 3-7 days/week for a total dose of 1-2.5 gms. Recommended IV hydration 250-1000 ml NS boluses pre- or post infusion (to limit renal toxicity).
With Flucytosine (optional)- 150 mg/kg/day, divided QID or Q 6 hrs.
Dosage adjustments must be made for impaired renal function. Pre-medication regimens are recommended with amphotericin infusions, especially in the faster 1-2 hr. infusion rates (diphenhydramine 25-50 mg with acetaminophen

650 mg; meperidine IV 25-50 mg for patients with either a history of or shaking chills or rigors). Infusion related phlebitis may be avoided by adding heparin (500-1000 units) and hydrocortisone (15-25 mg) directly to the amphotericin dose.

Laboratory monitoring:

Amphotericin - obtain baseline values then Lytes, BUN, Cr, Ca, Mg, 1-3 x/week, CBC w/diff, Plts, Alb, 1 x/week, LFTs every 1-2 weeks.

Adverse drug reactions:

Amphotericin - Renal toxicity, anemia, thrombocytopenia, fever, chills, transient hypotension, myalgias, nausea, vomiting (often related to infusion rate), hypokalemia, hypocalcemia, hypomagnesemia, phlebitis.

Drug-drug interactions:

Amphotericin - Renal toxic agents (aminoglycosides, pentamidine, foscarnet, vancomycin, TMP/SMX, acyclovir); corticosteroids (enhanced K^+ loss).

Infusion device system:

Amphotericin - Must be administered through infusion pump or disposable infusion device.

Drug dilutions:

Amphotericin - Admix with D5W (only) to a final concentration of 0.1 mg/ml for administration through a peripheral vascular access catheter, and to a final concentration of 0.25 mg/ml for administration through a central line. Both solutions are stable at refrigeration for 35 days.[54]

Histoplasmosis

Like coccdidioidomycosis, histoplasmosis is acquired by the respiratory route. In immunocompetent hosts, Histoplasma capsulatum usually causes asymptomatic infection but may cause an acute self-limiting pulmonary infection with no dissemination, whereas disseminated disease is the primary clinical presentation and is much more severe in AIDS patients.

Pathogen: Histoplasma capsulatum.

Site of infection: Lungs and cervical/hilar lymph nodes (non-disseminated), CNS, liver, spleen, GI tract, skin, and retina (disseminated).

Prophylaxis:

Amphotericin 1 mg/kg every 1-2 weeks, (low relapse rate), [57,58]

Ketoconazole 400 mg/day (relapse may occur within 6 months).

Treatment:

Amphotericin (IV) - 0.6 mg/kg/day, over 1-4 hrs., 3-7 days/week for a total dose of 2-3 gms. Recommended IV hydration 250-1000 ml NS boluses pre or post infusion (to limit renal toxicity).

With Flucytosine (optional) - 150 mg/kg/day, divided QID or Q 6 hrs. Dosage adjustments must be made for impaired renal function. Pre-medication regimens are recommended with amphotericin infusions, especially in the faster 1-2 hr. infusion rates (meperidine IV 25-50 mg for patients with a history of shaking chills or rigors). Infusion related phlebitis may be avoided by adding heparin (500-1000 units) and hydrocortisone (15-25 mg) directly to the amphotericin dose.

Laboratory monitoring:

Amphotericin - obtain baseline values then Lytes, BUN, Cr, Ca, Mg, 1-3 x/week, CBC w/diff, Plts, Alb, 1 x/week, LFTs every 1-2 weeks.

Adverse drug reactions:

Amphotericin - Renal toxicity, anemia, thrombocytopenia, fever, chills, transient hypotension, myalgias, nausea, vomiting (often related to infusion rate), hypokalemia, hypocalcemia, hypomagnesemia, phlebitis.

Drug-drug interactions:

Amphotericin - Renal toxic agents (aminoglycosides, pentamidine, foscarnet, vancomycin, TMP/SMX, acyclovir); corticosteroids (enhanced K+ loss).

Infusion device system:

Amphotericin - Must be administered through infusion pump or disposable infusion device.

Drug dilutions:

Amphotericin - Admix with D5W (only) to a final concentration of 0.1 mg/ml for administration through a peripheral vascular access catheter, and to a final concentration of 0.25 mg/ml for administration through a central line. Both solutions are stable at refrigeration for 35 days.[54]

BACTERIAL INFECTIONS

Mycobacterium avium Complex (MAC)

MAC represents two closely related organisms, Mycobacterium intracellular and Mycobacterium avium. MAC causes disseminated disease in up to 40% of patients with HIV in the United States.[59] Patients with a CD4 cell count < 100 and particularly < 50 are at a high risk for disseminated MAC infection.[60,61,62] MAC characteristically presents with severe clinical manifestations such as fever, sweats, weight loss, and anemia. Though effective antimicrobial treatment can decrease MAC bacteriemia and improve quality of life and duration of survival for HIV infected patients, treatment results for disseminated MAC infection remain poor.[63]

Pathogen: Mycobacterium avium or Mycobacterium intracellular.

Site of infection: Reticuloendothelial system, GI tract, liver, spleen, and bone marrow.

Prophylaxis: Rifabutin 300 mg QD for rest of life.[64]

Treatment:

Although studies have yet to determine an optimal regimen, the CDC recommends a combination of two of the following three agents, either azithromycin or clarithromycin with ethambutol. Practitioners have added one or more of the following as a multiple drug regimen; clofazamine, rifabutin, rifampin, ciprofloxacin, and IV amikacin; Amikacin dose - 7.5 mg/kg/dose over 30 mins., QD or Q 12 hrs., for first 4 weeks of therapy or for 2-4 weeks for acute exacerbations. Dosage is adjusted according to renal function.

Laboratory monitoring:

Obtain baseline values, then CBC w/diff, Plts, weekly; Lytes, BUN, Cr, 1-2 x/ week. Amikacin peak (15-30 ug/ml) and trough (5-10 ug/ml) levels with the Q 12 hr. regimen may be indicated, but intervention should be guided by patient clinical response. Baseline audio gram is recommended and repeated for signs and symptoms of ototoxicity.

Adverse drug reactions:

Renal toxicity, ototoxicity, tinitis, vertigo, neurotoxicity,

Drug-drug interactions:

Renal toxic agents (foscarnet, pentamidine, amphotericin, vancomycin, TMP/SMX, acyclovir); loop diuretics.

Infusion device system:

Gravity drip, infusion pump or disposable infusion device.

Drug dilutions:

Dose in 100-150 ml of D5W or NS (500 mg/100 ml), in viaflex, stable for 60 days under refrigeration.

OPPORTUNISTIC NEOPLASMS

Critical chemotherapy treatments can be expertly and safely provided in patients' homes. Tremendous advances have been made in the area of infusion device technology, vascular access device systems, and clinical expertise to allow home infusion services to provide home support for simple as well as complex chemotherapy regimens. Most of the following regimens described can easily be scheduled for home administration .

Kaposi's Sarcoma (KS)

Kaposi's sarcoma is the most common neoplasm in patients with AIDS and is almost exclusively confined to homosexual men with HIV infection.[66] Recent epidemiologic data suggests that a sexually transmitted agent may be responsible for the development of AIDS-related KS and that the percentage of patients with AIDS who develop KS is declining. KS can present in several clinical forms. The most common clinical manifestations of KS include one or more purplish-red cutaneous nodular lesions that vary in size and are not painful nor pruritic. Lesions may appear anywhere on the body, but the most frequent sites are the trunk, arms, head, neck, and frequently the hard palate. The lesions may be surrounded by bruising and edema. Local complications include lymphedema, bacterial infection, and superficial necrosis. Because a cure has not been developed for KS, treatment is a challenge and the goal of treatment is usually palliative. Chemotherapy and radiation may have good results in some patients; however due to the deleterious effects of treatment on the patient's immune function and overall clinical status, treatment selection should be individualized based on the invasiveness of the neoplasm and the patient's immune status. Systemic single agent (doxorubicin, vinblastine, etoposide) and multi-agent chemotherapy (vincristine+vinblastine, vincristine+ bleomycin, vincristine+bleomycin+doxorubicin) treatment with biologic agents (alpha-interferon, tumor necrosis factor), radiation, intralesional chemotherapy injections and topical liquid nitrogen are all viable conventional options for effective palliation of KS disease and associated clinical problems.

NON-HODGKIN'S LYMPHOMA (NHL)

NHL is a malignancy which may remain indolent (no therapy required) or progress aggressively with few long term survivors. HIV-infected patients are at increased risk for developing one of the non-Hodgkins's lymphomas. The most common sites of involvement are the GI tract, CNS, bone marrow, liver, and lung. Patients may present with symptoms of headache, nausea, dyspepsia, low-grade fever, chills, and weight loss. This presentation in HIV-infected patients is evidence of widespread disease at the time of diagnosis resulting in a poor prognosis with a median survival time of 4-7 months which may be prolonged if a positive response to intensive, multidrug chemotherapy regimens is achieved.

HEMATOPOIETIC GROWTH FACTORS

Erythropoietin (EPO)

Erythropoietin is a glycoprotein which stimulates red blood cell production. It is produced in the kidney and stimulates the division and differentiation of committed erythroid progenitors in the bone marrow. It is not uncommon for AIDS patients to develop hematologic abnormalities including anemia. Some patients require multiple palliative blood transfusions. The cause for anemia in AIDS patients may be related to decreased production of erythropoietin or release of iron binding proteins from neutrophils. Patients may also experience anemia as a result of toxicity from AZT or other cytotoxic drugs included in their regimen (i.e., TMP/SMX, gancyclovir, foscarnet, acyclovir). In addition, opportunistic infections in the HIV-infected patient can invade the bone marrow and impair erythropoiesis (i.e., M. tuberculosis, MAI, histoplasmosis, coccidioidomycosis, CMV, HSV).[67] Erythropoietin therapy can increase the mean hematocrit level and decrease the mean transfusion requirement in anemic patients with AIDS who are receiving AZT and have an endogenous erythropoietin level < 500 IU/L. Such a therapy is of no apparent benefit in patients whose endogenous erythropoietin levels are > 500 IU/L.[68] The starting recommended dose is 50-100 U/kg SQ or IV, 3 three times per week for 8 weeks then re-evaluate (equivalent to ~3,000-6,000 U T.I.W. for a 65 kg male). Plan to follow hematocrit level weekly to monitor response and prevent polycythemia. The dose should be titrated to maintain the desired response. If the hematocrit exceeds 40% the dose should be discontinued and restarted at 25% less dose. In clinical practice, the average dose will vary between 2,000 -10,000 U 2-3 times per week and changes are usually based on clinical judgement. Side effects in the HIV-infected population include fever, fatigue, headache, cough, diarrhea, rash, congestion, nausea, shortness of breath, skin reaction at medication site, and dizziness. An increase in the reticulocyte count is usually seen in 10 days, followed by an increase in RBCs, Hgb and Hct in 2-6 weeks.

Granulocyte Colony Stimulating Factor (G-CSF)

The colony stimulating factors are hematopoietic growth factors that regulate the proliferation and differentiation of hematopoietic precursor cells. The hematopoiesis cascade begins in the bone marrow with the pluripotent stem cell, which gives rise to progenitor cells. These progenitor cells, when exposed to various growth factors, differentiate into specific mature effector cells. G-CSF is a lineage-specific growth factor which acts to stimulate the growth of neutrophils, induce maturation and enhance neutrophil migration. HIV impairs hematopoiesis by an unknown mechanism, and this impairment in combination with drug induced myelotoxicity may place limits on the intensity and duration of therapy. G-CSF can reverse neutropenia induced by myelosuppressive drugs used in the treatment of AIDS, and it's manifestation (i.e., ganciclovir induced neutropenia.) Prior to the availability of G-CSF, sub-optimal dose changes were necessary to minimize severe neutropenia. The starting recommended dose is 5 mcg/kg/day SQ or IV 2-3 times per week (equivalent to approximately 2-3 x week for 300 mcg a 65 kg male). Plan to follow CBC w/diff at least weekly to monitor response and avoid complications of leucocytosis. As with EPO, the dose should be titrated to maintain the desired response. Parameters should be set for the highest acceptable neutrophil level and the G-CSF should be decreased or discontinued accordingly. In clinical practice the dose may vary between 300-600 mcg, 1-7 days per week. Significant side effects include skeletal pain (usually in pelvis, sternum, or back), myalgias, arthralgias, fever, anorexia, and diarrhea; others include rash, chest pain, splenomegaly, and increased alkaline phosphatase, lactic dehydrogenase, and uric acid.

WASTING SYNDROME

Malnutrition and progressive weight loss is a well recognized comorbidity factor in HIV infection and AIDS.[69] In Africa, AIDS was first recognized by a severe wasting condition preceding death described as "slim disease".[70] Malnutrition begins in the asymptomatic stages of HIV infection long before signs and symptoms are apparent. The CDC defines wasting syndrome as a profound involuntary weight loss greater than 10% of baseline body weight plus either chronic diarrhea (at least two loose stools per day for 30 days) or chronic weakness and documented fever (for 30 days intermittent or constant) in the absence of concurrent illness or condition other than HIV infection that could explain the findings (i.e., cancer, TB, cryptosporidiosis, or other specific enteritis).[71] Weight loss in AIDS may develop through several mechanisms, such as reduced dietary intake usually due to reduced appetite, gastrointestinal malabsorption, or HIV related alterations in metabolism. The weight loss of HIV infected patients is characterized by a predominant loss of body cell mass. Because protein constitutes most of body cell mass, this weight loss also results in protein wasting. The strategy to reverse wasting in AIDS is first to treat any secondary infections, then provide adequate amounts of all nutrients. The oral or enteral route is preferable to TPN for providing nutrition whenever possible. Megestrol acetate (Megace®) has been successfully used to stimulate appetite to increase weight.[72] Supplemental oral or enteral formulas should be lactose-free and low in fat (i.e., Sustacal®, Vital,®). Elemental diets are designed to provide maximum absorption with minimal digestion which is appropriate for patients with malabsorption and diarrhea (i.e., Vivonex T.E.N.®). Before implementing parenteral nutrition a complete nutritional assessment must be conducted. (See also Chapter 20.)

Malabsorption can be documented by performing a urine xylose test and obtaining GI culture results. Malnutrition is evidenced by hypoalbuminemia and at least a 10% weight loss. AIDS patients require more calories (1.5-2.0 x BEE) and proteins (1.5 - 2.0 gm/kg/day) than other TPN dependent patients to restore and maintain body cell mass. TPN may be indicated in patients who are infected with enteric pathogens (i.e., KS, cryptosporidiosis, MAC) resulting in large volume or secretory diarrhea, nausea, vomiting, and severe malabsorption unresponsive to antidiarrheals and oral or enteral nutritional supplementation. Octreotide (Sandostatin®) at a dose of 100 - 500 μg SQ every 8 hours has been successfully used to decrease stool frequencies in AIDS patients with refractory AIDS - associated diarrhea.[73] TPN may also be indicated for patients who experience severe nausea, vomiting, anorexia, and weight loss while undergoing radiation and/or chemotherapy treatments for AIDS related malignancies. For patients presenting with a clinical picture of unrelenting deterioration, parenteral nutrition does not alter the course of the disease and may actually increase mortality and morbidity secondary to TPN complications.[74,75] Ethical issues for the use of TPN in terminal patients who are in the final stages of their disease should be considered.

CONCLUSION

Increasingly, home infusion services are indicated for HIV patients to minimize hospital admissions, reduce health care costs, and optimize quality of life. For AIDS patients, most therapies are a matter of life or death, but insurance sponsorship or other means to pay for them are not available to many. HHC pharmacists should know that many pharmaceutical manufacturers offer indigent patient programs for oral and intravenous medications. These programs are accessed by contacting a local representative or calling the company directly.

Ultimately it is the HHC pharmacist's responsibility to provide safe and effective therapies in the home. Guidelines on the pharmacist's role in HHC are defined by ASHP[76] and standards of care are described by JCAHO.[77] The impact of the AIDS epidemic throughout the world with its social, political and financial effects is staggering. Prevention, treatment, and cure of AIDS and its clinical sequelae present an unparalleled challenge.

The author dedicates this chapter to her dear brother, Gregory George Wilson, to acknowledge his dauntless courage and inspiring attitude throughout his battle in fighting AIDS.

REFERENCES

1. Helper CD, Strand LM. Opportunities and responsibilities in pharmaceutical care. Am J Hosp Pharm. 1990; 47:539.
2. Centers for Disease Control. Pneumocystis pneumonia - - Los Angeles. MMWR 1981; 30:250-252.
3. Centers for Disease Control. Kaposi's sarcoma and pneumocystis pneumonia among homosexual men - New York and California. MMWR 1981; 30:305-308.
4. McDougal JS, Kennedy MS, Sligh JM, et al. Binding of HTLV-III/LAV to T4+ T cells by a complex of the 110K molecule and the T4 molecule. Science. 1985; 231:382-385.
5. Moss AR, Bacchetti P. Natural history of HIV infection. AIDS. 1989; 3:55-61.
6. Rutherford GW, Lifson AR, Hessol NA, et al. Course of HIV-1 in a cohort of homosexual and bisexual men: an 11 year follow-up study. Br Med J. 1990; 301:1183-1188.
7. Goedert JJ, Biggar RJ, Alosio CH, et al. Effect of T4 count and cofactors on the incidence of AIDS in homosexual men infected with human immunodeficiency virus. JAMA. 1987; 257:331-334.
8. Nicholson JKA, Spira TJ, Alosio CH, et al. Serial determinations of HIV-1 titers in HIV-infected homosexual men: association of rising titers with CD4 T cell depletion and progression to AIDS. AIDS Res Hum Retroviruses. 1989; 5:205-215.
9. Lang W, Perkins H, Anderson RE, et al. Patterns of T lymphocyte changes with human immunodeficiency virus infection: form seroconversion to the development of AIDS. J AIDS. 1989; 2:63-69.
10. Lange MA, deWolf F, Goudsmit J. Markers for progression of HIV infection. AIDS. 1989; 3(suppl.1):S153-160.
11. Taylor JM, Fahey JL, Detels R, et al. CD4 percentage, CD4 numbers, and CD4:CD8 ratio in HIV infection: which to choose and how to use. J AIDS. 1989; 2:114-124.
12. Chaisson RE, Stanton DL, Gallant JE, et al. Impact of the 1993 revision of the AIDS case definition on the prevalence of AIDS in a clinical setting. AIDS. 1993; 7:857-862.
13. Centers for Disease Control. 1993 revised classification system for HIV infection and expanded surveillance case definition for AIDS amongadolescents and adults. MMWR. 1992; 41:(RR-17):1-19.
14. Centers for Disease Control. AIDS Weekly Surveillance Report; Feb 2, 1987.
15. Wong RJ. Treating HIV infection: What pharmacists need to know. American Pharmacy. 1993; NS33(5):57-64.
16. Ninth International Conference on AIDS, Berlin, June 7-11, 1993. AIDS Report. 1993; 6(11):1-8.
17. Centers for Disease Control. Update: Mortality attributable to HIV infection/AIDS among persons aged 25-44 years - United States, 1990 and 1991. MMWR. 1993; 42(25):481-485.
18. Sarngadharan MG, Popovic M, Bruch L, et al. Antibodies reactive with human T-lymphotrophic retroviruses (HTLV-III) in the serum of patients with AIDS. Science. 1984; 224-506.
19. Pan LZ, Cheng-Mayer C, Levy JA. Patterns of antibody response in individuals infected with the human immunodeficiency virus. J Infect Dis. 1987; 155:626.
20. Centers for Disease Control. Update: Serologic testing for antibody to human immunodeficiency virus. MMWR. 1988; 39:833-840.
21. Reesink HW, Lelie PN, Huisman JG, et al. Evaluation of six enzyme immunoassays for antibody against human immunodeficiency virus. Lancet. 1986; ii:483-486.
22. Gallo RC, Salahuddin MG, Popovic M, et al. Frequent detection and isolation of cytopathic retroviruses (HTLV-III) from patients with AIDS and at risk for AIDS. Science. 1984; 224:500.
23. Richman DD, Fischl MA, Grieco MH, et al. The toxicity of azidothymidine (AZT) in the treatment of patients with AIDS and AIDS-related complex: A double blind, placebo-controlled trial. N Engl J Med. 1987; 317:192-197.
24. Volberding PA, Lagakos WS, Koch MA, et al. Zidovudine in asymptomatic human immunodeficiency virus infection. N Engl J Med. 1990; 322:941-949.
25. Yarchaan R, Pluda JM, Thomas R, et al. Long term toxicity/activity profile of 2'3'-dideoxyinosine in AIDS of AIDS-related complex. Lancet. 1990; 336:526-529.
26. Videx (didanosine) package insert. Princeton, NJ. Bristol-Myers Squibb Laboratories. 1991.
27. Meng TC, Fischl MA, Boota AM, et al. Combination therapy with zidovudine anddideoxycytidine in patients with advanced HIV infection: A phase I/II study. Ann Intern Med. 1991; 116:13-20.
28. Lane HC, Masur H, Gelmann EP, et al. Correlation between immunologic function and clinical subpopulations of patients with the acquired immune deficiency syndrome. Am J Med. 1985; 78:417.
29. Kaslow RA, Phair JP, Friedman HB, et al. Infection with the human immunodeficiency virus: Clinical manifestations and their relationship to immune deficiency. Ann Intern Med. 1987; 107:474.
30. Reider HR, Canthen GM, Bloch AB, et al. Tuberculosis and acquired immunodeficiency syndrome - Florida. Arch Intern Med. 1989; 149:1268.
31. Kapusnik-Uner JE. Acquired immunodeficiency syndrome (AIDS). In: Herfindal ET, Hirschman JL, eds. Clinical pharmacy and therapeutics. Baltimore MD: Williams and Wilkins. 1992; 1203-1218.
32. Collier AC, Meyers JD, Corey L, et al. Cytomegalovirus infection in homosexual men. Am J Med. 1987; 107:(2):133-138.
33. Jabs DA, Enger C, Bartlett JG. Cytomegalovirus retinitis and acquired immunodeficiency syndrome. Arch Ophthalmol. 1989; 107:75-80.

34. Jacobson MA. Foscarnet therapy for AIDS-related opportunistic herpes virus infections. In: Volberding P, Jacobson MA, eds. AIDS clinical review. New York, NY: Marcel Dekker, Inc. 1992; 173-189.
35. Katlama C, Dohin E, Caumes E, et al. Foscarnet induction therapy for cytomegalovirus retinitis in AIDS: Comparison of twice daily and three times daily regimens. J AIDS. 1992; 5(suppl.1):S18-S24.
36. Parasrampuria J, Li LC, Stelmach AH, et al. Stability of ganciclovir sodium in 5% dextrose injection and in 0.9% sodium chloride injection over 35 days. Am J Hosp Pharm. 1992; 49:116-118.
37. Outman WR, Mortland PM, Mitrano FP, et al. Stability and compatibility of diluted and undiluted foscarnet in polyvinyl chloride (PVC) containers when stored under refrigeration for 35 days. Drug News & New Drugs July 1, 1992. (Abstract presented at the 49th Annual Meeting of the ASHP, Washington, D.C.).
38. Siegal FP, Lopez C, Hammer GS, et al. Severe acquired immunodeficiency in male homosexuals manifested by chronic perianal ulcerative herpes simplex lesions. N Engl J Med. 1981; 305:1439-1444.
39. Erlich KS, Jacobson MA, Koehler JE, et al. Foscarnet therapy for severe acyclovir-resistant herpes simplex virus type-2 infections in patients with the acquired immunodeficiency syndrome (AIDS). Ann Intern Med. 1989; 110(9):710-713.
40. Safrin S, Crumpacker C, Chatis P, et al. A controlled trial comparing foscarnet with vidarabine for acyclovir-resistant mucocutaneous herpes simplex in the acquired immunodeficiency syndrome. N Engl J Med. 1991; 325(8):551-555.
41. Gupta VD, Pramar Y, Bethea C. Stability of acyclovir sodium in dextrose and sodium chloride injections. J Clin Pharm Ther. 1989; 14:451-456.
42. Hoppenjans WB, Bibler MR, Orme RL, et al. Prolonged cutaneous herpes zoster in acquired immunodeficiency syndrome. Arch Dermatol. 1990; 126:1048.
43. Jacobson MA, Berger TG, Fikrig S, et al. Acyclovir-resistant varicella zoster virus infection after chronic oral acyclovir therapy in patients with the acquired immunodeficiency syndrome (AIDS). Ann Intern Med. 1990; 112:187-191.
44. Safrin S, Berger TG, Gilson I, et al. Foscarnet therapy in five patients with AIDS and acyclovir-resistant varicella zoster infection. Ann Intern Med. 1991; 115:19-21.
45. Hopewell PC. Pneumocystis carinii pneumonia. In: Sande MA, Volberding PA, eds. The medical management of AIDS. Philadelphia, PA: W.B. Saunders Co. 1992; 261-283.
46. Conte JE, Chernoff D, Feigal DW, et al. Intravenous or inhaled pentamidine for treating Pneumocystis carinii pneumonia in AIDS. Ann Intern Med. 1990; 113:203-209.
47. Medina I, Mills J, Leoung G, et al. Oral therapy for Pneumocystis carinii pneumonia in the acquired immunodeficiency syndrome: A controlled trial of trimethoprim-sulfamethoxazole versus trimethoprim-dapsone. N Engl J Med. 1990; 323:776-782.
48. Toma E, Fournier S, Poisson M, et al. Clindamycin with primaquine for Pneumocystis carinii pneumonia. Lancet 1989; 1:1046.
49. The National Institutes of Health - University of California Expert Panel for Corticosteroids as Adjunctive Therapy for Pneumocystis Pneumonia: Consensus statement on the use of corticosteroids as adjunctive therapy for Pneumocystis pneumonia in the acquired immunodeficiency syndrome. N Engl J Med. 1990; 323:1500.
50. Kaufman MD, Scovone JM, Foley JJ. Stability of undiluted trimethoprim-sulfamethoxazole for injection in plastic wyringes. Am J Hosp Pharm. 1992; 49:2782-2783.
51. Kirschenbaum BE, Latiolais CJ, eds. Injectable medications, A guide to stability and reconstitution. NY,NY: McMahon Group. 1991.
52. Bozzette SA, Larsen R, Chiu J, et al. A placebo-controlled trial of maintenance therapy with fluconazole after treatment of cryptococcal meningitis in the acquired immunodeficiency syndrome. N Engl J Med. 1991; 324:580-584.
53. Larse RA, Leal ME, Chan LS. Floconazole compared with amphotericin B plus flucytosine for cryptococcal meningitis in AIDS. Ann Intern Med. 1990; 113:183-187.
54. Mitrano FP, Outman WR, Baptista RJ, et al. Chemical and visual stability of amphotericin B in 5% dextrose injection stored at 4°C for 35 days. Am J Hosp Pharm. 1991; 48:2635-2637.
55. Craven PC, et al. High-dose ketoconazole for treatment of fungal infections of the central nervous system. 1983; 98:160.
56. Galgiani JN. Fluconazole, a new antifungal agent (editorial). Ann Intern Med.1990; 113:177-179.
57. McKinsey DS, Gupta MR, Riddler SA, et al. Long-term amphotericin B therapy for disseminated histoplasmosis in patients with the acquired immunodeficiency syndrome (AIDS). Ann Intern Med. 1989; 111:655-659.
58. Salzman Sh, Smith RL, Aranda CP. Histoplasmosis in patients at risk for the acquired immunodeficiency syndrome in a nonendemic settin. Chest 1988; 93:916-921.
59. Havlik JA, Horsburgh CR, Metchock B, et al. Disseminated Mycobacterium avium complex infection: clinical identification and epidemiologic trends. J Infect Dis. 1992; 165:577-580.
60. Ellner JJ, Goldberger MJ, Parenti DM. Mycobacterium avium infection and AIDS: a therapeutic dilemma in rapid evolution. J Infect Dis. 1991; 163:1326-1335.
61. Horsburgh CR. Mycobacterium avium complex infection in the acquired immunodeficiency syndrome. N Engl J Med. 1991; 324:1332-1338.
62. Pitchenik AE, Fertel D. Tuberculosis and nontuberculous mycobacterial disease. Med Clin North Am. 1992; 76:121-171.
63. Peolquin CA. Controversies in the management of Mycobacterium avium complex infection in AIDS patients. Ann Pharmacother. 1993; 27:828-937.

64. Centers for Disease Control. Recommendations on prophylaxis and therapy for disseminated Mycobacterium avium complex for adults and adolescents infected with human immunodeficiency firus. MMWR. 1993; 42:(RR-9):18-20.
65. Northfelt DW, Volberding PA. AIDS-related Kaposi's sarcoma. Clinical presentation, biology, and therapy. Adv Oncol. 1991; 7:9-17.
66. Northfelt DW, Kahn JO, Vloberding PA. Treatment of AIDS-related Kaposi's sarcoma. Hematol Oncol Aspects of HIV Dis. 1991; 5:297-309.
67. Henry DH. Human recombinant erythropoietin in the treatment of severe anemia in patients with AIDS. Intern Med. 1989; 10:39-49.
68. Henry DH, Beall GN, Benson CA, et al. Recombinant human erythropoietin in the treatment of anemia associated with human immunodeficiency virus (HIV) infection and zidovudine therapy. Ann Intern Med. 1992; 117:739-748.
69. Kotler DP, Tierney AR, Francisco A, et.al. The magnitude of body cell mass depletion determines the timing of death from wasting in AIDS. Am J Clin Nutr.1989; 50:444-447.
70. Serwada D, Sewankambo NK, Carswell JW, et al. Slim disease: a new disease in Uganda and it association with HTLV- III infection. Lancet. 1985; ii:850-852.
71. Centers for Disease Control. Revision of the CDC surveillance case definition for acquired immunodeficiency syndrome. MMWR. 1987; 36(suppl. 2S):3S-15S.
72. Van Roenn JH, Murphy RL, Weber KM, et al. Megesteral acetate for the treatment of cachexia associated with human immunodeficiency virus infectional. Ann Intern Med. 1988; 109:840-841.
73. Cello JP, Grendell JH, Basuk P, et al. Effect of octreotide acetate on refractory AIDS associated diarrhea. Ann Intern Med. 1991; 115:705-710.
74. Shamberger RC, Brennan MF, Goodgame T, et al. A prospective randomized study of adjuvant parenteral nutrition in the treatment of sarcoma: results of metabolic and survival studies. Surger. 1984; 96:1-12.
75. Samual ML, Selig DE, Ogden S, et al. Hyperalimentation and chemotherapy for state III testicular cancer: a randomized study. Cancer Treat Rep. 1981;65:615-27.
76. ASHP guidelines on the pharmacist's role in home care. Am J Hosp Pharm. 1993; 50:1940-1944.
77. Pharmaceutical Services Standards. In: The 1993 Joint Commission on Accreditation of Healthcare Organizations, accreditation manual for home care. Oakbrook Terrace, IL. 1993.

Index